Current Research on HIV Drug Resistance

Current Research on HIV Drug Resistance

Editor

Hezhao Ji

MDPI • Basel • Beijing • Wuhan • Barcelona • Belgrade • Manchester • Tokyo • Cluj • Tianjin

Editor
Hezhao Ji
National Microbiology
Laboratory at JC Wilt
Infectious Diseases Research
Centre, Public Health Agency
of Canada
Canada

Editorial Office
MDPI
St. Alban-Anlage 66
4052 Basel, Switzerland

This is a reprint of articles from the Special Issue published online in the open access journal *Pathogens* (ISSN 2076-0817) (available at: https://www.mdpi.com/journal/pathogens/topical_collections/HIV_Drug_Resistance).

For citation purposes, cite each article independently as indicated on the article page online and as indicated below:

LastName, A.A.; LastName, B.B.; LastName, C.C. Article Title. *Journal Name* **Year**, *Volume Number*, Page Range.

ISBN 978-3-0365-5511-9 (Hbk)
ISBN 978-3-0365-5512-6 (PDF)

Contents

Hezhao Ji
Current Research on HIV Drug Resistance—A Topical Collection with *"Pathogens"*
Reprinted from: *Pathogens* **2022**, *11*, 966, doi:10.3390/pathogens11090966 1

Miaomiao Li, Shujia Liang, Chao Zhou, Min Chen, Shu Liang, Chunhua Liu, Zhongbao Zuo, Lei Liu, Yi Feng, Chang Song, Hui Xing, Yuhua Ruan, Yiming Shao and Lingjie Liao
HIV Drug Resistance Mutations Detection by Next-Generation Sequencing during Antiretroviral Therapy Interruption in China
Reprinted from: *Pathogens* **2021**, *10*, 264, doi:10.3390/pathogens10030264 5

Kaelo K. Seatla, Dorcas Maruapula, Wonderful T. Choga, Olorato Morerinyane, Shahin Lockman, Vladimir Novitsky, Ishmael Kasvosve, Sikhulile Moyo and Simani Gaseitsiwe
Limited HIV-1 Subtype C *nef* 3′PPT Variation in Combination Antiretroviral Therapy Naïve and Experienced People Living with HIV in Botswana
Reprinted from: *Pathogens* **2021**, *10*, 1027, doi:10.3390/pathogens10081027 19

Supang A. Martin, Patricia A. Cane, Deenan Pillay and Jean L. Mbisa
Coevolved Multidrug-Resistant HIV-1 Protease and Reverse Transcriptase Influences Integrase Drug Susceptibility and Replication Fitness
Reprinted from: *Pathogens* **2021**, *10*, 1070, doi:10.3390/pathogens10091070 29

Anneleen Kiekens, Idda H. Mosha, Lara Zlatić, George M. Bwire, Ally Mangara, Bernadette Dierckx de Casterlé, Catherine Decouttere, Nico Vandaele, Raphael Z. Sangeda, Omary Swalehe, Paolo Cottone, Alessio Surian, Japhet Killewo and Anne-Mieke Vandamme Factors Associated with HIV Drug Resistance in Dar es Salaam, Tanzania: Analysis of a Complex Adaptive System
Reprinted from: *Pathogens* **2021**, *10*, 1535, doi:10.3390/pathogens10121535 45

Yanink Caro-Vega, Fernando Alarid-Escudero, Eva A. Enns, Sandra Sosa-Rubí, Carlos Chivardi, Alicia Piñeirúa-Menendez, Claudia García-Morales, Gustavo Reyes-Terán, Juan G. Sierra-Madero and Santiago Ávila-Ríos
Retention in Care, Mortality, Loss-to-Follow-Up, and Viral Suppression among Antiretroviral Treatment-Naïve and Experienced Persons Participating in a Nationally Representative HIV Pre-Treatment Drug Resistance Survey in Mexico
Reprinted from: *Pathogens* **2021**, *10*, 1569, doi:10.3390/pathogens10121569 61

Claudia García-Morales, Daniela Tapia-Trejo, Margarita Matías-Florentino, Verónica Sonia Quiroz-Morales, Vanessa Dávila-Conn,Ángeles Beristain-Barreda, Miroslava Cárdenas-Sandoval, Manuel Becerril-Rodríguez, Patricia Iracheta-Hernández, Israel Macías-González, Rebecca García-Mendiola, Alejandro Guzmán-Carmona, Eduardo Zarza-Sánchez, Raúl Adrián Cruz, Andrea González-Rodríguez, Gustavo Reyes-Terán and SantiagoÁvila-Ríos
HIV Pretreatment Drug Resistance Trends in Mexico City, 2017–2020

Reprinted from: *Pathogens* **2021**, *10*, 1587, doi:10.3390/pathogens10121587 71

Soo-Yon Rhee, Michael Boehm, Olga Tarasova, Giulia Di Teodoro, Ana B. Abecasis, Anders Sönnerborg, Alexander J. Bailey, Dmitry Kireev, Maurizio Zazzi, the EuResist Network Study Group and Robert W. Shafer
Spectrum of Atazanavir-Selected Protease Inhibitor-Resistance Mutations
Reprinted from: *Pathogens* **2022**, *11*, 546, doi:10.3390/pathogens11050546 91

pathogens

MDPI

Editorial

Current Research on HIV Drug Resistance—A Topical Collection with "*Pathogens*"

Hezhao Ji [1,2]

1 National Microbiology Laboratory at JC Wilt Infectious Diseases Research Centre, Public Health Agency of Canada, Winnipeg, MB R3E 3R2, Canada; hezhao.ji@phac-aspc.gc.ca
2 Max Rady College of Medicine, University of Manitoba, Winnipeg, MB R3E 0J9, Canada

Viral drug resistance is an everlasting topic for HIV/AIDS professionals from clinical, laboratory and public health perspectives [1]. As one of the most challenging human viral pathogens, HIV is notorious for its significant genetic and antigenic diversity, both intra-host and inter-host, resulting from poor proofreading of the viral reverse transcriptase as the virus replicates coupled with its high replication rate [2–4]. Unsurprisingly, HIV drug resistance (HIVDR) was reported soon after the commercialization of the first antiretroviral drug [5]. Since then, HIVDR has been symbiotic with all HIV drugs currently applied in antiretroviral therapy (ART), although the genetic barriers for the resistance development again different drugs vary. *Pathogens* launched a topical collection of submissions in 2021 to catch the latest advances in HIVDR diagnosis, surveillance and research perspectives. While this collection remains open for new submissions, we already have ten excellent articles published thus far. This editorial piece provides a brief walkthrough of these articles and highlights their significant contributions to the HIVDR field in general.

Next-generation sequencing (NGS)-based HIVDR testing is a trending new standard for HIVDR typing, attributable to its high sensitivity and accuracy in semi-quantitative detection of HIVDR variants, especially those present at lower frequencies [6]. Li et al. applied NGS HIVDR testing in a cross-sectional study in China, revealing that HIVDR prevalence in patients under ART interruption is higher than in ART-naïve patients or those on ART therapy [7]. It provides more convincing evidence, reassuring the improved sensitivity of NGS in detecting lower abundance HIVDR mutations.

The application of integrase strand transfer inhibitor (INSTI)-based therapy is rising globally in first-line ART, attributable largely to the well-documented higher genetic barriers for resistance development against INSTIs. Two articles in this collection dealt with HIVDR against INSTIs. Seatla K et al. reported their findings in examining the correlation between 3′-polypurine tract (3′PPT) variations in the HIV-1 *nef* gene and failure of INSTI-based ART treatment [8]. Multiple HIV-1 genetic variations outside the *pol* gene have been reported to be associated with HIVDR occurrence, although they do not directly alter the coding of drug-targeted HIV enzymes [9–12]. One such viral genetic trait identified by in vitro breakthrough selection experiments is the 3′PPT variation in the HIV-1 *nef* gene, reported to be contributing to INSTI resistance [9]. However, several later studies failed to confirm this association in patients failing INSTI-based ART, but all reported the high genetic conservation of this region [13–15]. By examining the 3′PPT from 6009 HIV-1 subtype C sequences from Botswana, this study provides solid evidence of the high conservation of the 3′PPT sequence and rules out the causal connection between variations in this motif and INSTI resistance [8]. Martin et al. reported on the coevolution of the ART-targeted HIV-1 genes and the potential impacts of the co-evolved HIV-1 protease (PR) and reverse transcriptase (RT) genes on the HIV-1 viral fitness and its susceptibility to INSTIs [16]. This study highlights the close interactions of the ART-targeted viral enzymes/genes during ART, which necessitate the analysis of the whole HIV-1 *pol* gene, or even the entire genomes, to better decipher the mechanisms of HIVDR occurrence in the context of ART.

Citation: Ji, H. Current Research on HIV Drug Resistance—A Topical Collection with "*Pathogens*". *Pathogens* **2022**, *11*, 966. https://doi.org/10.3390/pathogens11090966

Received: 15 August 2022
Accepted: 22 August 2022
Published: 25 August 2022

HIVDR occurrence is, by all means, a multifactorial phenomenon involving many interconnected factors from social, economic, medical and behavioural perspectives. Kiekens et al. developed and presented a comprehensive local systems map that enables in-depth analysis and an understanding of HIVDR-relevant factors in a complex adaptive system [17]. While it was developed in a Tanzania-based study, this system could be easily adapted or adopted in other settings to better understand the local HIVDR situation and identify actionable strategies to combat HIVDR.

Population-level HIVDR surveillance provides valuable information in monitoring the HIVDR situation in the region, evaluating the impact of HIVDR-related policies and strategies and forming treatment guidelines to optimize clinical outcomes at population levels [1,18]. Two HIVDR surveillance studies from Mexico were included in this topical collection. García-Morales et al. presented a four-year observational study monitoring the pre-treatment HIVDR prevalence trend against protease inhibitor (PI), RT inhibitor (RTI) and INSTI in a large patient cohort from Mexico City during 2017~2020 [19]. Caro-Vega et al. presented a report describing the clinical outcomes of participants from a 2017 to 2018 national representative HIV PDR survey in Mexico [20]. Both articles exemplify large-scale HIVDR monitoring for a designated population or patient cohort and for the evaluation of its clinical significance.

Following the above is an excellent report on the spectrum of atazanavir-selected PI resistance mutation from Rhee et al. [21]. While ritonavir-boosted atazanavir is now an often-used second-line PI option in ART, especially in low- to middle-income countries (LMIC), there is a paucity of studies examining the PR mutations occurring in patients receiving atazanavir treatment. To fill this gap, the authors analyzed 1497 PR sequences from patients receiving boosted or unboosted atazanavir treatments and profiled all PR mutations selected by atazanavir in previously PI-naïve patients who failed atazanavir-containing regimens. I highly recommend this article for HIVDR researchers and clinicians in order to better understand the cross-resistance among commonly applied PIs for the optimal use of these drugs in clinical settings.

The last group of manuscripts in this collection includes three review or commentary articles summarizing the advances in three perspectives pertaining to HIVDR laboratory testing. Munyuza et al. reviewed the recent progress in applying a probe-capturing enrichment strategy for improved viral template recovery from samples containing degraded viral RNA/DNA or low viral loads for HIV and HCV genotyping [22]. Chua et al. summarized up-to-date advances in point-of-care test (POCT) technologies that may help boost the accessibility and simplicity of HIVDR assays with improved cost-effectiveness [23]. This information is valuable for promoting de-centralized HIVDR testing in LMIC where ART coverage is scaling up while HIVDR monitoring lags behind due to resource limitations. Ji and Sandstrom provided a comprehensive review of all clinical analytes that have been used in HIVDR testing thus far in both research and clinical settings [24]. It may assist in the optimal selection of specimens for different HIVDR testing needs.

Taken together, I hope this HIVDR topical collection will contribute to further advancements in basic research, laboratory testing and effective management pertaining to HIVDR. New submissions are always welcome when the collection is still open.

As the collection editor, I appreciate the collective efforts from all authors, reviewers, and editorial personnel of *Pathogens* who have made this topical collection a reality. Thank you!

Conflicts of Interest: The author declares no conflict of interest.

References

1. World Health Organization. *Global Action Plan on HIV Drug Resistance 2017–2021*; WHO: Geneva, Switzerland, 2017.
2. Coffin, J.M. HIV population dynamics in vivo: Implications for genetic variation, pathogenesis, and therapy. *Science* **1995**, *267*, 483–489. [CrossRef] [PubMed]
3. Ho, D.D. Perspectives series: Host/pathogen interactions. Dynamics of HIV-1 replication in vivo. *J. Clin. Investig.* **1997**, *99*, 2565–2567. [CrossRef] [PubMed]

4. Menendez-Arias, L. Targeting HIV: Antiretroviral therapy and development of drug resistance. *Trends Pharmacol. Sci.* **2002**, *23*, 381–388. [CrossRef]
5. Larder, B.A.; Darby, G.; Richman, D.D. HIV with reduced sensitivity to zidovudine (AZT) isolated during prolonged therapy. *Science* **1989**, *243*, 1731–1734. [CrossRef] [PubMed]
6. Ji, H.; Sandstrom, P.; Paredes, R.; Harrigan, P.R.; Brumme, C.J.; Avila, R.S.; Noguera-Julian, M.; Parkin, N.; Kantor, R. Are We Ready for NGS HIV Drug Resistance Testing? The Second "Winnipeg Consensus" Symposium. *Viruses* **2020**, *12*, 586. [CrossRef]
7. Li, M.; Liang, S.; Zhou, C.; Chen, M.; Liang, S.; Liu, C.; Zuo, Z.; Liu, L.; Feng, Y.; Song, C.; et al. HIV Drug Resistance Mutations Detection by Next-Generation Sequencing during Antiretroviral Therapy Interruption in China. *Pathogens* **2021**, *10*, 264. [CrossRef]
8. Seatla, K.K.; Maruapula, D.; Choga, W.T.; Morerinyane, O.; Lockman, S.; Novitsky, V.; Kasvosve, I.; Moyo, S.; Gaseitsiwe, S. Limited HIV-1 Subtype C nef 3′PPT Variation in Combination Antiretroviral Therapy Naive and Experienced People Living with HIV in Botswana. *Pathogens* **2021**, *10*, 1027. [CrossRef]
9. Malet, I.; Subra, F.; Charpentier, C.; Collin, G.; Descamps, D.; Calvez, V.; Marcelin, A.G.; Delelis, O. Mutations Located outside the Integrase Gene Can Confer Resistance to HIV-1 Integrase Strand Transfer Inhibitors. *mBio* **2017**, *8*, e00922-17. [CrossRef]
10. Dicker, I.B.; Samanta, H.K.; Li, Z.; Hong, Y.; Tian, Y.; Banville, J.; Remillard, R.R.; Walker, M.A.; Langley, D.R.; Krystal, M. Changes to the HIV long terminal repeat and to HIV integrase differentially impact HIV integrase assembly, activity, and the binding of strand transfer inhibitors. *J. Biol. Chem.* **2007**, *282*, 31186–31196. [CrossRef]
11. Rabi, S.A.; Laird, G.M.; Durand, C.M.; Laskey, S.; Shan, L.; Bailey, J.R.; Chioma, S.; Moore, R.D.; Siliciano, R.F. Multi-step inhibition explains HIV-1 protease inhibitor pharmacodynamics and resistance. *J. Clin. Investig.* **2013**, *123*, 3848–3860. [CrossRef]
12. Fun, A.; Wensing, A.M.; Verheyen, J.; Nijhuis, M. Human Immunodeficiency Virus Gag and protease: Partners in resistance. *Retrovirology* **2012**, *9*, 63. [CrossRef] [PubMed]
13. Malet, I.; Delelis, O.; Nguyen, T.; Leducq, V.; Abdi, B.; Morand-Joubert, L.; Calvez, V.; Marcelin, A.G. Variability of the HIV-1 3′ polypurine tract (3′PPT) region and implication in integrase inhibitor resistance. *J. Antimicrob. Chemother.* **2019**, *74*, 3440–3444. [CrossRef] [PubMed]
14. Wei, Y.; Sluis-Cremer, N. Mutations in the HIV-1 3′-Polypurine Tract and Integrase Strand Transfer Inhibitor Resistance. *Antimicrob. Agents Chemother.* **2021**, *65*, e02432-20. [CrossRef] [PubMed]
15. Acharya, A.; Tagny, C.T.; Mbanya, D.; Fonsah, J.Y.; Nchindap, E.; Kenmogne, L.; Jihyun, M.; Njamnshi, A.K.; Kanmogne, G.D. Variability in HIV-1 Integrase Gene and 3′-Polypurine Tract Sequences in Cameroon Clinical Isolates, and Implications for Integrase Inhibitors Efficacy. *Int. J. Mol. Sci.* **2020**, *21*, 1553. [CrossRef] [PubMed]
16. Martin, S.A.; Cane, P.A.; Pillay, D.; Mbisa, J.L. Coevolved Multidrug-Resistant HIV-1 Protease and Reverse Transcriptase Influences Integrase Drug Susceptibility and Replication Fitness. *Pathogens* **2021**, *10*, 1070. [CrossRef]
17. Kiekens, A.; Mosha, I.H.; Zlatic, L.; Bwire, G.M.; Mangara, A.; de Dierckx, C.B.; Decouttere, C.; Vandaele, N.; Sangeda, R.Z.; Swalehe, O.; et al. Factors Associated with HIV Drug Resistance in Dar es Salaam, Tanzania: Analysis of a Complex Adaptive System. *Pathogens* **2021**, *10*, 1535. [CrossRef]
18. World Health Organization. *HIV Drug Resistance Report 2021*; WHO: Geneva, Switzerland, 2021.
19. Garcia-Morales, C.; Tapia-Trejo, D.; Matias-Florentino, M.; Quiroz-Morales, V.S.; Davila-Conn, V.; Beristain-Barreda, A.; Cardenas-Sandoval, M.; Becerril-Rodriguez, M.; Iracheta-Hernandez, P.; Macias-Gonzalez, I.; et al. HIV Pretreatment Drug Resistance Trends in Mexico City, 2017–2020. *Pathogens* **2021**, *10*, 1587. [CrossRef]
20. Caro-Vega, Y.; Alarid-Escudero, F.; Enns, E.A.; Sosa-Rubi, S.; Chivardi, C.; Pineirua-Menendez, A.; Garcia-Morales, C.; Reyes-Teran, G.; Sierra-Madero, J.G.; Avila-Rios, S. Retention in Care, Mortality, Loss-to-Follow-Up, and Viral Suppression among Antiretroviral Treatment-Naive and Experienced Persons Participating in a Nationally Representative HIV Pre-Treatment Drug Resistance Survey in Mexico. *Pathogens* **2021**, *10*, 1569. [CrossRef]
21. Rhee, S.Y.; Boehm, M.; Tarasova, O.; Di, T.G.; Abecasis, A.B.; Sonnerborg, A.; Bailey, A.J.; Kireev, D.; Zazzi, M.; The EuResist Network Study Group; et al. Spectrum of Atazanavir-Selected Protease Inhibitor-Resistance Mutations. *Pathogens* **2022**, *11*, 546. [CrossRef]
22. Munyuza, C.; Ji, H.; Lee, E.R. Probe Capture Enrichment Methods for HIV and HCV Genome Sequencing and Drug Resistance Genotyping. *Pathogens* **2022**, *11*, 693. [CrossRef]
23. Chua, R.J.; Capina, R.; Ji, H. Point-of-Care Tests for HIV Drug Resistance Monitoring: Advances and Potentials. *Pathogens* **2022**, *11*, 724. [CrossRef] [PubMed]
24. Ji, H.; Sandstrom, P. Overview of the Analytes Applied in Genotypic HIV Drug Resistance Testing. *Pathogens* **2022**, *11*, 739. [CrossRef] [PubMed]

pathogens

MDPI

Article

HIV Drug Resistance Mutations Detection by Next-Generation Sequencing during Antiretroviral Therapy Interruption in China

Miaomiao Li [1], Shujia Liang [2], Chao Zhou [3], Min Chen [4], Shu Liang [5], Chunhua Liu [6], Zhongbao Zuo [1], Lei Liu [1], Yi Feng [1], Chang Song [1], Hui Xing [1], Yuhua Ruan [1], Yiming Shao [1] and Lingjie Liao [1,*]

1 National Center for AIDS/STD Control and Prevention, Chinese Center for Disease Control and Prevention, Beijing 102206, China; miaomiao_ana@163.com (M.L.); zuozhongbaocdc@163.com (Z.Z.); cdcliulei@163.com (L.L.); fengyi@chinaaids.cn (Y.F.); songchang604@163.com (C.S.); xingh09@163.com (H.X.); ruanyuhua92@163.com (Y.R.); yshao@bjmu.edu.cn (Y.S.)
2 Guangxi Center for Disease Control and Prevention, Nanning 530028, China; liangshujia@126.com
3 Chongqing Center for Disease Control and Prevention, Chongqing 400042, China; 2008zhch@163.com
4 Yunnan Center for Disease Control and Prevention, Kunming 650022, China; chenminyx@126.com
5 Sichuan Center for Disease Control and Prevention, Chengdu 610041, China; liangshu523@163.com
6 Henan Center for Disease Control and Prevention, Zhengzhou 450016, China; chunhua5167@163.com
* Correspondence: liaolj@chinaaids.cn

Abstract: Patients with antiretroviral therapy interruption have a high risk of virological failure when re-initiating antiretroviral therapy (ART), especially those with HIV drug resistance. Next-generation sequencing may provide close scrutiny on their minority drug resistance variant. A cross-sectional study was conducted in patients with ART interruption in five regions in China in 2016. Through Sanger and next-generation sequencing in parallel, HIV drug resistance was genotyped on their plasma samples. Rates of HIV drug resistance were compared by the McNemar tests. In total, 174 patients were included in this study, with a median 12 (interquartile range (IQR), 6–24) months of ART interruption. Most (86.2%) of them had received efavirenz (EFV)/nevirapine (NVP)-based first-line therapy for a median 16 (IQR, 7–26) months before ART interruption. Sixty-one (35.1%) patients had CRF07_BC HIV-1 strains, 58 (33.3%) CRF08_BC and 35 (20.1%) CRF01_AE. Thirty-four (19.5%) of the 174 patients were detected to harbor HIV drug-resistant variants on Sanger sequencing. Thirty-six (20.7%), 37 (21.3%), 42 (24.1%), 79 (45.4%) and 139 (79.9) patients were identified to have HIV drug resistance by next-generation sequencing at 20% (v.s. Sanger, $p = 0.317$), 10% (v.s. Sanger, $p = 0.180$), 5% (v.s. Sanger, $p = 0.011$), 2% (v.s. Sanger, $p < 0.001$) and 1% (v.s. Sanger, $p < 0.001$) of detection thresholds, respectively. K65R was the most common minority mutation, of 95.1% (58/61) and 93.1% (54/58) in CRF07_BC and CRF08_BC, respectively, when compared with 5.7% (2/35) in CRF01_AE ($p < 0.001$). In 49 patients that followed-up a median 10 months later, HIV drug resistance mutations at >20% frequency such as K103N, M184VI and P225H still existed, but with decreased frequencies. The prevalence of HIV drug resistance in ART interruption was higher than 15% in the survey. Next-generation sequencing was able to detect more minority drug resistance variants than Sanger. There was a sharp increase in minority drug resistance variants when the detection threshold was below 5%.

Keywords: HIV drug resistance; sanger sequencing; next-generation sequencing; interrupted antiretroviral therapy

Citation: Li, M.; Liang, S.; Zhou, C.; Chen, M.; Liang, S.; Liu, C.; Zuo, Z.; Liu, L.; Feng, Y.; Song, C.; et al. HIV Drug Resistance Mutations Detection by Next-Generation Sequencing during Antiretroviral Therapy Interruption in China. *Pathogens* **2021**, *10*, 264. https://doi.org/10.3390/pathogens10030264

Academic Editor: Hezhao Ji

Received: 22 January 2021
Accepted: 20 February 2021
Published: 25 February 2021

1. Introduction

The scale-up of antiretroviral therapy (ART) has reduced HIV-related deaths and prevented new HIV infections [1]. By the end of 2019, 25.4 million people globally had received ART, with an increase of 19 million when compared with 2009 [2]. However, while the number of patients with ART increases, so does the number of patients with treatment interruption. The rate of ART discontinuation ranges from 10% to 78% under different settings [3–6] and keeps rising with ART prolonged [7]. Patients with ART interruption have decreased CD4$^+$ T cell counts [8], a higher risk of AIDS or death [9] and are a potential source of HIV transmission.

The emergence of HIV drug resistance (HIVDR) results from the low fidelity of HIV reverse transcriptase, the rapid replication of the virus and the selective pressure of antiretroviral drugs [10]. It will compromise the efficacy of ART, lead to virological failure and hamper the progress of HIV/AIDS treatment and prevention [11]. Under ART interruption, HIVDR variants may persist, or revert to wild-type strains or to a resistant revertant like T215rev [12,13]. In addition, new HIVDR variants may be selected by residual drugs with longer half-lives in combined antiretroviral regimens [14].

HIVDR assays are usually carried out using Sanger sequencing (SS), which can detect minority variants at a 15%–20% frequency in HIV viral populations (quasi species) within patients [15]. Next-generation sequencing (NGS) has been increasingly valued in recent years, having the ability to detect lower-frequency mutants and thus more HIVDR variants [16], with increased throughput and higher cost-efficiency [17]. The HIVDR mutation frequencies detected by NGS, but not SS, concentrate between 1.1% and 21.3% [18]. NGS could identify HIV drug-resistant variants at a frequency as low as 0.4% [19]. When patients with low-frequency HIVDR mutations receive ART again, the minority drug-resistant strains may return as predominant ones under the selective pressure of the drug [20]. In addition, multiple studies have shown that the presence of low-frequency HIVDR mutations is often related to treatment failure [21,22].

In this study, we conducted a cross-sectional survey among patients under ART interruption, and compared the mutation detection between NGS and SS using plasma samples from patients with ART interruption, to provide more information about detecting low-frequency drug resistance mutations and further assistance in implementing ultrasensitive HIVDR surveillance in routine assays and to guide the choice of treatment regimen.

2. Results

2.1. Characteristics of the Study Population

A total of 174 patients were included in the survey in 2016 (Table 1). Only 60 (34.5%) patients were followed up a median 10 months later, with 49 still in ART interruption and 11 re-initiating ART. Among the 174 patients, 88.5% (154/174) were aged 30 and above; 66.1% (115/174) were male; 65.5% (114/174) were illiterate or had a primary school education; 67.2% (117/174) were married or living with a partner; 61.5% (107/174) and 4.0% (7/174) of the patients were infected through heterosexual and homosexual contacting, respectively and 27.6% (48/174) were infected through injection drug using. The numbers of patients with CRF01_AE, CRF07_BC and CRF08_BC HIV-1 strains were 35, 61 and 58 (20.1%, 35.1% and 33.3%), respectively. Seventy (40.2%) patients had a CD4$^+$ T cell count of <200 cells/mm^3 at investigation. A total of 150 (86.2%) patients had received non-nucleotide reverse transcriptase inhibitor (NNRTI)-based first-line antiretroviral regimens (stavudine (d4T)/azidothymidine (AZT)/tenofovir (TDF) + lamivudine (3TC) + efavirenz (EFV)/nevirapine (NVP)) before ART interruption. The median duration of treatment before ART interruption was 16 (interquartile range (IQR): 7–26) months, while the median duration of ART interruption was 12 (IQR: 6–24) months at survey.

2.2. Detected HIV Drug Resistance Mutations

Drug resistance mutations (DRMs) were detected at 12 positions in the partial *pol* region by Sanger sequencing (Figure 1), including one in the protease (PR) region, an accessory protease inhibitor (PI)-related resistance mutation (Q58E), and eleven in the reverse transcriptase (RT) region, including one nucleotide reverse transcriptase inhibitor (NRTI)-related (M184V), and ten others were NNRTI-related. The most common drug resistance mutation was K103N (13.2%), followed by V179D (6.3%) and E138AGK (3.5%). At the 20% detection threshold, NGS detected all the mutations identified by SS except a V106M mutation in one patient, as there were mixtures in the first (G to R) and third nucleotides (A to R) in the codon at Sanger sequencing. In addition, NGS detected three more mutations in three patients: Y188C, E138A and K103N, at frequencies of 22.96%, 27.38% and 43.68%, respectively. There were no additional DRMs detected at the frequencies between 15% and 20%. Low-frequency DRMs (<15% frequency) were only detected by NGS, but not by SS. K65R was the most common low-frequency DRM with frequencies between 1% and 9%, concentrated at frequencies from 2% to 5%. It is interesting that this low-frequency K65R mutation is significantly unevenly distributed among subtypes; 5.7% (2/35) in CRF01_AE, when compared with 95.1% (58/61) in CRF07_BC and 93.1% (54/58) in CRF08_BC ($p < 0.001$). Other low-frequency NRTI-related mutations were K70QE, F77L, T215AI and K219QE. M46LI was the common low-frequency PI-related mutation, with frequencies ranging from 1% to 13%. Other PI-related mutations such as L10F, I47V, I50V, F53L, I54VT and N83D have the mutation frequency of about 2%.

Table 1. Characteristics of participants with antiretroviral therapy (ART) interruption.

Characteristics	Number (%)
Total	174
Age	
18–30	20 (11.5)
30–50	78 (44.8)
≥50	76 (43.7)
Gender	
Male	115 (66.1)
Female	59 (33.9)
Education	
Illiterate and primary school	114 (65.5)
Secondary school and above	60 (34.5)
Marital status	
Married or living with partner	117 (67.2)
Single	32 (18.4)
Other	25 (14.4)
Route of HIV infection	
Heterosexual	107 (61.5)
Homosexual	7 (4.0)
Injecting drug using	48 (27.6)
Other	12 (6.9)
Subtype	
CRF01_AE	35 (20.1)
CRF07_BC	61 (35.1)
CRF08_BC	58 (33.3)
B′	16 (9.2)
Other [a]	4 (2.3)
$CD4^+$ T cell count at the time of investigation(per uL)	
<200	70 (40.2)
200–350	62 (35.6)
≥350	42 (24.2)
Antiretroviral regimen before discontinuation	
d4T+3TC+EFV/NVP	1 (0.6)
AZT+3TC+EFV/NVP	66 (37.9)
TDF+3TC+EFV/NVP	83 (47.7)
AZT/TDF+3TC+LPV/r	24 (13.8)
Duration of treatment before ART interruption(median, (IQR), months)	16 (7–26)
Duration of ART interruption at survey (median, (IQR), months)	12 (6–24)

[a] includes CRF 55_01B (2, 1.1%), CRF 62_BC (1, 0.6%), Unknown (1, 0.6%). HIV, Human immunodeficiency virus; ART, antiretroviral therapy; IQR, interquartile range; d4T, Stavudine; 3TC, Lamivudine; AZT, Azidothymidine; TDF, Tenofovir; EFV, Efavirenz; NVP, Nevirapine; LPV/r, Lopinavir/r.

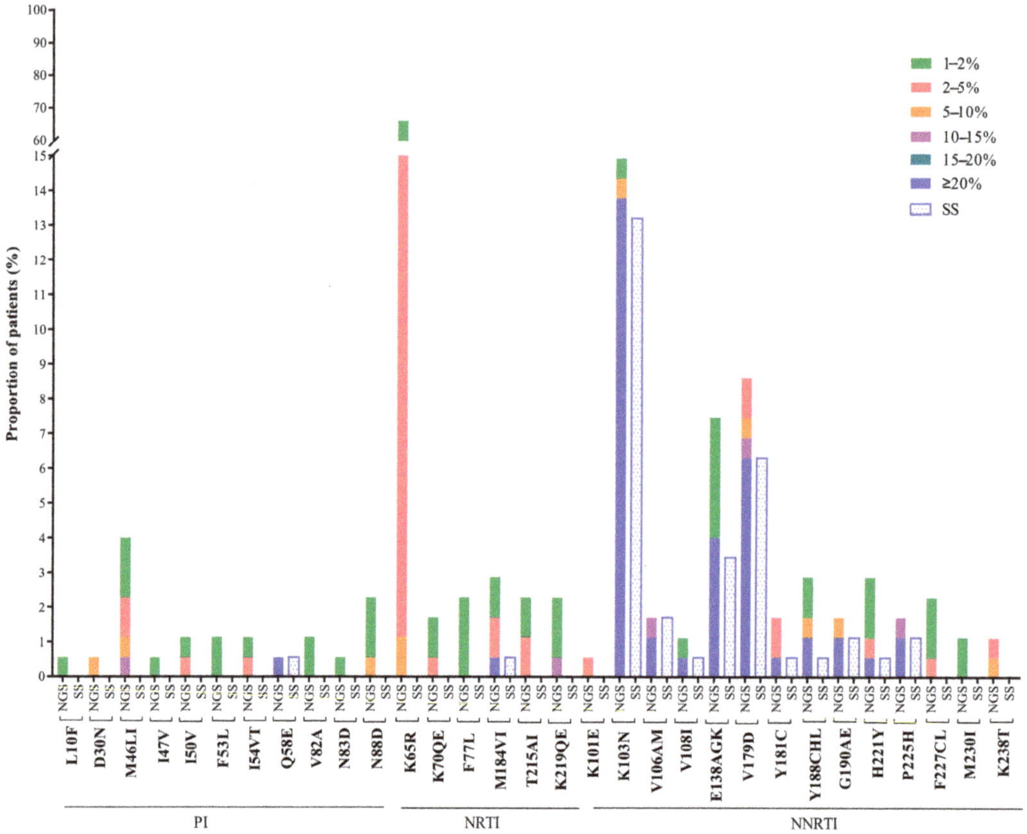

Figure 1. Frequency and pattern of HIV drug resistance (HIVDR) mutations detected by Sanger sequencing (SS) and next-generation sequencing (NGS) at different detection thresholds. Note: HIVDR, HIV drug resistance; SS, Sanger sequencing; NGS, Next-generation sequencing; PI, Protease inhibitor; NRTI, Nucleoside reverse-transcriptase inhibitor; NNRTI, non-nucleoside reverse-transcriptase inhibitor.

2.3. HIV Drug Resistance Interpretations

Based on Sanger sequencing, 19.5% (34/174) of the patients were shown to have drug resistance variants. With NGS, the rate of resistance was the same; 20.7% (36/174) at the detection thresholds 20% and 15%. It climbed up to 21.3% (37/174), 24.1% (42/174), 45.4% (79/174) and 79.9% (139/174) at thresholds 10%, 5%, 2% and 1%, respectively. Compared with SS, NGS got significantly higher rates of drug resistance at the 1%, 2% and 5% thresholds ($p < 0.05$). For PI and NRTI, the prevalence of HIVDR was the same at 0.6%, identified by SS and NGS at the 15% detection threshold. However, NGS at the 1% and 2% thresholds identified more NRTI-related drug resistance variants (69.0% and 24.7%, respectively) than SS. Compared with NGS, a slightly lower percentage of HIVDR was found by SS for NNRTI-related drug resistance (19.0%, Table 2). For the efavirenz (EFV) or nevirapine (NVP) in first-line NNRTI, the difference between NGS and SS in the identification of drug resistance levels was relatively small. EFV- or NVP-related resistance rates were identified in 15.5% (27/174) and 16.1% (28/174) of patients by SS and NGS (>15% frequencies), respectively.

Table 2. Prevalence of HIV drug resistance detected by SS and NGS.

	SS	20% NGS [a]		15% NGS [a]		10% NGS [a]		5% NGS [a]		2% NGS [a]		1% NGS [a]	
SS or NGS at Various Thresholds	N (%)	N (%)	*p* Value	N (%)	*p* Value	N (%)	*p* Value	N (%)	*p* Value	N (%)	*p* Value	N (%)	*p* Value
Any classes	34 (19.5)	36 (20.7)	0.317	36 (20.7)	0.317	37 (21.3)	0.180	42 (24.1)	0.011	79 (45.4)	<0.001	139 (79.9)	<0.001
PI-related	1 (0.6)	1 (0.6)	1.000	1 (0.6)	1.000	2 (1.2)	0.317	5 (2.9)	0.046	9 (5.2)	0.005	23 (13.2)	<0.001
NRTI-related	1 (0.6)	1 (0.6)	1.000	1 (0.6)	1.000	1 (0.6)	1.000	3 (1.7)	0.157	43 (24.7)	<0.001	120 (69.0)	<0.001
NNRTI-related	33 (19.0)	35 (20.1)	0.317	35 (20.1)	0.317	35 (20.1)	0.317	36 (20.7)	0.180	43 (24.7)	0.004	51 (29.3)	<0.001
EFV/NVP	27 (15.5)	28 (16.1)	0.564	28 (16.1)	0.564	29 (16.7)	0.317	31 (17.8)	0.103	37 (21.3)	0.004	46 (26.4)	<0.001

SS, Sanger sequencing; [a] NGS, next-generation sequencing at 1%, 2%, 5%, 10%, 15%, or 20% detection thresholds; PI, Protease inhibitor; NRTI, Nucleoside reverse-transcriptase inhibitor; NNRTI, non-nucleoside reverse-transcriptase inhibitor.

2.4. Relationship between CD4+ T Cell Count, Viral Load and HIVDR Mutation Frequency

The patients were divided into three groups across the mutation frequencies detected by NGS: 35 patients without HIVDR variants, 103 patients with mutation frequencies lower than 15% and 36 patients with mutation frequencies higher than 15%. Their median CD4+ T cell counts were 140 cell/mm^3 (18–289), 265 cell/mm^3 (IQR: 172–378) and 222 cell/mm^3 (IQR: 82–302), respectively ($p < 0.05$). In addition, their median viral loads were 4.6 $\log_{10}$ copies/mL (4.0–4.9), 4.3 $\log_{10}$ copies/mL (IQR: 3.6–4.7) and 4.0 $\log_{10}$ copies/mL (IQR: 3.6–4.4), respectively ($p < 0.05$). In addition, there was a statistically significant difference in the viral loads between patients with high-frequency variants and patients without variants ($p = 0.0198$, Figure 2).

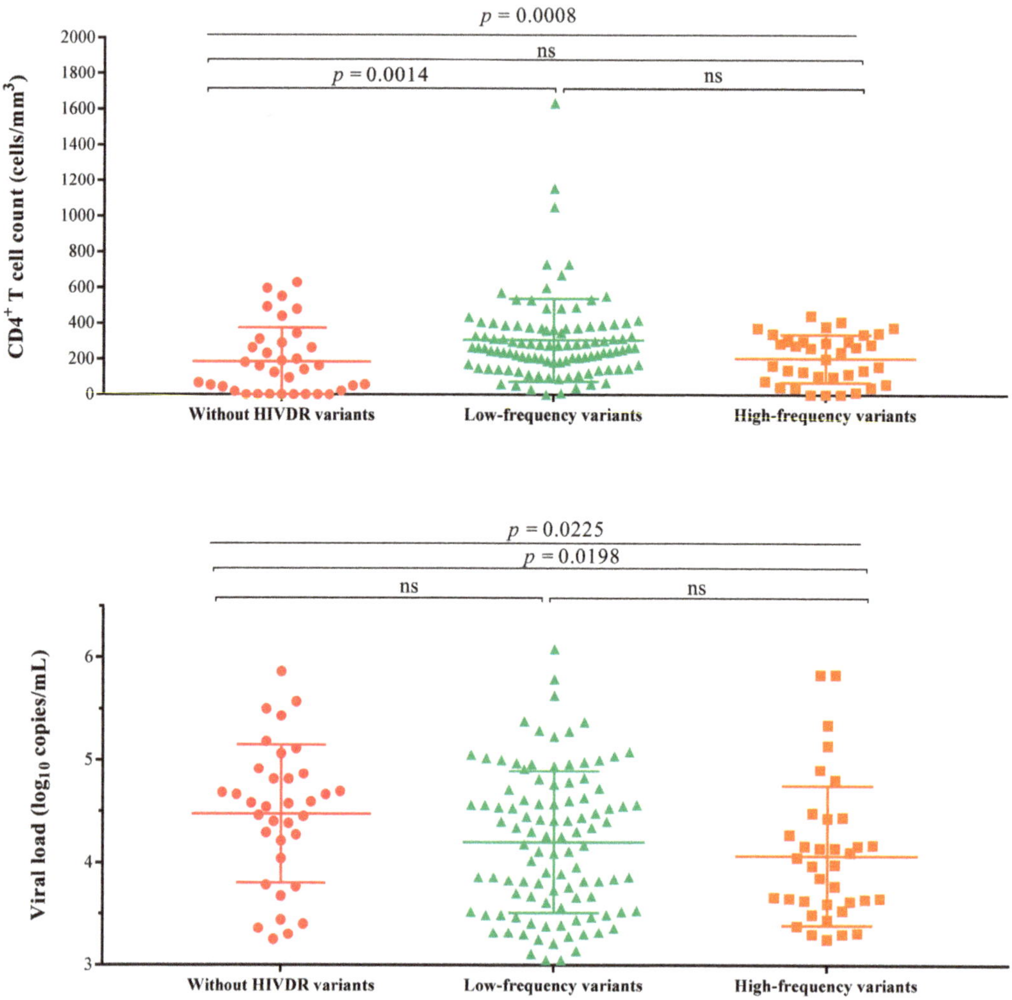

Figure 2. The relationship between the CD4+ T cell count, viral load and HIV drug resistance mutation frequency. Note: The patients were divided into three groups according to the mutation frequency detected by next-generation sequencing. High-frequency variants mean that their mutation frequencies were higher than 15% and low-frequency variants mean that their mutation frequencies were less than 15%. HIVDR, HIV drug resistance; ns, no significance.

2.5. Changes of HIVDR Mutations at Follow-Up

Forty-nine patients were still with ART interruption and were available for follow-up after the median of ten months (IQR: 8–11). At baseline, mutations with a frequency of 20% and above were NRTI-related, such as M184VI (2.0%, 1/49), and NNRTI-related like K103N (14.3%, 7/49), E138AG (4.1%, 2/49), V179D (2.0%, 1/49) and P225H (2.0%, 1/49). Although these variants still existed at follow-up, the frequencies of the mutations M184VI, K103N and P225H decreased over time, and most of them remained at frequencies of more than 20%. However, the frequency of K103N in one patient (GX064) had dropped from 43.7% to 15.3%, and the mutation K103N in another patient (CQ046) with a frequency of 36.9% disappeared (Supplementary Materials). Within a year, some minority DRMs at frequencies 1%–10% remained unchanged, including: PI-related D30N, M46LI, I54VT and N88D, NRTI-related K65R and NNRTI-related Y188CHL. Moreover, K65R was still the most common low-frequency mutation at the follow-up. However, some minority DRMs at frequencies of 1%–5% disappeared, including N83D with PI-related, K70E, T215A, and K219E with NRTI-related and K101E, Y181C, H221Y and K238T with NNRTI-related, while others emerged, such as NNRTI-related V106A in patient GX088 at a frequency of 8.7%, and L23I, I47V and I84V with PI-related, D67N and F77L with NRTI-related and L100V and F227L with NNRTI-related, which appeared at frequencies of 1%–5% (Figure 3).

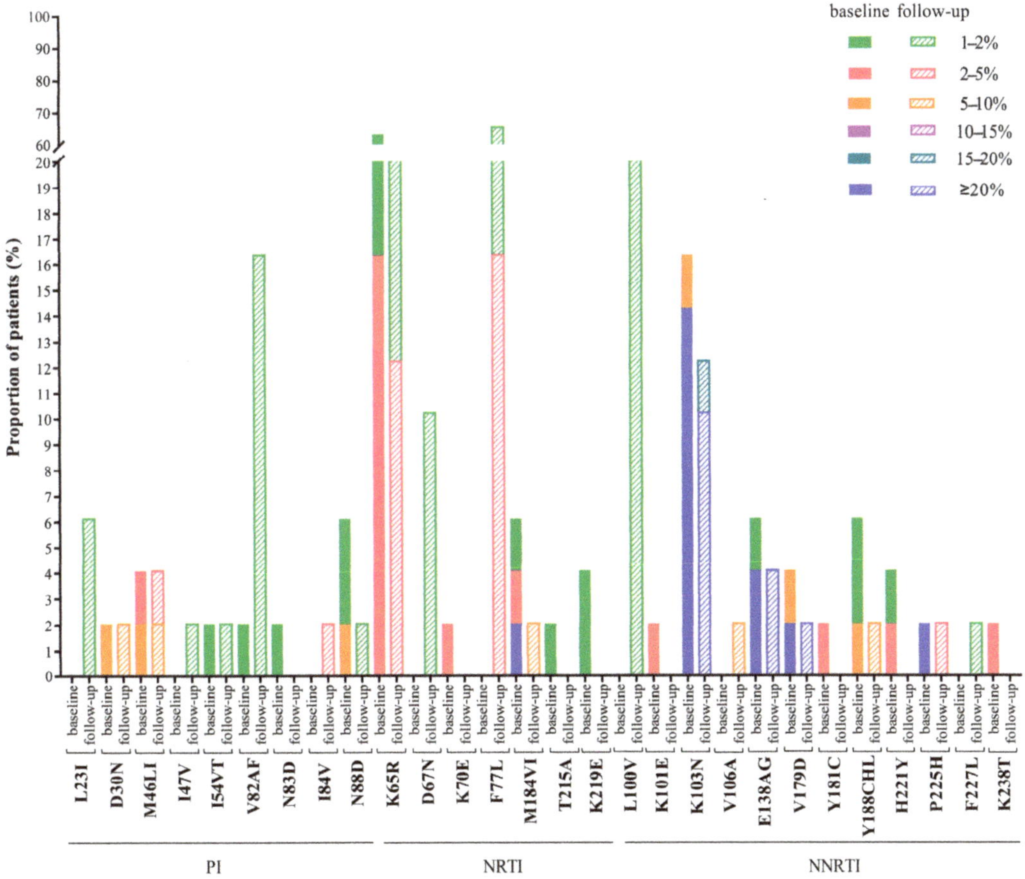

Figure 3. Changes of HIV drug resistance mutations during baseline and follow-up. Note: 49 of the 174 patients were followed up nearly a year later. Mutations and mutation frequency were detected by next-generation sequencing. PI, Protease inhibitor; NRTI, Nucleoside reverse-transcriptase inhibitor; NNRTI, non-nucleoside reverse-transcriptase inhibitor.

3. Discussion

In this study, a cross-sectional survey was conducted among 174 patients with ART interruption in five areas more heavily affected by HIV/AIDS in China. The prevalence of HIVDR was 19.5% at Sanger sequencing, which was obviously higher than a pretreatment HIVDR survey conducted among ART naïve patients in 2017 [23]. A cross-sectional survey of patients with a median of 13.9 months on antiretroviral therapy in eight provinces in China showed that the prevalence of HIVDR in patients receiving ART was 4.3% [24]. Other studies have also suggested that the prevalence of drug resistance in patients receiving ART in some areas of China during the same period is less than 5% [25–27]. Compared with patients who have been receiving antiretroviral therapy, patients whose ART has been interrupted have a higher HIVDR prevalence. Furthermore, the rate of resistance to EFV and/or NVP (15.5%) was more than three times that (4.6%) in those patients. These findings were consistent with those in other countries [28], providing more evidence that patients with ART interruption should consider substituting EFV/NVP for PI or integrase inhibitors when re-initiating antiretroviral treatment.

It was unexpected to get higher rates of HIVDR at NGS than through Sanger sequencing. However, the increase in HIVDR was not statistically significant until the detection threshold was lowered to 5%. Moreover, DRMs detected in protease would have limited impacts on such PIs as Lopinavir/r (LPV/r) in second-line regimens. Four DRMs including D30N (1), M46I (2) and N88D (1) were detected in protease in four participants at a 5%–15% frequency, in addition to one Q58E at a frequency above 90%. The former two confer high or intermediate resistance to Nelfinavir, which is seldomly used at present. N88D and Q58E are PI accessary resistance mutations. There were slight increases in NRTI and NNRTI resistance at the threshold of 5%, when compared with the threshold of 20% or SS, which was consistent with other previous studies [29,30].

Despite the same primer sets for reverse transcription and PCR amplification, there were three NNRTI DRMs in three patients with frequencies between 23% and 44% detected by NGS, not SS. These discrepancies were more likely to be PCR resampling produced at the first several rounds of amplification, and less likely to be the artifacts during NGS sequencing, as NGS artifacts had a <1% frequency and were randomly distributed. Compared with that at the threshold of 5%, the rates of HIVDR were almost doubled when the threshold decreased to 2%, and tripled when down to 1%, as very-low-frequency DRMs were dramatically increased between 1% and 5%. The minority mutations detected by NGS may have resulted from apolipoprotein B mRNA editing catalytic polypeptide (APOBEC)-mediated G-to-A hypermutation such as E138K, M184I and G190E in RT or spontaneous mutation during viral replication, or from PCR error, which was introduced by error-prone reverse transcriptase or PCR enzymes [31]. The sharp increase in low-frequency DRMs agrees with the 5% detection threshold mentioned in other studies [32,33]. At present, the optimal threshold for the NGS detection of low-frequency mutation sites is still inconclusive. Studies have shown that a 5% threshold can provide a reproducible clinically relevant treatment result [34], suggested using a detection threshold of 5% to minimize technical artifacts [31,35]. Using a 5% threshold to report low-frequency variation allows NGS to achieve a moderately increased sensitivity to detect low-frequency DRMs, without compromising sequence accuracy [36,37].

The most common NNRTI DRM above a 5% frequency was K103N (14.4%) in RT, which is consistent with the ART history of EFV/NVP-based first-line therapy. In NRTI DRMs, K65R was the highest (1.2%) at a >5% frequency, which was similar to other research results [29,38]. In addition, this mutation was dramatically increased to 20.7% at 2%–5% frequency. We also found that the distribution of the K65R mutation was related to the HIV subtypes CRF07_BC and CRF08_BC. The K65R mutation causes high-level resistance to tenofovir and intermediate resistance to lamivudine, which are the backbone of first- and second-line regimens. The minority K65R mutations may become major mutations when re-initiating ART, giving rise to virological failure. The subtype-specific differences in the K65R mutation distribution are mainly due to differences in codon usage [39], as it is subtype C in this region in the CRF07_BC and CRF08_BC strains.

The disease progression in patients with HIV is usually monitored by measuring their CD4$^+$ T cell counts. After the interruption of antiretroviral therapy, the CD4$^+$ T cell count drops rapidly in the first few months, then declines slowly [40,41]. A previous study did not find a significant difference in the CD4$^+$ T cell count between patients with and without HIVDR variants [42]. In this study, the patients were divided into three groups across mutation frequencies detected by NGS at a 15% threshold: patients without variants, patients with low-frequency variants and patients with high-frequency variants. Interestingly, the Kruskal–Wallis test found significant differences in the CD4$^+$ T cell counts among the three groups. After the interruption of ART, the viral load level increased exponentially, reaching a peak of 10^6 copies/mL. Then, the viral load usually drops to 10^3–10^5 copies/mL within a few weeks, which can remain relatively stable for many years [43]. In this study, the viral load of patients under ART interruption was above 10^3 copies/mL, and there were statistical differences in the viral loads among the three groups.

Generally speaking, the drug resistance rate will decrease over time in patients after ART interruption. This trend is mainly due to the fact that, in the absence of drug selection pressure, wild-type strains with high viral fitness replace resistant strains to become the main strains in patients [44]. Compared with the baseline, the HIVDR mutations, such as N88D, K65R, M184VI, K103N, E138AG, V179D and P225H, still existed but the frequency gradually decreased, consistent with earlier studies [18,42]. Nevertheless, we found new low-frequency mutations such as I84V, F77L and V106A at follow-ups in this study. A study also showed that new mutations emerge in the absence of drug selection pressure [18]. The emergence of new mutations may be due to the reason that, without the drug selection pressure, virus strains carrying resistance-related mutations may have reduced replication fitness, so they cannot become dominant strains. The results of this study show that new mutations emerge in the form of low frequency, but whether they will continue to exist as the main drug-resistant strains over time is still unknown, and further research is needed.

There are limitations to this study. Firstly, the number of participants was limited. The findings could not be simply extrapolated to other patients with ART interruption. However, the fall or rise in DRMs would be similar to the other settings without ART. The minority DRMs detected by NGS were consistent with other pre-treatment surveys. Secondly, the participants in this study mainly used NNRTI-based first-line regimens before ART interruption. Thus, the findings were not able to reflect the situations with the interruption of ART on PI or integrase inhibitors. Thirdly, the rate of follow-up was low, as patients with ART interruption also dropped out of the HIV care program and were reluctant to keep the follow-up appointments.

In conclusion, patients with ART interruption had higher HIVDR, especially to EFV/NVP. NGS is able to detect more DRMs in such patients than SS, but largely at frequencies of less than 5%. Studies have shown that the drug resistance reports based on a 5% threshold can predict the failure of ART [21,45]. Due to the limitations of this study, the optimal NGS threshold for predicting the failure of antiviral therapy has not yet been determined. Further studies are needed to define the NGS detection threshold for providing a predicative of ART failure.

4. Materials and Methods

4.1. Study Design and Study Participants

We conducted a cross-sectional study among adult patients with ART interruption between 1 January and 31 December 2016, in four provinces and one municipality of China, including Guangxi, Henan, Sichuan, Yunnan and Chongqing, where in China the HIV epidemic was more concentrated, as described previously [46]. Inclusion criteria were: patients aged eighteen years or older, had discontinued ART for at least one month at survey, had received ART for at least three months before ART interruption and had agreed to provide written informed consent. These patients were followed up in 2017. Plasma samples were handled locally and transported in dry ice to the laboratory at the National Center for AIDS/STD Control and Prevention (NCAIDS), Chinese Center for Disease Control and Prevention (China CDC), where the HIV viral load was measured, and HIV drug resistance was genotyped on samples with a viral load ≥1000 copies/mL.

4.2. HIV RNA Extraction and Sample Amplification

Viral RNA was extracted using the QIAamp viral RNA mini kit (Qiagen, Hilton, Germany), following the manufacturer's protocol. Extracted RNA was used for amplification of the PR region (4–99 amino acids) and the partial RT region (1–251 amino acids) of the HIV-1 *pol* gene region using an in-house method [47]. Briefly, the first-round PCR was performed in 25 μL volume reactions using the one-step RT-PCR kit (Promega, Madison, WI, USA) with the primers PRTM-F1 and RT-R1. The second-round PCR was performed in 50 μL volume reactions using the primers PRT-F2 and RT-R2.

4.3. Sanger Sequencing and Drug Resistance Analysis

The amplified products were sequenced using Sanger sequencer ABI 3730 (Applied Biosystems, Carlsbad, CA, USA). Obtained raw sequences were edited and assembled using Sequencher (version 4.10.1, Gene Codes Corporation, Ann Arbor, MI). The secondary peak threshold was set to 20%. The edited sequence was aligned with the HXB2 reference sequence through BioEdit (version 7.0.9, Informer Technologies Inc.). Sample contamination and other sequence quality controls were monitored using the WHO HIVDR QC tool (https://recall.bccfe.ca/who_qc/, accessed on 23 September 2019) and through constructing Neighbor joining phylogenetic trees using MEGA (version 6.06). HIV-1 subtypes were determined using reference sequences from HIV Databases (https://www.hiv.lanl.gov/content/index, accessed on 8 October 2019) through phylogenetic trees. The drug resistance mutations were identified and interpreted using the HIVdb version 8.9-1 (https://hivdb.stanford.edu/hivdb/, accessed on 10 October 2019).

4.4. Next-Generation Sequencing and Drug Resistance Analysis

Second-round amplicons were cleaned using KAPA PureBeads (Roche, Basel, Switzerland) and quantified using the Qubit dsDNA HS assay kit (Thermo Fisher Scientific, Carlsbad, CA, USA). Sequencing libraries were prepared using the 96-sample KAPA HyperPlus Kit (Roche, Basel, Switzerland). The samples were pooled in each run with a 40% Phix control library (v3, Illumina, San Diego, CA, USA) to increase the diversity of libraries and then sequenced on the Illumina Miseq system [48] using a v3 600-cycle reagent kit (Illumina, San Diego, CA, USA). The raw data were analyzed using the HyDRA Web tool (http://hydra.canada.ca/, accessed on 20 January 2020) according to *HyDRA Web User Guide* [49], producing lists and frequencies of drug resistance mutations, and then interpreted by using the HIVdb algorithm.

4.5. Statistical Analysis

DRMs were identified according to the 2019 International Antiviral Society (IAS) list. HIV drug resistance was defined as low-, intermediate- or high-levels of drug resistance according to the HIVdb algorithm 8.9-1. HIV drug resistance was determined based on NGS with detection thresholds of 20%, 15%, 10%, 5%, 2% and 1%, and was compared with that detected based on Sanger sequencing by the McNemar test, respectively. Quantitative data are presented as medians and were analyzed by the Kruskal–Wallis test. All data were analyzed using the Statistical Analysis System version 9.4 (SAS Institute Inc., Cary, NC, USA). Two-sided p values of <0.05 were considered statistically significant.

Supplementary Materials: The following are available online at https://www.mdpi.com/2076-0817/10/3/264/s1, Table S1: The HIV drug resistance mutations of each sample (n = 174) were detected by Sanger sequencing and the next-generation sequencing; Table S2: The drug resistance mutations of each sample (n = 49) at baseline and follow-up detected by the next-generation sequencing, and the value in brackets is the mutation frequencies.

Author Contributions: M.L., H.X., Y.R., Y.S. and L.L. (Lingjie Liao). were responsible for study design and planning. S.L. (Shujia Liang), C.Z., M.C., S.L. (Shu Liang) and C.L. contributed to data collection. M.L., L.L. (Lei Liu), Z.Z., Y.F., C.S., H.X., Y.R., Y.S. and L.L. (Lingjie Liao) contributed to data analysis and interpretation. M.L., H.X., Y.R., Y.S. and L.L. (Lingjie Liao) contributed to writing the manuscript. All authors read and approved the final version of the manuscript.

Funding: This work was supported by National Natural Science Foundation of China (11971479), the Ministry of Science and Technology of China (grant 2017ZX10201101, 2018ZX10721102-006), the State Key Laboratory of Infectious Disease Prevention and Control, the Department of Science and Technology of Guangxi Zhuang Autonomous Region (AB16380213), the Key technical posts for HIV/AIDS prevention and control of Guangxi Bagui scholars, and special funds for AIDS prevention and control. The fund providers had no role in the study design, data collection and analysis, decision to publish, or preparation of the manuscript.

Institutional Review Board Statement: Institutional review board approval was granted by the National Center for AIDS/STD Control and Prevention, Chinese Center for Disease Control and Prevention.

Informed Consent Statement: Informed consent was obtained from all subjects involved in the study.

Data Availability Statement: Data are contained within the article.

Conflicts of Interest: The authors declare that there are no conflict of interest.

References

1. Poorolajal, J.; Hooshmand, E.; Mahjub, H.; Esmailnasab, N.; Jenabi, E. Survival rate of AIDS disease and mortality in HIV-infected patients: A meta-analysis. *Public Health* **2016**, *139*, 3–12. [CrossRef] [PubMed]
2. UNAIDS. Latest Global and Regional Statistics on the Status of the AIDS Epidemic. 2020. Available online: https://www.unaids.org/sites/default/files/media_asset/UNAIDS_FactSheet_en.pdf (accessed on 27 September 2020).
3. Touloumi, G.; Pantazis, N.; Antoniou, A.; Stirnadel, H.A.; Walker, S.A.; Porter, K. Highly Active Antiretroviral Therapy Interruption. *JAIDS J. Acquir. Immune Defic. Syndr.* **2006**, *42*, 554–561. [CrossRef]
4. Olsen, C.H.; Mocroft, A.; Kirk, O.; Vella, S.; Blaxhult, A.; Clumeck, N.; Fisher, M.; Katlama, C.; Phillips, A.; Lundgren, J.; et al. Interruption of combination antiretroviral therapy and risk of clinical disease progression to AIDS or death. *HIV Med.* **2007**, *8*, 96–104. [CrossRef]
5. Kavasery, R.; Galai, N.; Astemborski, J.; Lucas, G.M.; Celentano, D.D.; Kirk, G.D.; Mehta, S.H. Nonstructured Treatment Interruptions Among Injection Drug Users in Baltimore, MD. *JAIDS J. Acquir. Immune Defic. Syndr.* **2009**, *50*, 360–366. [CrossRef] [PubMed]
6. Zhu, H.; Napravnik, S.; Eron, J.; Cole, S.; Ma, Y.; Wohl, D.; Dou, Z.; Zhang, Y.; Liu, Z.; Zhao, D.; et al. Attrition among Human Immunodeficiency Virus (HIV)- Infected Patients Initiating Antiretroviral Therapy in China, 2003–2010. *PLoS ONE* **2012**, *7*, e39414. [CrossRef]
7. Alvarez-Uria, G.; Naik, P.K.; Pakam, R.; Midde, M. Factors associated with attrition, mortality, and loss to follow up after antiretroviral therapy initiation: Data from an HIV cohort study in India. *Glob. Health Action* **2013**, *6*, 21682. [CrossRef]
8. Ananworanich, J.; Gayet-Ageron, A.; Le Braz, M.; Prasithsirikul, W.; Chetchotisakd, P.; Kiertiburanakul, S.; Munsakul, W.; Raksakulkarn, P.; Tansuphasawasdikul, S.; Sirivichayakul, S.; et al. CD4-guided scheduled treatment interruptions compared with continuous therapy for patients infected with HIV-1: Results of the Staccato randomised trial. *Lancet* **2006**, *368*, 459–465. [CrossRef]
9. Hogg, R.S.; Heath, K.; Bangsberg, D.; Yip, B.; Press, N.; O'Shaughnessy, M.V.; Montaner, J.S.G. Intermittent use of triple-combination therapy is predictive of mortality at baseline and after 1 year of follow-up. *AIDS* **2002**, *16*, 1051–1058. [CrossRef] [PubMed]
10. Pereira-Vaz, J.; Duque, V.; Trindade, L.; Saraiva-Da-Cunha, J.; Meliço-Silvestre, A. Detection of the protease codon 35 amino acid insertion in sequences from treatment-naïve HIV-1 subtype C infected individuals in the Central Region of Portugal. *J. Clin. Virol.* **2009**, *46*, 169–172. [CrossRef]
11. World Health Organization. Global Action Plan on HIV Drug Resistance 2017–2021. Available online: https://www.who.int/hiv/pub/drugresistance/hivdr-action-plan-2017-2021/en/ (accessed on 15 September 2020).
12. Devereux, H.L.; Youle, M.; Johnson, M.A.; Loveday, C. Rapid decline in detectability of HIV-1 drug resistance mutations after stopping therapy. *Aids* **1999**, *13*, F123–F127. [CrossRef]

13. Lawrence, J.; Mayers, D.L.; Hullsiek, K.H.; Collins, G.; Abrams, D.I.; Reisler, R.B.; Crane, L.R.; Schmetter, B.S.; Dionne, T.J.; Saldanha, J.M.; et al. Structured Treatment Interruption in Patients with Multidrug-Resistant Human Immunodeficiency Virus. *N. Engl. J. Med.* **2003**, *349*, 837–846. [CrossRef]
14. Taylor, S.; Jayasuriya, A.; Fisher, M.; Allan, S.; Wilkins, E.; Gilleran, G.; Heald, L.; Fidler, S.; Owen, A.; Back, D.; et al. Lopinavir/ritonavir single agent therapy as a universal combination antiretroviral therapy stopping strategy: Results from the STOP 1 and STOP 2 studies. *J. Antimicrob. Chemother.* **2011**, *67*, 675–680. [CrossRef]
15. Casadellà, M.; Paredes, R. Deep sequencing for HIV-1 clinical management. *Virus Res.* **2017**, *239*, 69–81. [CrossRef] [PubMed]
16. Arias, A.; López, P.; Sánchez, R.; Yamamura, Y.; Rivera-Amill, V. Sanger and Next Generation Sequencing Approaches to Evaluate HIV-1 Virus in Blood Compartments. *Int. J. Environ. Res. Public Health* **2018**, *15*, 1697. [CrossRef] [PubMed]
17. John, E.P.S.; Simen, B.B.; Turenchalk, G.S.; Braverman, M.S.; Abbate, I.; Aerssens, J.; Bouchez, O.; Gabriel, C.; Izopet, J.; Meixenberger, K.; et al. A Follow-Up of the Multicenter Collaborative Study on HIV-1 Drug Resistance and Tropism Testing Using 454 Ultra Deep Pyrosequencing. *PLoS ONE* **2016**, *11*, e0146687. [CrossRef]
18. Nouchi, A.; Nguyen, T.; Valantin, M.A.; Simon, A.; Sayon, S.; Agher, R.; Calvez, V.; Katlama, C.; Marcelin, A.G.; Soulie, C. Dynamics of drug resistance-associated mutations in HIV-1 DNA reverse tran-scriptase sequence during effective ART. *J. Antimicrob. Chemother.* **2018**, *73*, 2141–2146. [CrossRef]
19. Kozal, M.J.; Chiarella, J.; John, E.P.S.; Moreno, E.A.; Simen, B.B.; Arnold, T.E.; Lataillade, M. Prevalence of low-level HIV-1 variants with reverse transcriptase mutation K65R and the effect of antiretroviral drug exposure on variant levels. *Antivir. Ther.* **2011**, *16*, 925–929. [CrossRef] [PubMed]
20. Metzner, K.J.; Giulieri, S.G.; Knoepfel, S.A.; Rauch, P.; Burgisser, P.; Yerly, S.; Gunthard, H.F.; Cavassini, M. Minority Quasispecies of Drug-Resistant HIV-1 That Lead to Early Therapy Failure in Treatment-Naive and -Adherent Patients. *Clin. Infect. Dis.* **2009**, *48*, 239–247. [CrossRef]
21. Mbunkah, A.H.; Bertagnolio, S.; Hamers, R.L.; Hunt, G.; Inzaule, S.; De Wit, T.F.R.; Paredes, R.; Parkin, N.T.; Jordan, M.R.; Metzner, K.J.; et al. Low-Abundance Drug-Resistant HIV-1 Variants in Antiretroviral Drug-Naive Individuals: A Systematic Review of Detection Methods, Prevalence, and Clinical Impact. *J. Infect. Dis.* **2019**, *221*, 1584–1597. [CrossRef]
22. Inzaule, S.C.; Hamers, R.L.; Noguera-Julian, M.; Casadellà, M.; Parera, M.; Kityo, C.; Steegen, K.; Naniche, D.; Clotet, B.; De Wit, T.F.R.; et al. Clinically relevant thresholds for ultrasensitive HIV drug resistance testing: A multi-country nested case-control study. *Lancet HIV* **2018**, *5*, e638–e646. [CrossRef]
23. Kang, R.-H.; Liang, S.-J.; Ma, Y.-L.; Liang, S.; Xiao, L.; Zhang, X.-H.; Lu, H.-Y.; Xu, X.-Q.; Luo, S.-B.; Sun, X.-G.; et al. Pretreatment HIV drug resistance in adults initiating antiretroviral therapy in China, 2017. *Infect. Dis. Poverty* **2020**, *9*, 1–9. [CrossRef]
24. Zuo, Z.; Liang, S.; Sun, X.; Bussell, S.; Yan, J.; Kan, W.; Leng, X.; Liao, L.; Ruan, Y.; Shao, Y.; et al. Drug Resistance and Virological Failure among HIV-Infected Patients after a Decade of Antiretroviral Treatment Expansion in Eight Provinces of China. *PLoS ONE* **2016**, *11*, e0166661. [CrossRef] [PubMed]
25. Lin, B.; Sun, X.; Su, S.; Lv, C.; Zhang, X.; Lin, L.; Wang, R.; Fu, J.; Kang, D. HIV drug resistance in HIV positive individuals under antiretroviral treatment in Shandong Province, China. *PLoS ONE* **2017**, *12*, e0181997. [CrossRef]
26. Wang, J.; He, C.; Hsi, J.H.; Xu, X.; Liu, Y.; He, J.; Ling, H.; Ding, P.; Tong, Y.; Zou, X.; et al. Virological Outcomes and Drug Resistance in Chinese Patients after 12 Months of 3TC-Based First-Line Antiretroviral Treatment, 2011–2012. *PLoS ONE* **2014**, *9*, e88305. [CrossRef] [PubMed]
27. Xing, H.; Wang, X.; Liao, L.; Ma, Y.; Su, B.; Fu, J.; He, J.; Chen, L.; Pan, X.; Dong, Y.; et al. Incidence and Associated Factors of HIV Drug Resistance in Chinese HIV-Infected Patients Receiving Antiretroviral Treatment. *PLoS ONE* **2013**, *8*, e62408. [CrossRef]
28. World Health Organization. HIV Drug Resistance Report 2019. Available online: https://www.who.int/hiv/pub/drugresistance/hivdr-report-2019/en/ (accessed on 28 August 2020).
29. Moscona, R.; Ram, D.; Wax, M.; Bucris, E.; Levy, I.; Mendelson, E.; Mor, O. Comparison between next-generation and Sanger-based sequencing for the detection of transmitted drug-resistance mutations among recently infected HIV-1 patients in Israel, 2000–2014. *J. Int. AIDS Soc.* **2017**, *20*, 21846. [CrossRef]
30. Taylor, T.; Lee, E.R.; Nykoluk, M.; Enns, E.; Liang, B.; Capina, R.; Gauthier, M.-K.; Van Domselaar, G.; Sandstrom, P.; Brooks, J.; et al. A MiSeq-HyDRA platform for enhanced HIV drug resistance genotyping and surveillance. *Sci. Rep.* **2019**, *9*, 1–11. [CrossRef] [PubMed]
31. Tzou, P.L.; Ariyaratne, P.; Varghese, V.; Lee, C.; Rakhmanaliev, E.; Villy, C.; Yee, M.; Tan, K.; Michel, G.; Pinsky, B.A.; et al. Comparison of anIn VitroDiagnostic Next-Generation Sequencing Assay with Sanger Sequencing for HIV-1 Genotypic Resistance Testing. *J. Clin. Microbiol.* **2018**, *56*, e00105-18. [CrossRef] [PubMed]
32. Stelzl, E.; Pröll, J.; Bizon, B.; Niklas, N.; Danzer, M.; Hackl, C.; Stabentheiner, S.; Gabriel, C.; Kessler, H.H. Human immunodeficiency virus type 1 drug resistance testing: Evaluation of a new ultra-deep sequencing-based protocol and comparison with the TRUGENE HIV-1 Genotyping Kit. *J. Virol. Methods* **2011**, *178*, 94–97. [CrossRef] [PubMed]
33. Chen, N.-Y.; Kao, S.-W.; Liu, Z.-H.; Wu, T.-S.; Tsai, C.-L.; Lin, H.-H.; Wong, W.-W.; Chang, Y.-Y.; Chen, S.-S.; Ku, S.W.-W. Shall I trust the report? Variable performance of Sanger sequencing revealed by deep sequencing on HIV drug resistance mutation detection. *Int. J. Infect. Dis.* **2020**, *93*, 182–191. [CrossRef] [PubMed]
34. Ávila-Ríos, S.; Parkin, N.; Swanstrom, R.; Paredes, R.; Shafer, R.; Ji, H.; Kantor, R. Next-Generation Sequencing for HIV Drug Resistance Testing: Laboratory, Clinical, and Implementation Considerations. *Viruses* **2020**, *12*, 617. [CrossRef]

35. Trabaud, M.-A.; Icard, V.; Ramière, C.; Tardy, J.-C.; Scholtes, C.; André, P. Comparison of HIV-1 drug-resistance genotyping by ultra-deep sequencing and sanger sequencing using clinical samples. *J. Med. Virol.* **2017**, *89*, 1912–1919. [CrossRef] [PubMed]
36. Fogel, J.M.; Bonsall, D.; Cummings, V.; Bowden, R.; Golubchik, T.; De Cesare, M.; Wilson, E.A.; Gamble, T.; Del Rio, C.; Batey, D.S.; et al. Performance of a high-throughput next-generation sequencing method for analysis of HIV drug resistance and viral load. *J. Antimicrob. Chemother.* **2020**, *75*, 3510–3516. [CrossRef] [PubMed]
37. Dessilly, G.; Goeminne, L.; Vandenbroucke, A.-T.; Dufrasne, F.E.; Martin, A.; Kabamba-Mukabi, B. First evaluation of the Next-Generation Sequencing platform for the detection of HIV-1 drug resistance mutations in Belgium. *PLoS ONE* **2018**, *13*, e0209561. [CrossRef]
38. Liu, T.F.; Shafer, R.W. Web Resources for HIV Type 1 Genotypic-Resistance Test Interpretation. *Clin. Infect. Dis.* **2006**, *42*, 1608–1618. [CrossRef]
39. Clutter, D.S.; Jordan, M.R.; Bertagnolio, S.; Shafer, R.W. HIV-1 drug resistance and resistance testing. *Infect. Genet. Evol.* **2016**, *46*, 292–307. [CrossRef]
40. Mocroft, A.; Phillips, A.N.; Gatell, J.; Ledergerber, B.; Fisher, M.; Clumeck, N.; Losso, M.; Lazzarin, A.; Fätkenheuer, G.; Lundgren, J.D. Normalisation of CD4 counts in patients with HIV-1 infection and maximum virological suppression who are taking combination antiretroviral therapy: An observational cohort study. *Lancet* **2007**, *370*, 407–413. [CrossRef]
41. El-Sadr, W.; Lundgren, J.D.; Neaton, J.D.; Gordin, F.; Abrams, D.; Arduino, R.C.; Babiker, A.; Burman, W.J.; Clumeck, N.; Cohen, C.; et al. $CD4^+$ Count–Guided Interruption of Antiretroviral Treatment. *N. Engl. J. Med.* **2006**, *355*, 2283–2296. [CrossRef]
42. E Iarikov, D.; Irizarry-Acosta, M.; Martorell, C.; A Rauch, C.; Hoffman, R.P.; Skiest, D.J. Use of HIV Resistance Testing After Prolonged Treatment Interruption. *JAIDS J. Acquir. Immune Defic. Syndr.* **2010**, *53*, 333–337. [CrossRef]
43. Hill, A.L.; Rosenbloom, D.I.S.; Nowak, M.A.; Siliciano, R.F. Insight into treatment of HIV infection from viral dynamics models. *Immunol. Rev.* **2018**, *285*, 9–25. [CrossRef]
44. Paredes, R.; Sagar, M.; Marconi, V.C.; Hoh, R.; Martin, J.N.; Parkin, N.T.; Petropoulos, C.J.; Deeks, S.G.; Kuritzkes, D.R. In Vivo Fitness Cost of the M184V Mutation in Multidrug-Resistant Human Immunodeficiency Virus Type 1 in the Absence of Lamivudine. *J. Virol.* **2008**, *83*, 2038–2043. [CrossRef]
45. Mohamed, S.; Ravet, S.; Camus, C.; Khiri, H.; Olive, D.; Halfon, P. Clinical and analytical relevance of NNRTIs minority mutations on viral failure in HIV-1 infected patients. *J. Med. Virol.* **2014**, *86*, 394–403. [CrossRef]
46. Lei, L.; Zhong-Bao, Z.; Ling-Jie, L.; Shu-Jia, L.; Yan-Ling, M.; Guo-Hui, W.; Shu, L.; Sui-An, T.; Jian-Mei, H.; Yi-Ming, S.; et al. The drug resistance in HIV/AIDS patients who had stopped ART in 2016. *China Trop. Med.* **2018**, *18*, 1613–1618.
47. Inzaule, S.; Yang, C.; Kasembeli, A.; Nafisa, L.; Okonji, J.; Oyaro, B.; Lando, R.; Mills, L.A.; Laserson, K.; Thomas, T.; et al. Field Evaluation of a Broadly Sensitive HIV-1 In-House Genotyping Assay for Use with both Plasma and Dried Blood Spot Specimens in a Resource-Limited Country. *J. Clin. Microbiol.* **2012**, *51*, 529–539. [CrossRef]
48. Ravi, R.K.; Walton, K.; Khosroheidari, M. MiSeq: A Next Generation Sequencing Platform for Genomic Analysis. In *Methods in Molecular Biology*; Springer Science and Business Media LLC: Berlin/Heidelberg, Germany, 2018; Volume 1706, pp. 223–232.
49. Nykoluk, M.; Taylor, T.; Enns, E.; Ji, H. HyDRA Web User Guide. 2016. Available online: https://hydra.canada.ca/pages/about?lang=en-CA (accessed on 20 August 2019).

pathogens

MDPI

Article

Limited HIV-1 Subtype C *nef* 3′PPT Variation in Combination Antiretroviral Therapy Naïve and Experienced People Living with HIV in Botswana

Kaelo K. Seatla [1,2,*], Dorcas Maruapula [1,2], Wonderful T. Choga [1,3], Olorato Morerinyane [1], Shahin Lockman [1,4], Vladimir Novitsky [5,6], Ishmael Kasvosve [2], Sikhulile Moyo [1,4] and Simani Gaseitsiwe [1,4]

1 Botswana Harvard AIDS Institute Partnership, Gaborone, Botswana; dmaruapula@bhp.org.bw (D.M.); wchoga@bhp.org.bw (W.T.C.); omorerinyane@bhp.org.bw (O.M.); slockman@hsph.harvard.edu (S.L.); smoyo@bhp.org.bw (S.M.); sgaseitsiwe@bhp.org.bw (S.G.)
2 Faculty of Health Sciences, School of Allied Health Professions, University of Botswana, Gaborone, Botswana; kasvosvei@ub.ac.bw
3 Division of Human Genetics, Department of Pathology, Faculty of Health Sciences, University of Cape Town, Cape Town 7925, South Africa
4 Department of Immunology & Infectious Diseases, Harvard T.H. Chan School of Public Health, Boston, MA 02115, USA
5 The Warren Alpert Medical School of Brown University, Providence, RI 12321, USA; vnovi@hsph.harvard.edu
6 Division of Infectious Diseases, The Miriam Hospital, Providence, RI 23324, USA
* Correspondence: kseatla@bhp.org.bw; Tel.: +267-390-2671; Fax: +267-390-284

Citation: Seatla, K.K.; Maruapula, D.; Choga, W.T.; Morerinyane, O.; Lockman, S.; Novitsky, V.; Kasvosve, I.; Moyo, S.; Gaseitsiwe, S. Limited HIV-1 Subtype C *nef* 3′PPT Variation in Combination Antiretroviral Therapy Naïve and Experienced People Living with HIV in Botswana. *Pathogens* **2021**, *10*, 1027. https://doi.org/10.3390/pathogens10081027

Academic Editor: Hezhao Ji

Received: 28 May 2021
Accepted: 11 August 2021
Published: 13 August 2021

Abstract: Dolutegravir (DTG) is a potent anti-HIV drug that is used to treat HIV globally. There have been reports of mutations in the HIV-1 3′-polypurine tract (3′PPT) of the *nef* gene, contributing to DTG failure; however, there are limited 'real-world' data on this. In addition, there is a knowledge gap on the variability of 3′PPT residues in patients receiving combination antiretroviral therapy (cART) with and without viral load (VL) suppression. HIV-1 subtype C (HIV-1C) whole-genome sequences from cART naïve and experienced individuals were generated using next-generation sequencing. The *nef* gene sequences were trimmed from the generated whole-genome sequences using standard bioinformatics tools. In addition, we generated separate integrase and *nef* gene sequences by Sanger sequencing of plasma samples from individuals with virologic failure (VF) while on a DTG/raltegravir (RAL)-based cART. Analysis of 3′PPT residues was performed, and comparison of proportions computed using Pearson's chi-square test with p-values < 0.05 was considered statistically significant. A total of 6009 HIV-1C full genome sequences were generated and had a median $\log_{10}$ HIV-1 VL (Q1, Q3) copies/mL of 1.60 (1.60, 2.60). A total of 12 matching integrase and *nef* gene sequences from therapy-experienced participants failing DTG/ RAL-based cART were generated. HIV-1C 3′PPT *nef* gene sequences from therapy-experienced patients failing DTG cART (n = 12), cART naïve individuals (n = 1263), and individuals on cART with and without virological suppression (n = 4696) all had a highly conserved 3′PPT motif with no statistically significant differences identified. Our study confirms the high conservation of the HIV-1 *nef* gene 3′PPT motif in 'real-world' patients and showed no differences in the motif according to VL suppression or INSTI-based cART failure. Future studies should explore other HIV-1 regions outside of the pol gene for associations with DTG failure.

Keywords: HIV-1; *nef*; Botswana; drug resistance mutations; 3′-polypurine tract; dolutegravir

1. Introduction

Dolutegravir (DTG) is a widely used second-generation integrase strand transfer inhibitor (INSTI) with a high genetic barrier to resistance [1–5]. It prevents the HIV integrase enzyme from incorporating viral DNA into the host cell genome [1]. However, resistance mutations within the integrase enzyme can cause reduced susceptibility to

DTG [1,6]. Most major DTG resistance mutations amongst therapy-experienced individuals are usually located within the HIV-1 catalytic core domain of the integrase region [1,7]. However, a handful of studies have suggested associations between DTG failure and mutations outside the integrase region in the 3′-polypurine tract (3′PPT) of the HIV-1 *nef* gene [8,9].

The *nef* gene of HIV-1 is a small accessory protein of about 206 amino acids that contributes to HIV disease progression mainly by downregulating the expression of CD4 and major histocompatibility complex class I molecules, amongst other functions [10–13]. It has a highly conserved purine-dominated 15-nucleotide sequence (3′PPT) that is involved in the reverse transcription process, resulting in the production of double-stranded viral DNA, enabling the integration into the host cell genome [14–16].

Malet et al. unexpectedly cultured a virus that had mutations in the 3′PPT motif conferring resistance to DTG [8]. Similar mutations were identified in the guanine-tract (G-tract) motif at the 3′ end of 3′PPT of one patient with virologic failure (VF) while on a DTG monotherapy trial [9].

A subsequent study by Malet et al. with a larger number of individuals failing INSTI-based regimens revealed a highly conserved 3′PPT with no associations with DTG failure discernible [17]. Further in vitro work went on to confirm this [18]. A recent study from Cameroon amongst INSTI-naïve individuals also showed a highly conserved 3′PPT region [19]. Furthermore, analysis of publicly available HIV-1 *nef* gene sequences from the Los Alamos HIV-1 database reveals a highly conserved 3′PPT region across various subtypes [17].

Given these inconsistent study results and the fact that there are limited 'real-world' data on the contribution of 3′PPT to failure of DTG-based regimens, we conducted this study to address these knowledge gaps. In our study, we sought to determine the diversity of 3′PPT of the HIV-1 subtype C (HIV-1C) *nef* gene amongst cART-naïve and cART-treated individuals with and without VF. We also assessed whether HIV-1C mutations in 3′PPT contribute to VF amongst individuals failing INSTI-based cART regimens regardless of the presence of mutations in the integrase region.

2. Materials and Methods

2.1. Selection of Study Population and HIV-1 Genotyping

Participant samples were obtained from two studies conducted in Botswana. The first study consisted of sequences generated from residual plasma specimens obtained from therapy-experienced individuals experiencing VF while on DTG- or raltegravir (RAL)-based cART described elsewhere (BOSELE study; Figure 1) [7]. VF was defined as two or more consecutive plasma HIV-1 RNA levels (viral loads (VL)) > 400 copies/mL as per standard of care guidelines in Botswana. The HIV-1 integrase region was amplified using nested reverse transcription-polymerase chain reactions (RT-PCRs) where necessary and sequenced using a BigDye™ Terminator v3.1 Cycle Sequencing Kit (Applied Biosystems, Carlsbad, CA, USA) on a 3130xl Genetic Analyser (Life Technologies Corporation, Applied Biosystems, Carlsbad, CA, USA) as previously described [7,20]. Sequencing of the *nef* gene was attempted from the same HIV-1 extracts that integrase sequences were successfully generated from. Briefly, products of about 620 base pairs were amplified using nested RT-PCRs where necessary using the following primers numbered relative to HIV-1 reference strain (HxB2) nucleotide positions (shown in brackets): NEF8683F_pan TAGCAGTAGCTGRGKGRACAGATAG (8683–8707), NEF9536R_pan TACAGGCAAAAAGCAGCTGCTTATATGYAG (9507–9536), NEF8746_SgrI_AscI_F AGAGCACCGGCGCGCCTCCACATACCTASAAGAATMAGACARG (8736–8772), and NEF9474_SacII_ClaI_R GCCTCCGCGGATCGATCAGGCCACRCCTCCCTGGAAASKCCC (9449–9491) [21]. Amplicons were bidirectionally Sanger-sequenced as described above. The Sequencher software, version 5.0 (Gene Codes Corporation, Ann Arbor, MI, USA), was used to manually edit our electropherograms and form contigs with further downstream analysis carried using the BioEdit software.

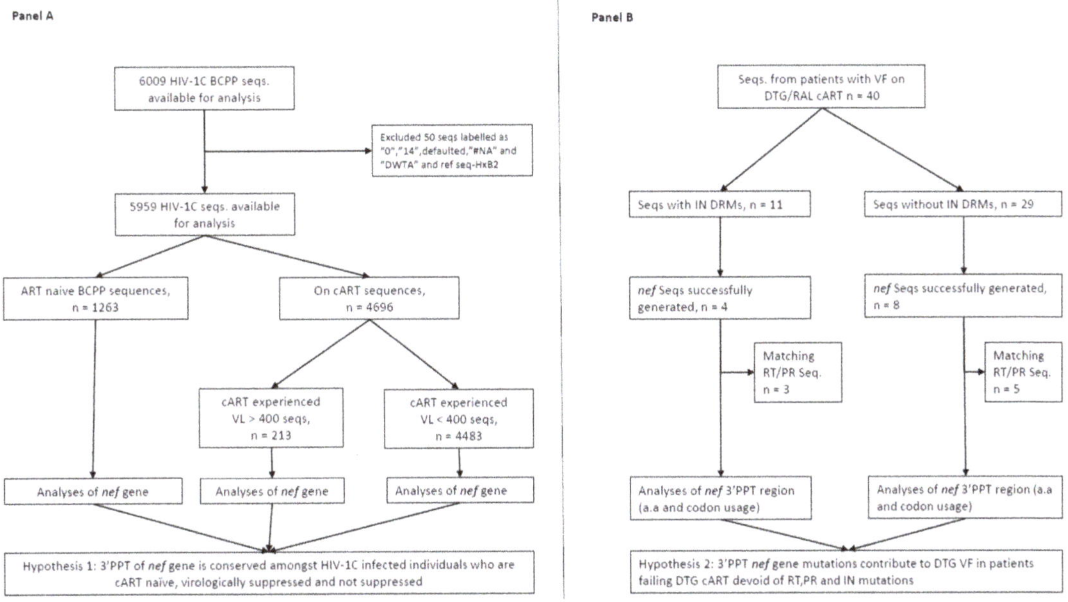

Figure 1. Study schema depicting the selection of study sequences. (**A**), selection and analysis of 3′PPT *nef* gene sequences according to participant cART status and HIV-1 RNA levels; (**B**), selection and analysis of 3′PPT of *nef* gene amongst individuals with VF while on DTG/RAL-based cART. Seqs, sequences; PID, participant identification number; VL, viral load; VF, virologic failure; RAL, raltegravir; DTG, dolutegravir; cART, combination antiretroviral therapy; 3′PPT, 3′-polypurine tract; RT, reverse transcriptase HIV-1 gene; PR, protease HIV-1 gene; DRMs, drug resistance mutations; HIV-1C, HIV-1 subtype C.

The second group consisted of full-genome HIV-1C sequences obtained from participants enrolled in a large community-randomised HIV-1 prevention trial described elsewhere (BCPP study) [22,23]. The sequences were aligned to the HIV reference strain (HxB2) at the nucleotide level using virulign [24] and block-trimmed to the *nef* gene of HxB2 in the BioEdit, version 7.2.0, software [25]. We included two nucleotides before and one nucleotide after the 3′PPT *nef* gene sequence to have a complete amino acid coding for the 3′PPT tails. The sequences were assessed for hypermutations using the Hypermut tool at the Los Alamos National Laboratory HIV Database website (http://www.hiv.lanl.gov/ accessed on 8 March 2021). All sequences were exported to Microsoft® Excel® for Microsoft 365 MSO (16.0.13901.20148) 32-bit for further downstream analysis, and graphs were created. Additional statistical computations were performed using Stata version 14 (Stata Corporation, College Station, TX, USA) and R version 4.0.3; Pearson's chi-square test was used to compare the proportion of 3′PPT of *nef* gene mutations per position by ART status and VL suppression. p-Values < 0.05 were considered statistically significant.

The Abbott RealTime HIV-1 assay, Cobas TaqMan/Cobas AmpliPrep HIV test (Roche Molecular Systems, Branchburg, NJ, USA), or Aptima HIV-1 Quant assay on Panther Systems (Hologic Inc., San Diego, CA, USA) was used to quantify HIV-1 RNA levels.

2.2. Ethical Statement

Both study protocols were approved by the health research and development division of the Botswana Ministry of Health and Wellness (Botswana's IRB of authority). For the BOSELE study participants, a waiver of informed consent was obtained, and for the BCPP study, all the participants provided informed consent. The BCPP study was approved by the IRB at the U.S. Centers for Disease Control and Prevention and is registered at

ClinicalTrials.gov (NCT01965470). All studies were conducted according to the principles stated in the Declaration of Helsinki.

3. Results

A total of 6021 HIV-1C *nef* gene sequences were available for analysis from both studies, and their basic demographics are shown in Table 1.

Table 1. Basic demographics of 6009 HIV-1C diagnosed, cART-naïve, and cART-experienced individuals.

Basic Characteristics		* HIV-1C Diagnosed Participant Sequences Available for Analysis (n = 6009)	** Sequences from Participants with VF on DTG cART (n = 40)
Age (years), median (Q1, Q3)		40 (33, 48)	41 (26, 45)
† Gender	Female n (%)	4241 (71%)	15 (44%)
	Male n (%)	1757 (29%)	19 (56%)
	Unknown n (%)	11 (0.2%)	** N/A
Median log $_{10}$ HIV-1 RNA (Q1, Q3) copies/mL		1.60 (1.60, 2.60)	4.53 (3.98, 5.10)

* Participants from BCPP study, ** We generated 40 sequences representing 34 'unique' individuals from an ongoing study characterizing therapy-experienced participants experiencing VF while on DTG/RAL cART. † Analysable gender data available for 5998 individuals; rest of dataset contained 'ND' shown as 'Unknown'. ND, not documented; VF, virologic failure; DTG, dolutegravir; cART, combination antiretroviral therapy; BCPP, Botswana Combination Prevention Project. Column 3 of this table is the same dataset represented in Column 3 of Table 1 of Seatla et al. [7]. This table has been modified with permission from Seatla et al. [7].

We included two nucleotides before (HxB2 nct position 9067 and 9068) and one nucleotide after 3′PPT (HxB2 nct position 9084) in our analysis of the 15-nucleotide 3′PPT region (5′ AAAAGAAAAGGGGGG 3′-HXB2 numbering 9069 to 9083) to complete the amino acid translation of the flanking regions of 3′PPT (Table 2, Figure 2).

All nucleotide positions of our HIV-1C *nef* gene 3′PPT sequences were highly conserved regardless of whether cART-naïve (n = 1263), on ART with VL < 400 (n = 4483) copies/mL, or on cART with VL ≥ 400 copies/mL (n = 213) groups (Figure 2). In addition, there was no statistically significant difference between 'cART naïve' and 'on cART' groups (p = 0.81), 'on cART < 400′ and 'on cART ≥ 400′ groups (p = 0.88), 'ART naïve' and 'on cART < 400′ groups (p = 0.72), 'cART naïve' and 'on cART ≥ 400′ groups (p = 0.99), 'on cART and cART < 400′ groups (p = 0.86), 'on cART and cART ≥ 400′ groups (p = 0.92), and 'on ART' and individuals with VF while on DTG/RAL cART group (p = 0.81). Analysis of sequences derived from buffy coat (n = 6009) adjusted for hypermutations (n = 2992) also revealed highly conserved *nef* 3′PPT residues with no statistically significant difference determined. The terminal six guanine stretch of 3′PPT also showed a high degree of conservation with all nucleotide residues having a mean rate of 99.47% (Figure 2, Supplementary Materials).

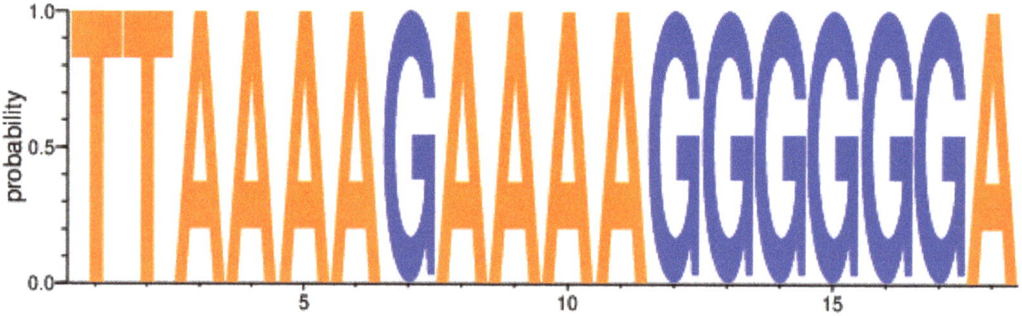

Figure 2. HIV-1C *nef* gene 3′PPT variability amongst 6009 sequences from individuals on cART and not on cART. 3′PPT, 3′polypurine tract; cART, combination antiretroviral therapy; HIV-1C, HIV-1 subtype C.

Table 2. HIV-1C *nef* 3′PPT variability amongst 12 therapy-experienced individuals experiencing VF while on DTG/RAL cART.

	[B] Major DRMs			3′PPT of the HIV-1 *nef* Gene																	
HxB2_nct_positions				9067	9068	9069	9070	9071	9072	9073	9074	9075	9076	9077	9078	9079	9080	9081	9082	9083	9084
HxB2_NEF_nct position				271	272	273	274	275	276	277	278	279	280	281	282	283	284	285	286	287	288
HXB2_NEF_gene_seqs.	RT (NRTI; NNRTI)	PI	INSTI	T	T	A	A	A	A	G	A	A	A	A	G	G	G	G	G	G	A
[¥] 139-0001-8	M41L, D67N, K70KR, V75M, M184V, L210W, T215Y, K219E; A98G, Y181C, G190A	M46I, I47V, I54L, L76V, I84V, Q58E, N83D	E138K, S147G, Q148R, N155H, (E157Q)	T	T	A	A	A	A	G	A	A	A	A	G	G	G	G	G	G	A
[¥] 139-0002-8	[±] K70R, M184V;K219N/Y181C (20APRIL2009) [±] D67N, K70R, M184V/NONE (18AUG2016)	[±] V32I, I47V, I54L, I84V (20 APRIL2009) [±] V32I, I47V, I54L, I84V (18AUG2016)	E138K, G140A, S147G, Q148R, (T97A)	T	T	A	A	A	A	G	A	A	A	A	G	G	G	G	G	G	A
[¥] 139-0004-6	[±] M41L, T69G, K70R, M184V, T215C, K219E; A98G, K101E	[±] M46I, I54V, L76V, V82A	T66A, G118R, E138EAKT	T	T	A	A	A	A	G	A	A	A	A	G	G	G	G	G	G	A
139-0005-3	* M184V; A98G	* Q58E	* ND	T	T	A	A	A	A	G	A	A	A	A	G	G	G	G	G	G	A
[¥] 139-0012-9	[±] M184V, M41L, T215Y; ND (9 June 2010)	[±] M46I,V82A Accessory; L10F, L24I (9 June 2010)	N155NH (D232DN)	T	T	A	A	A	A	G	A	A	A	A	G	G	G	G	G	G	A
139-0013-0	[±] M184V, A62V, M41L (28 July 2011); [±] E138K (3 February 2016), [±] * E138K (24 January 2018)	[±] V11IV (28 July 2011)	ND	T	T	A	A	A	A	G	A	A	A	A	G	G	G	G	G	G	A
139-0015-4	* ND	* ND	* ND	T	T	A	A	A	A	G	A	A	A	A	G	G	G	G	G	G	A
139-0017-2	* ND	* ND	* ND	T	T	A	A	A	A	G	A	A	A	A	G	G	G	G	G	G	A
139-0018-3	[±] D67G, K70E, M184V; Y181C, G190A	* ND	* ND	T	T	A	A	A	A	G	A	A	A	A	G	G	G	G	G	G	A
139-0021-4	* K65N; V179D	* ND	* ND	T	T	A	A	A	A	G	A	A	A	A	G	G	G	G	G	G	A
139-0026-8	* ND	* ND	* ND	T	T	A	A	A	A	G	A	A	A	A	G	G	G	G	G	G	A
139-0119-5	* ND; K103N, P225H	* ND	* ND	T	T	A	A	A	A	G	A	A	A	A	G	G	G	G	G	G	A
				Leucine, Leu, L			Lysine, Lys, K			Glutamic acid, Glu, E			Lysine, Lys, K			Glycine, Gly, G			Glycine, Gly, G		

[B] Major DRMs assessed by using the Stanford HIV drug resistance database; * denotes that RT-PCR testing for IN, RT, and PR was performed on the same (unique) sample from each patient. [±] Historical DRMs denoted with '±' retrieved from electronic databases and/or patients' medical charts. Mutations listed within brackets '()' are accessory mutations. [¥] denotes the same participants as listed in Table 2 of Seatla et al. [7]. ND, no mutations detected; cART, combination antiretroviral therapy; GRT, genotypic resistance testing; RT, reverse transcriptase; NRTI, nucleoside/nucleotide reverse transcriptase inhibitors; NNRTI, non-nucleoside reverse transcriptase inhibitors; PR, protease; PI, protease inhibitor; HxB2, HIV reference sequence_K03455; INSTI, integrase strand transfer inhibitors; DRMs, drug resistance mutations. Light blue colour depicts the 3′PPT of the HIV-1 *nef* gene, yellow and orange colours depict the amino acid translation of the 3-nucleotide sequence. Adapted from Figure 2a of Malet et al. [8], Figure 1 of Malet I et al. [17], and with permission from Table 2 of Seatla et al. [7].

4. Discussion

We analysed 12 HIV-1C *nef* 3′PPT sequences (eight had paired integrase sequences without INSTI drug resistance mutations and four had paired IN sequences with INSTI drug resistance mutations) from patients with VF while on DTG/RAL-based cART to search for changes in 3′PPT sequence that could be linked to DTG VF as previously reported, and we did not find any. Amongst the eight patients who were failing an INSTI-based regimen but who did not have INSTI resistance mutations in the integrase region, all had a 100% conservation in their 3′PPT sequences (they had no mutations at the nucleotide or amino acid level). In addition, we analysed 1263 3′PPT sequences from patients who were cART naïve to investigate HIV-1C 3′PPT variability. We further analysed 4696 3′PPT sequences from patients on cART (but not on a DTG-based regimen) stratified according to virological suppression and found no 3′PPT region variability.

Malet et al. found some significant variability at position 9071 (25% and 10% in HIV-1 subtype B and CRF01, respectively) [17] and position 9075 (10% variability in HIV-1 subtype D). In our analysis, position 9071 revealed a variability of 0.29% (n = 6009) and 0% (n = 12) of sequences from patients not exposed to DTG cART and those failing DTG/RAL cART, respectively. Position 9075 was also conserved with a variability of 0.4% (n = 6009) and 0% (n = 12) amongst the two groups. Perhaps this difference in variability could be explained by the different HIV-1 subtypes—all our sequences were HIV-1C.

We observed a high conservation amongst the six nucleotides of the G-tract residues of 3′PPT (mean of 99.47%) similar to what others have found (99.95%) [8,17–19].

We did not explore the entire HIV-1C genome (5′ long terminal repeat (LTR), gag, protease, reverse transcriptase, vif, vpr, vpu, envelope, and 3′ LTR) for other mutations that could be linked to INSTI resistance. We did not measure plasma DTG or RAL levels to check whether issues of nonadherence could be contributing to VF.

In conclusion, we conducted one of the largest analyses of the HIV-1C 3′PPT region, showing great conservation of the region at the nucleotide and amino acid level. Although we did not detect any association of 3′PPT mutations with VF on INSTI-based cART, our data were limited on the number of 3′PPT sequences generated from patients failing an INSTI-containing regimen without INSTI mutations. However, our data add to a growing list of studies that have found no association of 3′PPT mutations with INSTI resistance [17,18]. Future studies should also investigate the role of other HIV-1 genes outside of Pol as this might enhance our understanding of mechanisms associated with INSTI resistance.

Supplementary Materials: The following are available online at https://www.mdpi.com/article/10.3390/pathogens10081027/s1, Table S1: HIV-1C nef 3′PPT variability amongst 12 therapy experienced individuals experiencing VF while on DTG/RAL ART. We included the two proximal and last distal nct positions to the 3′PPT to complete aminoacid picture of the region; 3′polypurine tract, 3′PPT; nct, nucleotide; VL, viral load; seqs., sequences; VF, virological failure; DTG, dolutegravir; RAL, raltegravir; cART, combination antiretroviral therapy, Adapted from Figure 2a of Malet I et al. [7]; Figure S1: HIV-1C nef 3′PPT variability amongst sequences from individuals on cART and not on ART, n = 5959. cART, combination antiretroviral therapy; 3′PPT, 3′polypurine tract; Figure S2: HIV-1C nef 3′PPT variability amongst cART naive individuals, n = 1263; Figure S3: HIV-1C nef 3′PPT variability amongst individuals on ART with VL $\leq$ 400 copies/mL, n = 4483; Figure S4: HIV-1C nef 3′PPT variability amongst individuals on ART with VL > 400 copies/mL, n = 213; Figure S5: HIV-1C nef 3′PPT variability amongst sequences from individuals on ART and not on ART, n = 2992 (hypermutations removed); Figure S6: HIV-1C nef 3′PPT variability amongst ART naive individuals, n = 762 (hypermutations removed); Figure S7: HIV-1C nef 3′PPT variability amongst individuals on ART with VL $\leq$ 400 copies/mL, n = 2074 (hypermutations removed); Figure S8: HIV-1C nef 3′PPT variability amongst individuals on ART with VL > 400 copies/mL, n = 119 (hypermutations removed).

Author Contributions: Writing–original draft preparation, K.K.S.; conceptualization, S.G., K.K.S.; investigation, K.K.S.; writing—reviewing and editing, K.K.S., S.G., I.K., S.L., S.M., O.M., V.N., D.M., W.T.C., data curation, K.K.S., S.G.; formal analysis, K.K.S., O.M., S.M., S.G.; project administration, S.G., S.L.; supervision, S.G., I.K; funding acquisition, S.G., K.K.S., S.L. All authors have read and agreed to the published version of the manuscript.

Funding: This publication was made possible with help from the Harvard University Center for AIDS Research (CFAR), an NIH-funded program (P30 AI060354), which is supported by the following NIH cofunding and participating institutes and centres: National Institute of Allergy and Infectious Diseases; National Cancer Institute; Eunice Kennedy Shriver National Institute of Child Health and Human Development; National Heart, Lung, and Blood Institute; National Institute on Drug Abuse; National Institute of Mental Health; National Institute on Aging; National Institute of Diabetes and Digestive and Kidney Diseases; National Institute of General Medical Sciences; National Institute on Minority Health and Health Disparities; National Institute of Dental and Craniofacial Research; Office of AIDS Research; and Fogarty International Center. The content is solely the responsibility of the authors and does not necessarily represent the official views of the National Institutes of Health. This work was supported through the Sub-Saharan African Network for TB/HIV Research Excellence (SANTHE), a DELTAS Africa Initiative (grant # DEL-15-006). The DELTAS Africa Initiative is an independent funding scheme of the African Academy of Sciences' (AAS) Alliance for Accelerating Excellence in Science in Africa (AESA) and supported by the New Partnership for Africa's Development Planning and Coordinating Agency (NEPAD Agency) with funding from the Wellcome Trust (grant # 107752/Z/15/Z) and the UK government. The views expressed in this publication are those of the author(s) and not necessarily those of AAS, NEPAD Agency, Wellcome Trust, or the UK government. 'Research reported in this publication was supported by the Fogarty International Center and National Institute of Mental Health of the National Institutes of Health under Award Number D43 TW010543. The content is solely the responsibility of the authors and does not necessarily represent the official views of the National Institutes of Health.' S.L. was supported by the National Institutes of Health (NIH)/National Institute of Allergy and Infectious Diseases K24 mentoring grant—NIH K24 AI131928. All funders had no role in the study design, data collection and analysis, decision to publish, or preparation of the manuscript. The Botswana Combination Prevention Project Impact Evaluation was supported by the President's Emergency Plan for AIDS Relief (PEPFAR) through the Centers for Disease Control and Prevention (CDC) under the terms of cooperative agreements U01 GH000447 and U2G GH001911. The contents of this article are solely the responsibility of the authors and do not necessarily represent the official positions of the funding agencies.

Institutional Review Board Statement: Both study protocols were approved by the health research and development division of the Botswana Ministry of Health and Wellness (Botswana's IRB of authority). For the BOSELE study participants, a waiver of informed consent was obtained, and for the BCPP study, all the participants provided informed consent. The BCPP study was approved by the IRB at the U.S. Centers for Disease Control and Prevention and is registered at ClinicalTrials.gov (NCT01965470). All studies were conducted according to the principles stated in the Declaration of Helsinki.

Informed Consent Statement: For the BOSELE study participants, a waiver of informed consent was obtained, and for the BCPP study, all the participants provided informed consent.

Data Availability Statement: Sequences available at national centre for biotechnology information (NCBI) GenBank, accession numbers MW690052-MW690089, MG989443.1, MG989444.

Acknowledgments: We thank our patients and the staff of all infectious disease care clinics (PMH IDCC) that we visited throughout Botswana. We thank the Botswana Harvard HIV Reference Laboratory staff, Botswana Harvard Partnership, and Botswana Ministry of Health and Wellness for their collaboration. We thank the study participants from both study cohorts without whom this study would not have been possible.

Conflicts of Interest: All authors have no conflict of interest to declare.

References

1. Anstett, K.; Brenner, B.; Mesplede, T.; Wainberg, M.A. HIV drug resistance against strand transfer integrase inhibitors. *Retrovirology* **2017**, *14*, 36. [CrossRef]
2. DHHS; Panel on Antiretroviral Guidelines for Adults and Adolescents. Guidelines for the Use of Antiretroviral Agents in Adults and Adolescents with HIV; Department of Health and Human Services. 2021. Available online: https://clinicalinfo.hiv.gov/en/guidelines/adult-and-adolescent-arv/whats-new-guidelines (accessed on 13 August 2021).
3. MoHW. Handbook of the Botswana 2016 Integrated HIV Clinical Care Guidelines. Available online: https://www.moh.gov.bw/Publications/Handbook_HIV_treatment_guidelines.pdf (accessed on 15 April 2020).
4. Raffi, F.; Rachlis, A.; Stellbrink, H.J.; Hardy, W.D.; Torti, C.; Orkin, C.; Bloch, M.; Podzamczer, D.; Pokrovsky, V.; Pulido, F.; et al. Once-daily dolutegravir versus raltegravir in antiretroviral-naive adults with HIV-1 infection: 48 week results from the randomised, double-blind, non-inferiority SPRING-2 study. *Lancet* **2013**, *381*, 735–743. [CrossRef]
5. WHO. *Update of Recommendations on First- and Second-Line Antiretroviral Regimens*; (WHO/CDS/HIV/19.15); Licence: CC BY-NC-SA 3.0 IGO; World Health Organization: Geneva, Switzerland, 2019.
6. Oliveira, M.; Ibanescu, R.I.; Anstett, K.; Mesplede, T.; Routy, J.P.; Robbins, M.A.; Brenner, B.G.; The Montreal Primary HIV (PHI) Cohort Study Group. Selective resistance profiles emerging in patient-derived clinical isolates with cabotegravir, bictegravir, dolutegravir, and elvitegravir. *Retrovirology* **2018**, *15*, 56. [CrossRef]
7. Seatla, K.K.; Maruapula, D.; Choga, W.T.; Ntsipe, T.; Mathiba, N.; Mogwele, M.; Kapanda, M.; Nkomo, B.; Ramaabya, D.; Makhema, J.; et al. HIV-1 Subtype C Drug Resistance Mutations in Heavily Treated Patients Failing Integrase Strand Transfer Inhibitor-Based Regimens in Botswana. *Viruses* **2021**, *13*, 594. [CrossRef]
8. Malet, I.; Subra, F.; Charpentier, C.; Collin, G.; Descamps, D.; Calvez, V.; Marcelin, A.G.; Delelis, O. Mutations Located outside the Integrase Gene Can Confer Resistance to HIV-1 Integrase Strand Transfer Inhibitors. *mBio* **2017**, *8*, e00922-17. [CrossRef]
9. Wijting, I.E.A.; Lungu, C.; Rijnders, B.J.A.; van der Ende, M.E.; Pham, H.T.; Mesplede, T.; Pas, S.D.; Voermans, J.J.C.; Schuurman, R.; van de Vijver, D.; et al. HIV-1 Resistance Dynamics in Patients With Virologic Failure to Dolutegravir Maintenance Monotherapy. *J. Infect. Dis.* **2018**, *218*, 688–697. [CrossRef]
10. Anderson, S.J.; Lenburg, M.; Landau, N.R.; Garcia, J.V. The cytoplasmic domain of CD4 is sufficient for its down-regulation from the cell surface by human immunodeficiency virus type 1 Nef. *J. Virol.* **1994**, *68*, 3092–3101. [CrossRef]
11. Garcia, J.V.; Miller, A.D. Serine phosphorylation-independent downregulation of cell-surface CD4 by nef. *Nature* **1991**, *350*, 508–511. [CrossRef]
12. Schwartz, O.; Maréchal, V.; Le Gall, S.; Lemonnier, F.; Heard, J.-M. Endocytosis of major histocompatibility complex class I molecules is induced by the HIV–1 Nef protein. *Nat. Med.* **1996**, *2*, 338–342. [CrossRef]
13. Watkins, R.L.; Zou, W.; Denton, P.W.; Krisko, J.F.; Foster, J.L.; Garcia, J.V. In vivo analysis of highly conserved Nef activities in HIV-1 replication and pathogenesis. *Retrovirology* **2013**, *10*, 125. [CrossRef]
14. Das, A.T.; Berkhout, B.; Paraskevis, D. How Polypurine Tract Changes in the HIV-1 RNA Genome Can Cause Resistance against the Integrase Inhibitor Dolutegravir. *mBio* **2018**, *9*, e00006-18. [CrossRef]
15. Julias, J.G.; McWilliams, M.J.; Sarafianos, S.G.; Alvord, W.G.; Arnold, E.; Hughes, S.H. Effects of Mutations in the G Tract of the Human Immunodeficiency Virus Type 1 Polypurine Tract on Virus Replication and RNase H Cleavage. *J. Virol.* **2004**, *78*, 13315–13324. [CrossRef]
16. Jones, F.D.; Hughes, S.H. In vitro analysis of the effects of mutations in the G-tract of the human immunodeficiency virus type 1 polypurine tract on RNase H cleavage specificity. *Virology* **2007**, *360*, 341–349. [CrossRef]
17. Malet, I.; Delelis, O.; Nguyen, T.; Leducq, V.; Abdi, B.; Morand-Joubert, L.; Calvez, V.; Marcelin, A.G. Variability of the HIV-1 3′ polypurine tract (3′PPT) region and implication in integrase inhibitor resistance. *J. Antimicrob. Chemother.* **2019**, *74*, 3440–3444. [CrossRef]
18. Wei, Y.; Sluis-Cremer, N. Mutations in the HIV-1 3′-Polypurine Tract and Integrase Strand-Transfer Inhibitor Resistance. *Antimicrob. Agents Chemother.* **2021**, *65*, e02432-20. [CrossRef]
19. Acharya, A.; Tagny, C.T.; Mbanya, D.; Fonsah, J.Y.; Nchindap, E.; Kenmogne, L.; Jihyun, M.; Njamnshi, A.K.; Kanmogne, G.D. Variability in HIV-1 Integrase Gene and 3′-Polypurine Tract Sequences in Cameroon Clinical Isolates, and Implications for Integrase Inhibitors Efficacy. *Int. J. Mol. Sci.* **2020**, *21*, 1553. [CrossRef]
20. Seatla, K.K.; Choga, W.T.; Mogwele, M.; Diphoko, T.; Maruapula, D.; Mupfumi, L.; Musonda, R.M.; Rowley, C.F.; Avalos, A.; Kasvosve, I.; et al. Comparison of an in-house 'home-brew' and commercial ViroSeq integrase genotyping assays on HIV-1 subtype C samples. *PLoS ONE* **2019**, *14*, e0224292. [CrossRef]
21. Jones, B.R.; Miller, R.L.; Kinloch, N.N.; Tsai, O.; Rigsby, H.; Sudderuddin, H.; Shahid, A.; Ganase, B.; Brumme, C.J.; Harris, M.; et al. Genetic Diversity, Compartmentalization, and Age of HIV Proviruses Persisting in CD4(+) T Cell Subsets during Long-Term Combination Antiretroviral Therapy. *J. Virol.* **2020**, *94*, e01786-19. [CrossRef]
22. Gaolathe, T.; Wirth, K.E.; Holme, M.P.; Makhema, J.; Moyo, S.; Chakalisa, U.; Yankinda, E.K.; Lei, Q.; Mmalane, M.; Novitsky, V.; et al. Botswana's progress toward achieving the 2020 UNAIDS 90-90-90 antiretroviral therapy and virological suppression goals: A population-based survey. *Lancet HIV* **2016**, *3*, e221–e230. [CrossRef]
23. Makhema, J.; Wirth, K.E.; Pretorius Holme, M.; Gaolathe, T.; Mmalane, M.; Kadima, E.; Chakalisa, U.; Bennett, K.; Leidner, J.; Manyake, K.; et al. Universal Testing, Expanded Treatment, and Incidence of HIV Infection in Botswana. *N. Engl. J. Med.* **2019**, *381*, 230–242. [CrossRef]

24. Libin, P.J.K.; Deforche, K.; Abecasis, A.B.; Theys, K. VIRULIGN: Fast codon-correct alignment and annotation of viral genomes. *Bioinformatics* **2018**, *35*, 1763–1765. [CrossRef] [PubMed]
25. Hall, T.A. BioEdit: A User-Friendly Biological Sequence Alignment Editor and Analysis Program for Windows 95/98/NT. *Proc. Nucleic Acids Symp. Ser.* **1999**, *41*, 95–98.

pathogens

Article

Coevolved Multidrug-Resistant HIV-1 Protease and Reverse Transcriptase Influences Integrase Drug Susceptibility and Replication Fitness

Supang A. Martin [1], Patricia A. Cane [1], Deenan Pillay [2] and Jean L. Mbisa [1,*]

[1] Antiviral Unit, Virus Reference Department, Public Health England, London NW9 5EQ, UK; supang.martin@gmail.com (S.A.M.); pat.cane@phe.gov.uk (P.A.C.)
[2] Division of Infection and Immunity, University College London, London WC1E 6BT, UK; d.pillay@ucl.ac.uk
* Correspondence: tamyo.mbisa@phe.gov.uk

Abstract: Integrase strand transfer inhibitors (InSTIs) are recommended agents in first-line combination antiretroviral therapy (cART). We examined the evolution of drug resistance mutations throughout HIV-1 *pol* and the effects on InSTI susceptibility and viral fitness. We performed single-genome sequencing of full-length HIV-1 *pol* in a highly treatment-experienced patient, and determined drug susceptibility of patient-derived HIV-1 genomes using a phenotypic assay encompassing full-length *pol* gene. We show the genetic linkage of multiple InSTI-resistant haplotypes containing major resistance mutations at Y143, Q148 and N155 to protease inhibitor (PI) and reverse transcriptase inhibitor (RTI) resistance mutations. Phenotypic analysis of viruses expressing patient-derived IN genes with eight different InSTI-resistant haplotypes alone or in combination with coevolved protease (PR) and RT genes exhibited similar levels of InSTI susceptibility, except for three haplotypes that showed up to 3-fold increases in InSTI susceptibility ($p \leq 0.032$). The replicative fitness of most viruses expressing patient-derived IN only significantly decreased, ranging from 8% to 56% ($p \leq 0.01$). Interestingly, the addition of coevolved PR + RT significantly increased the replicative fitness of some haplotypes by up to 73% ($p \leq 0.024$). Coevolved PR + RT contributes to the susceptibility and viral fitness of patient-derived IN viruses. Maintaining patients on failing cART promotes the selection of fitter resistant strains, and thereby limits future therapy options.

Keywords: HIV-1; single genome sequencing; drug resistance; integrase strand transfer inhibitors; replication fitness

Citation: Martin, S.A.; Cane, P.A.; Pillay, D.; Mbisa, J.L. Coevolved Multidrug-Resistant HIV-1 Protease and Reverse Transcriptase Influences Integrase Drug Susceptibility and Replication Fitness. *Pathogens* **2021**, *10*, 1070. https://doi.org/10.3390/pathogens10091070

Academic Editors: Lawrence S. Young and Jochen Bodem

Received: 23 June 2021
Accepted: 12 August 2021
Published: 24 August 2021

1. Introduction

Since the introduction of combination antiretroviral therapy (cART) against HIV-1 in the late 1990s, the number of overall new HIV infections and AIDS-related deaths has decreased [1]. Despite this, the development of resistance to antiretrovirals (ARVs) remains a barrier to the treatment of HIV infection, especially in low- and middle-income countries, and work is ongoing to produce drugs that target novel steps of the viral life cycle. One of the later classes of drugs to be approved for clinical use targets the integration of the virus into the host cell genome, specifically the DNA strand transfer reaction [2,3]. To date, there are five licensed integrase strand transfer inhibitors (INSTIs), raltegravir (RAL), elvitegravir (EVG), dolutegravir (DTG), bictegravir (BIC) and cabotegravir (CAB), that are available singly or as combination pills with RTIs [4].

Originally, RAL was used as part of a second-line treatment or salvage regimen for those failing previous lines of therapy [5]. However, InSTIs are now recommended for use as a third agent in a nucleos(t)ide reverse transcriptase inhibitor (NRTI)-based first-line therapy [6,7]. Thus, it is highly likely that patients going onto InSTI-containing treatment will develop alongside or harbour viruses containing protease inhibitor (PI) and RTI resistance mutations. However, little is known about the full effects and coevolution of drug resistance in the full-length HIV-1 *pol* gene, the target of the four main classes of ARVs used in cART: PIs, NRTIs, non-nucleoside reverse transcriptase inhibitors (NNRTIs) and InSTIs. This is because routine genotypic resistance testing in HIV-infected patients normally involves standard "bulk" population sequencing of viral genes of interest; usually protease (PR) and the N terminal of RT, or the catalytic core domain of integrase (IN) separately, or, alternatively, short read (75 to 300 bp) next-generation sequencing is used [8,9]. In addition, most phenotypic drug susceptibility assays have been developed to study the drug susceptibility of smaller patient-derived *gag-pol* fragments [10–13]. A limited number of studies have investigated the drug susceptibility of patient-derived full-length *pol* genes [14–16]. Consequently, not much is known about the effects of different combinations of PI, RTI and InSTI resistance mutations on overall drug susceptibility and viral fitness. These data may be important in informing how best to use drugs targeting all three genes in clinical practice. Here, we use a full-length *pol* single-genome sequencing assay to investigate the development, evolution and linkage of PI, RTI and InSTI resistance mutations in a patient undergoing InSTI-containing therapy. We also investigate the effect on InSTI susceptibility and viral fitness of patient-derived *IN* only or in combination with coevolved *PR* and *RT*, using a single-replication-cycle drug susceptibility assay.

2. Results

2.1. Single-Genome Sequencing of Full-Length HIV-1 pol Gene in Longitudinal Samples from a Patient Failing RAL-Containing Therapy

Single genomes were generated from five out of six samples over a 16-month period (Table 1). A total of 117 single genomes were generated at the following time points: before initiation of RAL therapy (preRAL; n = 16), 4 and 5 months after initiation of RAL therapy (4RAL and 5RAL; n = 26 and 23, respectively), 4 months after cessation of RAL therapy (4post; n = 39) and 2 weeks after re-initiation of RAL therapy (reRAL; n = 13).

Table 1. Clinical history of patient.

Patient	Months Before or After Initiation of RAL Therapy	Viral Load (Copies/mL)	CD4 Count (Cells/mm^3)	Antiretroviral Treatment	Number of Single Genomes
A	−3 (preRAL)	59,000	150	LPVr, 3TC	16
	2 (2RAL)	140	230	DRVr, ETR, RAL	Na [a]
	4 (4RAL)	39,000	280	DRVr, ETR, RAL	26
	5 (5RAL)	63,000	200	DRVr, ETR, RAL	23
	9 (4post)	77,300	140	TDF, 3TC	39
	14 (ReRAL)	1900	140	DRVr, TDF, FTC, ETR, RAL	13

[a] na = no amplification, possibly due to low viral load.

Analysis of the 16 single genomes before exposure to RAL (preRAL) revealed no RAL resistance mutations, except for the presence of an amino acid substitution (G163E) in a single genome at a position associated with RAL resistance (Figure 1). On the other hand, all single genomes generated after initiation of RAL treatment (4RAL and 5RAL; n = 49) contained RAL resistance mutations at all the three major RAL resistance positions at 4RAL, with these being: Y143R/C (n = 15), Q148R (n = 10) and N155H (n = 1). The major RAL resistance pathways were reduced to two at 5RAL, with these being: Y143R/C (n = 16) and Q148R (n = 7). None of the three major RAL resistance-associated mutations at positions 143, 148 and 155 observed at 4RAL were found on the same genome. However, all three major RAL resistance mutations were found to be linked to one of the following accessory mutations: E92Q, T97A, G140A, V151I and G163R/K. Analysis of the genetic linkage of the major and accessory resistance mutations revealed seven different RAL-associated haplotypes in the 49 single genomes during the first round of RAL treatment

(4RAL and 5RAL), with these being: Y143R + G163R (n = 27), Y143R + G163K (n = 1), Y143C + E92Q (n = 1), Y143C + G163R (n = 1), Y143C + T97A (n = 1), Q148R + G140A (17) and N155H + V151I (n = 1). Six of the haplotypes were present at 4RAL, and this number decreased to three a month later at 5RAL. However, at both time points, two haplotypes, Y143R + G163R and Q148R + G140A, dominated the population constituting 46.2% and 38.5% of the population at 4RAL and 65.2% and 30.4% at 5RAL, respectively.

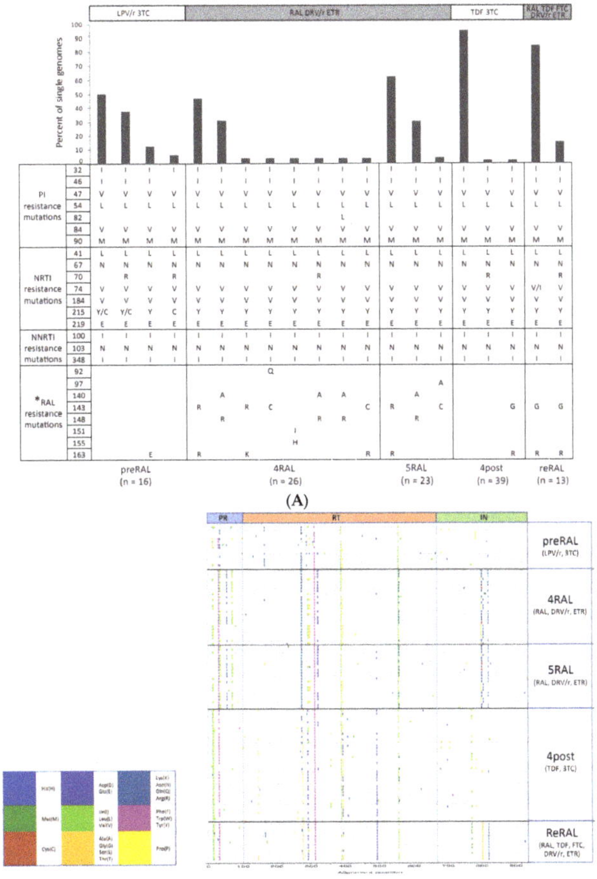

(A)

(B)

Figure 1. Genetic linkage of drug resistance mutations in PR, RT and IN genes from patient failing RAL-containing therapy. (**A**) Genetically linked major PI, NRTI, NNRTI and RAL resistance mutations identified by single genome sequencing in longitudinal samples are shown in columns. The percent of single genomes containing the linked resistance mutations at each time point are shown in bar graphs above the mutation columns. The details of treatment are indicated above the bar graphs and the number of single genomes generated at each time point is indicated below each figure. The bar graph on the right-hand side shows the frequency of the mutations in the Stanford HIV Drug Resistance Database in treatment-experienced patients infected with subtype B. (**B**) Highlighter plot of amino acid differences throughout the pol gene of the patient single genomes during the different time points and treatment regimens. The differences are in reference to the ancestral single genome at the preRAL time point. preRAL = before initiation of RAL therapy; 4RAL, 5RAL and 8RAL = 4, 5 and 8 months after initiation of RAL therapy, respectively; 1post, 3post and 4post = 1, 3 and 4 months after stopping RAL therapy; reRAL = 0.5 months after reinitiating RAL therapy; * = accessory RAL resistance mutations included; ** = L74V only; *** = T215Y only; **** = Y143R and Y143C only.

Within four months following the withdrawal of RAL treatment (4 post), 97.4% (38/39) of the single genomes contained no RAL resistance-associated mutations, with only one single genome still harbouring the G163R mutation and a novel substitution at major resistance position 143 (Y to G). This minor variant was not detected in any of the single genomes at 4RAL or 5RAL. Two weeks after RAL therapy was re-initiated (ReRAL), this novel Y143G + G163R mutant dominated the viral population with all of the single genomes (n = 13) containing the double mutation.

2.2. *The Development and Linkage of Drug Resistance Mutations in Full-Length HIV-1 pol Gene*

We investigated the linkage of RAL resistance mutations in IN to drug resistance mutations in PR and RT. We found little variation in the composition of PI and RTI resistance mutations over the sampling period. All 117 amplified single genomes contained numerous PI (V32I, I47V, I54L, I84V, and L90M), NRTI (M41L/I, D67N, L74V/I, M184V, T215Y/C and K219E) and NNRTI (L100I, K103N and N348I) resistance mutations (Figure 1). This is consistent with the extensive ART experience of the patient.

These PI and RTI resistance mutations were maintained in the viral population, even in the absence of the respective drugs. For example, the PI resistance mutations in the preRAL time point were still present at the 4post time point when the patient was no longer on PIs (Figure 1). We observed the genetic linkage of drug resistance mutations across the full-length *pol* gene in 100% (n = 64) of single genomes that contained RAL resistance mutations (Figure 1A). Analysis of the Stanford HIV Drug Resistance Database showed that these mutations were identified in a significant proportion of patient samples infected with subtype B, except for the PI V82L, NRTI L74I and T215C, and InSTI Y143G (Figure 1A). However, the frequency of linkage of the mutations could not be verified, as the data were from population-based Sanger sequencing, and not single-genome sequencing.

Although the major PI and RTI resistance mutations were maintained throughout the study period, regardless of treatment regimen, there was selection for or against the major RAL resistance mutations and other mutations in all three gene regions, depending on the treatment regimen (Figure 1B).

2.3. *Intrapatient Evolution of InSTi Susceptibility*

We investigated the effect of the different drug resistance-associated mutations identified during the development of RAL resistance on RAL susceptibility. We generated nine recombinant virus vectors expressing patient-derived *IN* genes with eight different RAL-resistant haplotypes and a wild-type sequence that were identified by single genome sequencing (Figure 2). As expected, the RAL EC_{50} of the virus expressing the patient-derived wild-type *IN* from the pre-RAL time-point (ptA_WT*IN*) was equivalent to that of the wild-type control virus (p8.9NSX) at 4.2 $\pm$ 0.11 vs. 4.5 $\pm$ 0.37 nM (p = 0.76; Figure 3A). In contrast, all viruses containing patient-derived *IN* from single genomes sampled during RAL treatment exhibited significant decreases in RAL susceptibility of up to 200-fold. compared to that of the wild-type *IN* control with EC_{50} values ranging from 84.6 $\pm$ 10.5 to 900 $\pm$ 145.2 nM ($p \leq 0.0001$). Interestingly, the major RAL-resistant haplotype at 4RAL and 5RAL, Y143R + G163R, had the highest decrease in RAL susceptibility (200-fold), compared to a moderate decrease in RAL susceptibility of 50-fold for the Y143G + G163R haplotype, that emerged during re-initiation of RAL therapy.

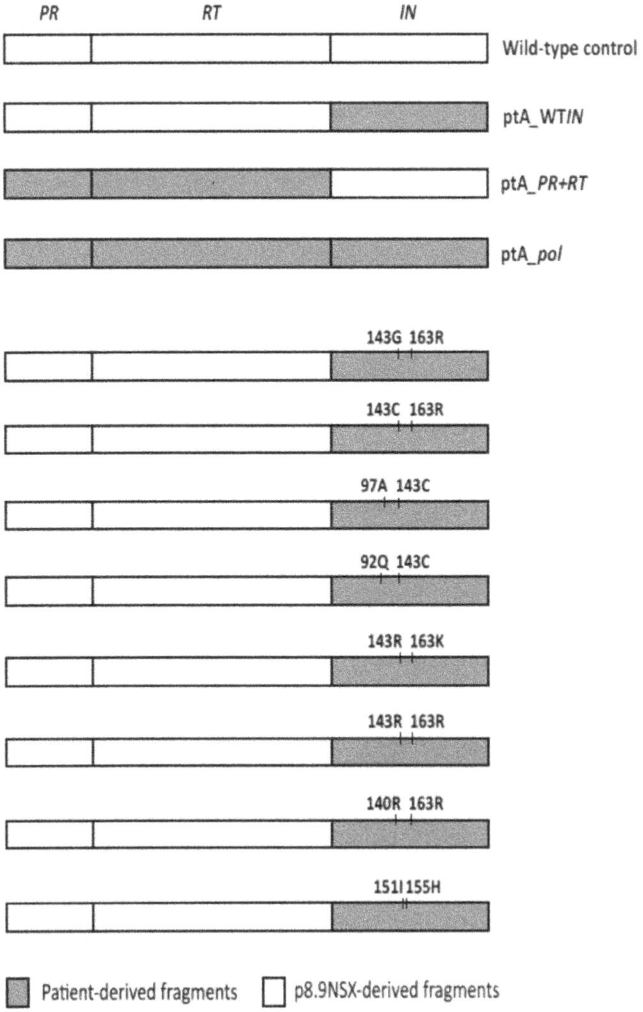

Figure 2. A schematic representation of recombinant viral vectors used in phenotypic drug susceptibility and viral fitness assays. Patient-derived *IN* genes containing different RAL-resistant haplotypes or wild-type only were sub-cloned into p8.9NSX vector. Patient-derived full-length *pol* vectors were generated by subcloning the patient-derived *IN* genes into a vector expressing the PR + RT fragment from the patient. The patient-derived *PR* + *RT* fragment contained the PI resistance mutations L10F, V32I, I47V, I54L, A71T, I84V and L90M, and RTI resistance mutations M41L, D67N, I74V, M184V, T215Y, K219E, L100I, K103N and N348I. Wild-type control = p8.9NSX wild-type subtype B; ptA_WT*IN* = patient-derived wild-type in *IN*; ptA_*PR* + *RT* = patient-derived *PR* and *RT*; ptA_*pol* = patient-derived full-length *pol*, wild-type in *IN*. Vectors with patient-derived full-length *pol* containing RAL-resistant haplotypes are not shown.

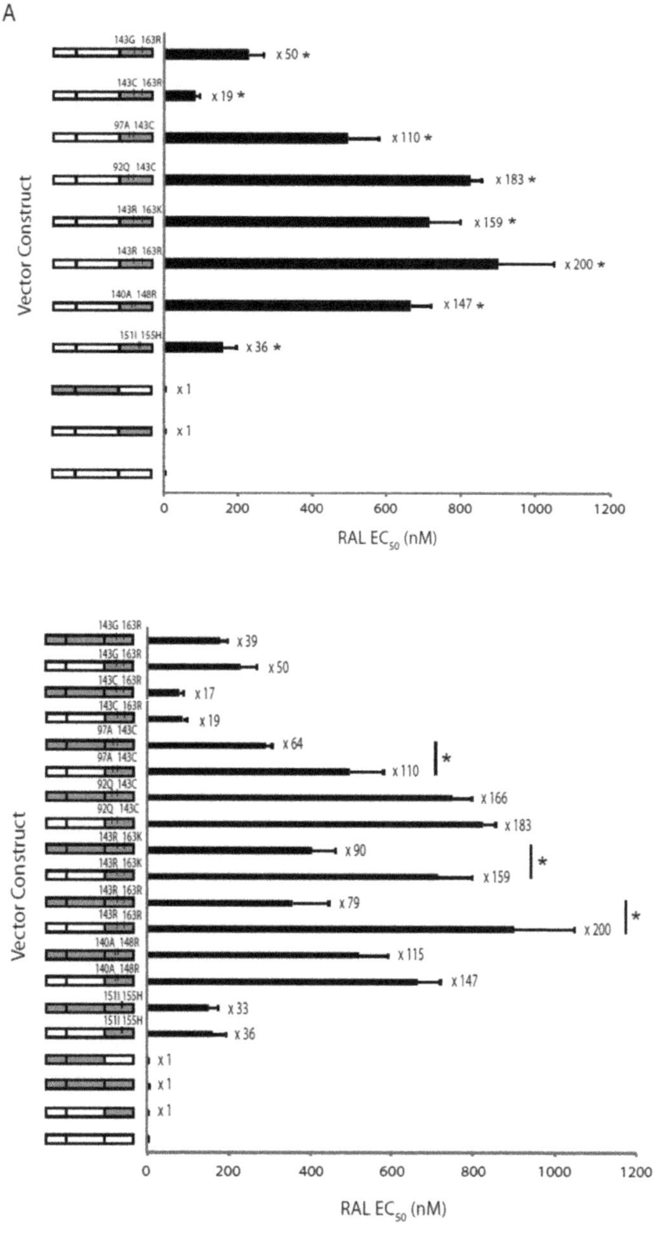

Figure 3. Susceptibility to RAL exhibited by recombinant viruses expressing patient-derived HIV-1 gene fragments. (**A**) Susceptibility to RAL exhibited by recombinant viruses expressing patient-derived *IN* genes only. (**B**) Comparison of RAL susceptibilities exhibited by recombinant viruses expressing patient-derived *IN* genes only or full-length *pol* genes. Error bars represent standard error of the mean of 6 to 12 independent experiments. Fold change in EC_{50} values compared to the p8.9NSX wild-type control are indicated next to each bar. Viruses exhibiting a significantly higher RAL EC_{50} ($p < 0.05$) compared to wild-type control (**A**) or their full-length *pol* counterpart (**B**) are indicated with *.

Next, we investigated the susceptibility of the viruses expressing patient-derived fragments against a different InSTI, EVG. Interestingly, the EVG EC_{50} of the virus expressing the patient-derived wild-type *IN* from pre-RAL time point (ptA_WT*IN*) was significantly higher compared to the wild-type control (p8.9NSX) at 0.24 ± 0.026 vs. 0.1 ± 0.016 nM ($p = 0.0002$; Figure 4A). This is consistent with other studies, that have shown a 2- to 3-fold increase in EVG EC_{50} for viruses expressing *IN* genes from InSTI-naïve patients compared to wild-type controls [17,18]. Two viruses expressing patient-derived *IN* containing the RAL resistance mutations, Y143C + G163R and Y143G + G163R, also exhibited EVG EC_{50} values similar to that of the wild-type control at 0.06 ± 0.022 and 0.22 ± 0.088 nM, respectively ($p \geq 0.12$). The remaining six viruses expressing patient-derived *IN* only were found to have significantly higher EVG EC_{50} values compared to the wild-type control, ranging from 0.48 ± 0.064 to 23.31 ± 0.69 nM ($p < 0.05$). This includes the virus expressing the Y143R + G163R mutation combination, which exhibited the highest fold change in RAL EC_{50} (200-fold), but which only resulted in a 5-fold change in EVG susceptibility. The highest fold change in EVG susceptibility (227-fold) was exhibited by the virus expressing the Q148R + G140A mutation combination, which also resulted in a very high fold change in RAL susceptibility (147-fold).

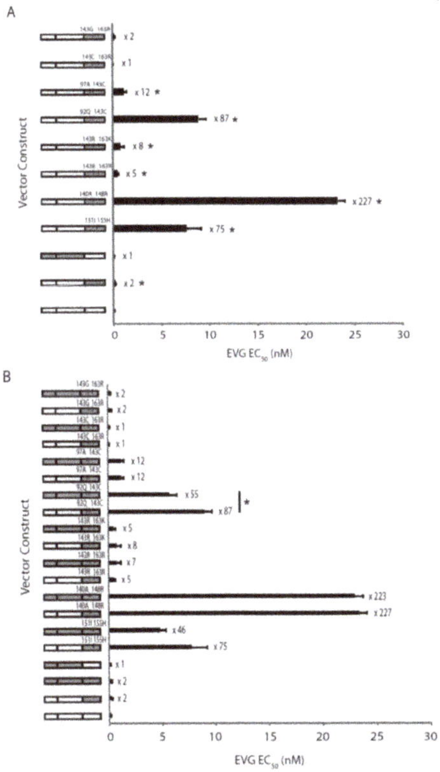

Figure 4. Cross-resistance to EVG exhibited by recombinant viruses expressing patient-derived HIV-1 gene fragments. (**A**) Susceptibility to EVG exhibited by recombinant viruses expressing patient-derived *IN* genes only. (**B**) Comparison of EVG susceptibilities exhibited by recombinant viruses expressing patient-derived *IN* genes only or full-length *pol* genes. Error bars represent standard error of the mean of 6 to 12 independent experiments. Fold change in EC_{50} values, compared to the p8.9NSX wild-type control are indicated next to each bar. Viruses exhibiting a significantly higher EVG EC_{50} ($p < 0.05$) compared to wild-type control (**A**) or their full-length *pol* counterpart (**B**) are indicated with *.

2.4. The Effects of Coevolved PR and RT Genes on Susceptibility to InSTIs

To determine if the coevolved *PR* and *RT* genes influence the susceptibility to the InSTIs RAL and EVG, we generated recombinant vectors expressing patient-derived full-length *pol* gene. The virus expressing the patient-derived full-length *pol* with resistance mutations in *PR* and *RT* but wild-type in *IN* (designated ptA_*pol*), as well as the virus expressing the patient-derived *PR* and *RT* only (designated ptA_*PR* + *RT*) had RAL susceptibilities comparable to that of the wild-type control virus (p8.9NSX) with EC_{50} values of 5.5 ± 1.1 nM, 4.1 ± 0.48 and 4.5 ± 0.37 nM, respectively ($p \geq 0.30$; Figure 3B). Overall, the viruses expressing patient-derived full-length *pol* from time points during RAL treatment exhibited RAL susceptibilities that were similar to viruses expressing respective patient-derived *IN* only, except for the Y143R + G163R, Y143R + G163K and Y143C + T97A mutation combinations. For these three viruses, the patient-derived *IN* only showed significantly greater decreases in RAL susceptibilities than the respective full-length *pol* ($p \leq 0.032$). This suggests that the coevolved *PR* and *RT* can confer a negative effect on resistance to RAL, which is dependent on the combination of resistance mutations in *IN*.

To determine if the coevolved *PR* and *RT* also influences EVG susceptibility, we investigated the EVG susceptibilities of viruses expressing patient-derived full-length *pol* (Figure 4B). Similar to the virus expressing patient-derived wild-type *IN* gene only (ptA_WT*IN*), the virus expressing patient-derived full-length *pol* with resistant *PR* and *RT* genes but wild-type *IN* gene (ptA_*pol*) also exhibited a significantly higher EVG EC_{50} compared to wild-type control virus at 0.18 ± 0.033 vs. 0.1 ± 0.016 nM ($p = 0.03$). Overall, the EVG EC_{50} values of viruses expressing patient-derived full-length *pol* were similar to that of viruses expressing patient-derived *IN* gene only, with the exception of the virus expressing Y143C + E92Q mutations, which showed a significant decrease in EVG susceptibility for patient-derived *IN* gene only compared to full-length *pol* gene ($p = 0.0064$). Again, this may indicate that the patient coevolved *PR* and *RT* genes' influence on the susceptibility to EVG is dependent on the combination of InSTI resistance mutations; however, this effect is different between EVG and RAL.

2.5. The Effects of Patient-Derived pol Gene Fragments on Viral Replicative Fitness

Next, we tested the replicative fitness of the viruses expressing patient-derived full-length *pol* or *IN* gene only (Figure 5). Using a single-replication-cycle assay, the wild-type control virus, the virus expressing patient-derived *PR* + *RT* (ptA_*PR* + *RT*) and the virus expressing patient-derived full-length *pol* with wild-type *IN* showed similar replicative fitness to the virus expressing patient-derived wild-type *IN* only (ptA_WT*IN*; set to 100%) at 110.5 ± 7.7%, 109.7 ± 12.3% and 102.9 ± 8%, respectively ($p \geq 0.39$).

Interestingly, the only other virus that showed replicative fitness comparable to that of ptA_WT*IN* was the patient-derived full-length *pol* or *IN* only virus, expressing the rare *IN* Y143G + G163R mutation combination at 86.9 ± 7.6 and 102 ± 6.6%, respectively ($p = 0.28$ and 0.85). All other viruses expressing patient-derived full-length *pol* or *IN* only had significantly lower replicative fitness than ptA_WT*IN*, ranging from 12.9 ± 0.6 to 72.9 ± 3.4% ($p \leq 0.01$).

In general, the replicative fitness of viruses expressing full-length *pol* was greater than or comparable to that of viruses expressing the respective *IN* gene only. The viruses showing significantly increased replicative fitness upon expression of patient-derived full-length *pol* relative to *IN* gene only were those with the following RAL resistance mutation combinations: Q148R + G140A ($p = 0.0023$), Y143R + G163R ($p = 0.024$), Y143R + G163K ($p \leq 0.0001$) and Y143C + G163R ($p = 0.013$). Furthermore, viruses that dominated the population during the two RAL treatment phases had both high levels of RAL resistance and replication fitness (Figure 6).

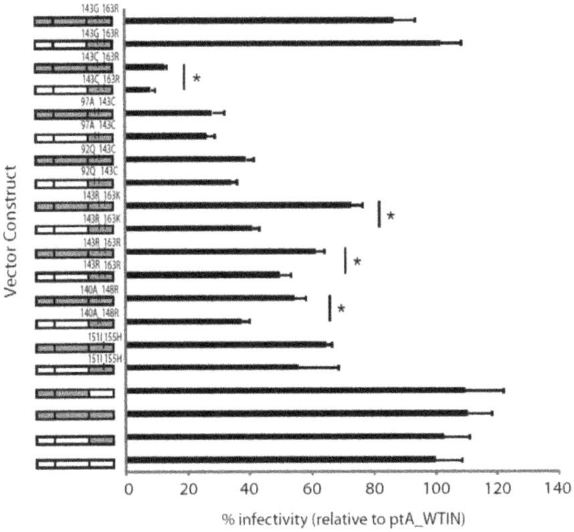

Figure 5. The effect on viral replicative fitness of patient-derived *IN* gene only or full-length *pol* gene. Viral infectivity in a single-replication-cycle assay was used to determine the replicative fitness of recombinant viruses expressing patient-derived *IN* gene only or full-length *pol* genes. The replicative fitness relative to ptA_WT*IN* control (vector containing patient-derived *IN* only from the pre-RAL time point), set at 100%, is shown for each virus. Significant differences ($p < 0.05$) between patient-derived *IN* only viruses and their full-length *pol* counterparts are indicated with *. The error bars represent standard error of the mean of six independent experiments.

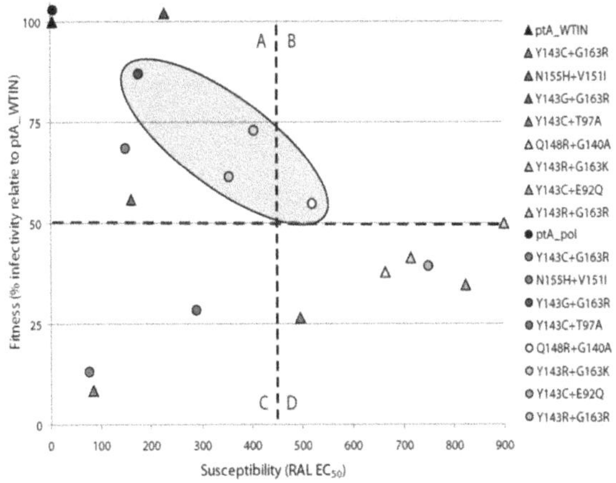

Figure 6. Relationship between the replicative fitness and RAL susceptibility exhibited by recombinant viruses from ptA. A graph plotting the relationship between replicative fitness and RAL susceptibility of recombinant viruses expressing either patient-derived *IN* gene only or full-length *pol* gene. The graph is equally divided into four hypothetical quadrants: (**A**) high replicative fitness (>50%) and low RAL resistance (<450 nM), (**B**) high replicative fitness (>50%) and RAL resistance (>450 nM), (**C**) low replicative fitness (<50%) and RAL resistance (>450 nM), (**D**) low replicative fitness (<50%) and high RAL resistance (<450 nM). Triangles represent viruses expressing patient-derived *IN* gene only; circles represent the respective viruses expressing full-length *pol* gene. The shaded oval represents viruses that dominated the viral population during RAL-containing salvage therapy at 4RAL, 5RAL and reRAL.

3. Discussion

InSTIs are a preferred third agent in NRTI-based regimen. Consequently, some patients on an InSTI-containing regimen will or have previously failed therapies containing PIs and RTIs, especially in low- and middle-income countries. Thus, it is important to understand the interaction and development of drug resistance mutations in the context of patient-derived full-length *pol* gene. In this study, we used a full-length HIV-1 *pol* gene SGS assay to demonstrate the genetic linkage of drug resistance mutations throughout the *pol* gene. We showed that drug resistance mutations in IN are linked to those in PR and RT, and that different combinations of InSTI resistance mutations can develop concurrently linked to the same PR and RT drug resistance mutations. This is consistent with another study showing the linkage of EVG resistance mutations in IN to drug resistance mutations in PR and RT [15].

Our data also revealed the simultaneous presence of mutations at all three major InSTI drug resistance positions (Q148, Y143 and N155) during treatment failure, albeit on different genomes, which is also consistent with previous findings [19–23]. In this study, the major InSTI resistance mutations were always linked to accessory mutations. This may be due to a longer period between initiation of RAL therapy and first sampling, which was at least 4 months. It is well established that major RAL resistance mutations can appear rapidly (sometimes within a month) after initiation of RAL treatment, with accessory mutations developing subsequently to compensate for fitness loss and/or to increase drug resistance [19–29]. The genetic linkage of major and accessory mutations suggests that the accessory mutations compensate for fitness loss and/or increase drug resistance of a viral variant through cis-acting mechanisms. This has been confirmed for the Q148H + G140S double mutant, in which it was demonstrated that the catalytic properties of IN were greatly impaired by the single mutants. However, the double mutant could fully restore the catalytic properties of IN only when the two mutations were present on the same IN polypeptide [28].

Our findings also shed light on the complexities of the intrapatient evolution of the Y143 resistance pathway, and the effects of accessory mutations linked to this pathway. Previous studies suggest that the accessory mutations linked to the Y143 mutations play a positive role in IN activity and/or RAL resistance [21,24,30]. In this study, we observed that different accessory mutations combined with a particular substitution at position Y143 differentially influenced the levels of susceptibility to RAL. For example, we observed the development of the Y143C resistance mutation, linked to three different accessory mutations (E92Q, T97A and G163R), differentially decreased RAL susceptibility from 19- to 183-fold, as well as viral fitness by 8 to 35% compared to wild-type virus. All three of the accessory mutations are found in the vicinity of the catalytic active site of *IN* [31]; therefore, it is envisioned that they could be affecting susceptibility and replicative fitness by directly influencing the structure of the active site.

The differential effect on RAL susceptibility and viral fitness also extended to different substitutions at primary resistance position 143 (R, C or G), linked to the same accessory mutation (G163R). This finding is contrary to another study which showed that the RAL susceptibilities of both the Y143R and Y143C mutants were similar [30]. However, in this study, the Y143 mutants were not linked to the G163R accessory mutation, which may partially explain the different observations. These data suggest that accessory mutations linked to Y143 mutations affect both the replicative fitness and InSTI susceptibility of the mutant viruses, and that a balance between the two could play a role in determining the development and evolution of resistance. Consistent with this observation, the Y143G + G163R mutant, that was present as a minority variant after RAL treatment was stopped, emerged as the dominant viral variant upon the re-initiation of RAL therapy. This variant exhibited a significantly higher RAL EC_{50} than the Y143C + G163R mutant, and had a significantly higher replicative fitness compared to the Y143R + G163R and Y143C + G163R mutants. The replicative fitness of Y143G + G163R was in fact the highest of all RAL resistant variants identified in this patient, and was comparable to that of wild-type virus. It is therefore likely that the subsequent outgrowth of this viral variant after the re-initiation of RAL therapy may be due to its higher replicative fitness compared to the other RAL resistant viruses present in the patient. The late and rare development of the Y143G substitution could be due to a high genetic barrier. The wild-type codon for position 143 in IN in this patient was TAC. One nucleotide change was required for the Y to C substitution (TAC to TGC), whilst two nucleotide changes were needed to generate the G substitution (TAC to GGC) or R substitution (TAC to CGC). The second change required for the Y to R substitution (T to C) is a transition which occurs at a higher frequency compared to the T to G transversion required for the Y to G substitution. Thus, although more advantageous to the virus in terms of fitness, the Y143G substitution is likely to occur less frequently compared to Y143R/C substitutions. This is supported by analysis of data available from the Stanford HIV Drug Resistance Database, which showed no instances of Y143G mutation in InSTI-experienced subtype B infected patients (Figure 1B). This also illustrates that continuous selective drug pressure during a failing regimen will force the virus to continue evolving towards a fitter resistant virus, that is then more likely to persist in the absence of drug pressure [32,33].

A limitation of the study is that the analysis, although in depth, is from one patient. Future studies will focus on investigating this phenomenon in a large group of patients, and include investigation of resistance to second generation InSTIs, such as DTG and use of full-length genome clones. Nonetheless, the data show that the coevolved *PR* and *RT* genes affect the susceptibility and replicative fitness of an *IN* gene harbouring InSTI resistance mutations by up to three-fold. This concurs with another study, that showed an effect on viral fitness and susceptibility to EFV and RAL for certain combinations of NNRTI and InSTI resistance mutations [34]. On the other hand, other studies have shown that mutations in PR and RT have little effect on the susceptibility to InSTIs, but can reduce viral replicative fitness of a resistant *IN* gene [35]. Different experimental approaches, such as the use of site-directed mutants compared to patient-derived fragments, or differences in the combination of resistance mutations and/or accessory mutations, could explain the contradictory outcomes. Therefore, further comprehensive studies coupling biological and biochemical investigations are required to elucidate the interactions between mutations in full-length HIV-1 *pol* gene and their effects on susceptibility and viral fitness, including that to the new InSTIs DTG, BIC and CAB. However, taken together, these data suggest that analysis of only part of the HIV-1 genome is probably not sufficient to gauge the true dynamics in the evolution and extent of drug resistance in the era of cART, as shown by recent studies linking InSTI resistance to env and cPPT regions [33,36,37]. The use of assays encompassing full-length *pol* gene or more of the viral genome may provide useful insights into drug resistance mechanisms, and help devise better treatment strategies as well as improve the prediction of the emergence of drug resistance and subsequent treatment failure.

4. Materials and Methods

4.1. Clinical Samples

The plasma samples used in this study were obtained from a patient attending the Mortimer Market Clinic, UCLH, who was infected with subtype B virus and initiated on RAL salvage therapy (600 mg daily) in September 2007. They continued RAL in combination with darunavir/ritonavir (DRV/r) and etravirine (ETR) until February 2008, when the patient experienced virological failure. The patient was then switched onto therapy containing tenofovir (TDF) and lamivudine (3TC), but experienced virological failure again 2 months later (April 2008). RAL treatment was then re-started in combination with TDF/emtricitabine (FTC), DRV/r and ETR in September 2008. Six samples were obtained, and these were: pre-RAL therapy (preRAL); 2, 4 and 5 months on RAL (2RAL, 4RAL and 5RAL, respectively); 4 months after RAL was stopped (4post); and 0.5 months after RAL was re-started (reRAL) [23]. Informed consent was obtained in the context of routine resistance testing as a part of clinical protocol.

4.2. Single-Genome Sequencing

A previously described, single genome sequencing assay [38] was modified by designing new antisense primers at the end of *IN*, and used to sequence full-length *pol* from sequential samples. cDNA synthesis and single genome PCR reactions were carried out as described, but using the antisense primer KVL069 (5′-TTCTTCCTGCCATAGGARATGCCT AAG-3′) [39] followed by a nested PCR reaction using either 5095- (5′-TAATCCTCATCCTG TCTACYTGCCACAC-3′), KVL084 (5′-TCCTGTATGCARACCCCAATATG-3′) [39] or 5222-deg (5′-TGTCTATAAAACCATCCTYTAGC-3′) antisense primers.

4.3. Single-Replication Cycle Drug Susceptibility Assay

To study phenotypic drug susceptibility, we used a previously described three plasmid-based retroviral vector system, utilising luciferase expression as a measure of infectivity [13,40]. The p8.9NSX *gag-pol* expression vector, which contains a unique *Apa*I restriction site in *gag* (upstream of the *PR* start codon) and an *Eco*RI restriction site in *vif* (downstream of the *IN* stop codon), was modified by introducing a unique *Cla*I restriction site at the beginning of *IN* (flanking amino acids 4/5), creating the p8.9NSXClaI+ vector. In parallel, mutagenesis was used to introduce the same *Cla*I and *Eco*RI sites in nine of the single genomes amplified from the patient in the single genome assay. The nine single genome variants were selected from different on- and off-RAL treatment time points, which included all the different RAL resistance mutation combinations observed in the patient, with these being: N155H + V151I, Q148R + G140A, Y143R + G163R, Y143R + G163K, Y143C + E92Q, Y143C + T97A, Y143C + G163R, Y143G + G163R as well as a wild-type *IN* from the pre-RAL time point (used as a control and designated ptA_WT*IN*).

In addition, the *Apa*I restriction site in *gag* and the *Cla*I restriction site at the beginning of *IN* were introduced into a single genome containing L10F, V32I, L33F, M46I, I47V, I54L, A71T, I84V, L89V and L90M in *PR*, and M41L, D67N, L74V, M184V, T215Y, K219E, L100I, K103N and N348I in *RT*. These resistance mutations were present in all single genomes chosen for the analysis. The unique restriction sites were then used for the subcloning of patient-derived *PR* + *RT* (*Apa*I and *Cla*I) or *IN* (*Cla*I and *Eco*RI) into p8.9NSXClaI+, to generate ptA_*PR* + *RT* and patient-derived *IN* only vectors, respectively (Figure 2). The generation of full-length *pol* vectors was achieved by subcloning patient-derived *IN* fragments into ptA_*PR* + *RT*, using the *Cla*I and *Eco*RI restriction sites. All mutagenesis was carried out using the QuikChange Lightning Multi Site-Directed Mutagenesis kit or QuikChange II XL Site-Directed Mutagenesis kit (Agilent Technologies), according to the manufacturer's protocol. The presence of mutations was verified by sequencing.

The two other vectors used in this assay are the retroviral expression vector, pCSFLW, which encodes the firefly luciferase reporter gene, and pMDG, which encodes the vesicular stomatitis virus G protein. Viruses were generated by cotransfection of 293T cells as previously described, and then used to infect fresh 293T cells in the presence of serially diluted RAL or EVG [41,42]. The replication fitness of the virus was determined by p24 ELISA (Genscreen™ HIV-1 Ag Assay, Bio-Rad) and expressed as a percent of the ptA_WT*IN* control, as described previously [13].

4.4. Antiretroviral Drugs

RAL and EVG (repository references ARP980 and ARP991, respectively) were obtained from the National Institute for Biological Standards and Control.

4.5. Statistical Analyses

Differences in EC_{50} values and replicative fitness were calculated using the Student's *t* test tool, available on www.graphpad.com (accessed on 10 June 2021). *p* values which were <0.05 were regarded as significant.

4.6. Nucleotide Sequence Accession Numbers

The single-genome sequences generated and used in this study have been submitted to GenBank and assigned the accession numbers MH663797-MH663975.

Author Contributions: Conceptualisation, P.A.C., D.P. and J.L.M.; data curation, S.A.M. and D.P.; formal analysis, S.A.M., P.A.C., D.P. and J.L.M.; funding acquisition, J.L.M.; investigation, S.A.M., P.A.C., D.P. and J.L.M.; methodology, S.A.M. and J.L.M.; project administration, J.L.M.; resources, D.P. and J.L.M.; supervision, P.A.C., D.P. and J.L.M.; writing—original draft, S.A.M. and J.L.M.; writing—review and editing, P.A.C., D.P. and J.L.M. All authors have read and agreed to the published version of the manuscript.

Funding: This research was funded by a PHE PhD Studentship. The views expressed in this publication are those of the author(s) and not necessarily those of the NHS, the Department of Health and Social Care or PHE.

Institutional Review Board Statement: All experiments were performed in accordance with the "Guidance on Conducting Research in Public Health England" (Version 3, October 2015: Document code RD001A). This study uses samples and data collected as part of standard of care with informed consent, therefore specific approval was not necessary. The samples were anonymised by removal of any patient identifiable information and assignment of a non-specific project number prior to genetic characterization.

Informed Consent Statement: Informed consent was obtained in the context of routine resistance testing as a part of clinical protocol. Therefore, no ethical approval was required.

Data Availability Statement: Sequence data generated by the study is available through NCBI GenBank and assigned the accession numbers MH663797-MH663975.

Acknowledgments: We would like to thank Bridget Ferns of the University College London Hospitals (UCLH) NHS Foundation Trust and all members of the Antiviral Unit at Public Health England (PHE) for their support.

Conflicts of Interest: The authors declare no conflict of interest.

References

1. UNAIDS Joint United Nations Programme on HIV/AIDS. *UNAIDS Data 2020*; UNAIDS: Geneva, Switzerland, 2020.
2. Grobler, J.A.; Stillmock, K.; Hu, B.; Witmer, M.; Felock, P.; Espeseth, A.S.; Wolfe, A.; Egbertson, M.; Bourgeois, M.; Melamed, J.; et al. Diketo acid inhibitor mechanism and HIV-1 integrase: Implications for metal binding in the active site of phosphotransferase enzymes. *Proc. Natl. Acad. Sci. USA* **2002**, *99*, 6661–6666. [CrossRef] [PubMed]
3. Marchand, C.; Johnson, A.A.; Karki, R.G.; Pais, G.C.; Zhang, X.; Cowansage, K.; Patel, T.A.; Nicklaus, M.C.; Burke, T.R., Jr.; Pommier, Y. Metal-dependent inhibition of HIV-1 integrase by beta-diketo acids and resistance of the soluble double-mutant (F185K/C280S). *Mol. Pharmacol.* **2003**, *64*, 600–609. [CrossRef]
4. Arribas, J.R.; Eron, J. Advances in antiretroviral therapy. *Curr. Opin. HIV AIDS* **2013**, *8*, 341–349. [CrossRef] [PubMed]
5. Steigbigel, R.T.; Cooper, D.A.; Teppler, H.; Eron, J.J.; Gatell, J.M.; Kumar, P.N.; Rockstroh, J.K.; Schechter, M.; Katlama, C.; Markowitz, M.; et al. Long-term efficacy and safety of Raltegravir combined with optimized background therapy in treatment-experienced patients with drug-resistant HIV infection: Week 96 results of the BENCHMRK 1 and 2 Phase III trials. *Clin. Infect. Dis.* **2010**, *50*, 605–612. [CrossRef]
6. Churchill, D.; Waters, L.; Ahmed, N.; Angus, B.; Boffito, M.; Bower, M.; Dunn, D.; Edwards, S.; Emerson, C.; Fidler, S.; et al. British HIV Association guidelines for the treatment of HIV-1-positive adults with antiretroviral therapy 2015. *HIV Med.* **2016**, *17* (Suppl. 4), s2–s104. [CrossRef]
7. European AIDS Clinical Society. Guidelines 2018. Available online: https://www.eacsociety.org/files/2018_guidelines-9.1-english.pdf (accessed on 4 November 2019).
8. Mbisa, J.L. Antiviral Resistance Testing. eLS. 2013. Available online: https://onlinelibrary.wiley.com/doi/abs/10.1002/9780470015902.a0024795 (accessed on 10 June 2021).
9. Avila-Rios, S.; Parkin, N.; Swanstrom, R.; Paredes, R.; Shafer, R.; Ji, H.; Kantor, R. Next-Generation Sequencing for HIV Drug Resistance Testing: Laboratory, Clinical, and Implementation Considerations. *Viruses* **2020**, *12*, 617. [CrossRef]
10. Hertogs, K.; de Bethune, M.P.; Miller, V.; Ivens, T.; Schel, P.; Van Cauwenberge, A.; Van Den Eynde, C.; Van Gerwen, V.; Azijn, H.; Van Houtte, M.; et al. A rapid method for simultaneous detection of phenotypic resistance to inhibitors of protease and reverse transcriptase in recombinant human immunodeficiency virus type 1 isolates from patients treated with antiretroviral drugs. *Antimicrob. Agents Chemother.* **1998**, *42*, 269–276. [CrossRef]

11. Kellam, P.; Larder, B.A. Recombinant virus assay: A rapid, phenotypic assay for assessment of drug susceptibility of human immunodeficiency virus type 1 isolates. *Antimicrob. Agents Chemother.* **1994**, *38*, 23–30. [CrossRef]
12. Petropoulos, C.J.; Parkin, N.T.; Limoli, K.L.; Lie, Y.S.; Wrin, T.; Huang, W.; Tian, H.; Smith, D.; Winslow, G.A.; Capon, D.J.; et al. A novel phenotypic drug susceptibility assay for human immunodeficiency virus type 1. *Antimicrob. Agents Chemother.* **2000**, *44*, 920–928. [CrossRef]
13. Parry, C.M.; Kohli, A.; Boinett, C.J.; Towers, G.J.; McCormick, A.L.; Pillay, D. Gag determinants of fitness and drug susceptibility in protease inhibitor-resistant human immunodeficiency virus type 1. *J. Virol.* **2009**, *83*, 9094–9101. [CrossRef] [PubMed]
14. Weber, J.; Vazquez, A.C.; Winner, D.; Rose, J.D.; Wylie, D.; Rhea, A.M.; Henry, K.; Pappas, J.; Wright, A.; Mohamed, N.; et al. Novel method for simultaneous quantification of phenotypic resistance to maturation, protease, reverse transcriptase, and integrase HIV inhibitors based on 3'Gag(p2/p7/p1/p6)/PR/RT/INT-recombinant viruses: A useful tool in the multitarget era of antiretroviral therapy. *Antimicrob. Agents Chemother.* **2011**, *55*, 3729–3742.
15. Winters, M.A.; Lloyd, R.M., Jr.; Shafer, R.W.; Kozal, M.J.; Miller, M.D.; Holodniy, M. Development of elvitegravir resistance and linkage of integrase inhibitor mutations with protease and reverse transcriptase resistance mutations. *PLoS ONE* **2012**, *7*, e40514. [CrossRef]
16. Van Baelen, K.; Rondelez, E.; Van Eygen, V.; Arien, K.; Clynhens, M.; Van den Zegel, P.; Winters, B.; Stuyver, L.J. A combined genotypic and phenotypic human immunodeficiency virus type 1 recombinant virus assay for the reverse transcriptase and integrase genes. *J. Virol. Methods* **2009**, *161*, 231–239. [CrossRef]
17. Low, A.; Prada, N.; Topper, M.; Vaida, F.; Castor, D.; Mohri, H.; Hazuda, D.; Muesing, M.; Markowitz, M. Natural polymorphisms of human immunodeficiency virus type 1 integrase and inherent susceptibilities to a panel of integrase inhibitors. *Antimicrob. Agents Chemother.* **2009**, *53*, 4275–4282. [CrossRef]
18. Garrido, C.; Villacian, J.; Zahonero, N.; Pattery, T.; Garcia, F.; Gutierrez, F.; Caballero, E.; Van Houtte, M.; Soriano, V.; de Mendoza, C.; et al. Broad phenotypic cross-resistance to elvitegravir in HIV-infected patients failing on raltegravir-containing regimens. *Antimicrob. Agents Chemother.* **2012**, *56*, 2873–2878. [CrossRef]
19. Charpentier, C.; Karmochkine, M.; Laureillard, D.; Tisserand, P.; Belec, L.; Weiss, L.; Si-Mohamed, A.; Piketty, C. Drug resistance profiles for the HIV integrase gene in patients failing raltegravir salvage therapy. *HIV Med.* **2008**, *9*, 765–770. [CrossRef]
20. Malet, I.; Delelis, O.; Soulie, C.; Wirden, M.; Tchertanov, L.; Mottaz, P.; Peytavin, G.; Katlama, C.; Mouscadet, J.F.; Calvez, V.; et al. Quasispecies variant dynamics during emergence of resistance to raltegravir in HIV-1-infected patients. *J. Antimicrob. Chemother.* **2009**, *63*, 795–804. [CrossRef] [PubMed]
21. Reigadas, S.; Anies, G.; Masquelier, B.; Calmels, C.; Stuyver, L.J.; Parissi, V.; Fleury, H.; Andreola, M.L. The HIV-1 integrase mutations Y143C/R are an alternative pathway for resistance to Raltegravir and impact the enzyme functions. *PLoS ONE* **2010**, *5*, e10311. [CrossRef] [PubMed]
22. Fransen, S.; Gupta, S.; Danovich, R.; Hazuda, D.; Miller, M.; Witmer, M.; Petropoulos, C.J.; Huang, W. Loss of raltegravir susceptibility by human immunodeficiency virus type 1 is conferred via multiple nonoverlapping genetic pathways. *J. Virol.* **2009**, *83*, 11440–11446. [CrossRef] [PubMed]
23. Ferns, R.B.; Kirk, S.; Bennett, J.; Cook, P.M.; Williams, I.; Edwards, S.; Pillay, D. The dynamics of appearance and disappearance of HIV-1 integrase mutations during and after withdrawal of raltegravir therapy. *AIDS* **2009**, *23*, 2159–2164. [CrossRef]
24. Canducci, F.; Marinozzi, M.C.; Sampaolo, M.; Boeri, E.; Spagnuolo, V.; Gianotti, N.; Castagna, A.; Paolucci, S.; Baldanti, F.; Lazzarin, A.; et al. Genotypic/phenotypic patterns of HIV-1 integrase resistance to raltegravir. *J. Antimicrob. Chemother.* **2010**, *65*, 425–433. [CrossRef] [PubMed]
25. Baldanti, F.; Paolucci, S.; Gulminetti, R.; Brandolini, M.; Barbarini, G.; Maserati, R. Early emergence of raltegravir resistance mutations in patients receiving HAART salvage regimens. *J. Med. Virol.* **2010**, *82*, 116–122. [CrossRef] [PubMed]
26. Fun, A.; Van Baelen, K.; van Lelyveld, S.F.; Schipper, P.J.; Stuyver, L.J.; Wensing, A.M.; Nijhuis, M. Mutation Q95K enhances N155H-mediated integrase inhibitor resistance and improves viral replication capacity. *J. Antimicrob. Chemother.* **2010**, *65*, 2300–2304. [CrossRef] [PubMed]
27. Delelis, O.; Malet, I.; Na, L.; Tchertanov, L.; Calvez, V.; Marcelin, A.G.; Subra, F.; Deprez, E.; Mouscadet, J.F. The G140S mutation in HIV integrases from raltegravir-resistant patients rescues catalytic defect due to the resistance Q148H mutation. *Nucleic Acids Res.* **2009**, *37*, 1193–1201. [CrossRef]
28. Metifiot, M.; Maddali, K.; Naumova, A.; Zhang, X.; Marchand, C.; Pommier, Y. Biochemical and pharmacological analyses of HIV-1 integrase flexible loop mutants resistant to raltegravir. *Biochemistry* **2010**, *49*, 3715–3722. [CrossRef] [PubMed]
29. Nakahara, K.; Wakasa-Morimoto, C.; Kobayashi, M.; Miki, S.; Noshi, T.; Seki, T.; Kanamori-Koyama, M.; Kawauchi, S.; Suyama, A.; Fujishita, T.; et al. Secondary mutations in viruses resistant to HIV-1 integrase inhibitors that restore viral infectivity and replication kinetics. *Antivir. Res.* **2009**, *81*, 141–146. [CrossRef]
30. Delelis, O.; Thierry, S.; Subra, F.; Simon, F.; Malet, I.; Alloui, C.; Sayon, S.; Calvez, V.; Deprez, E.; Marcelin, A.G.; et al. Impact of Y143 HIV-1 integrase mutations on resistance to raltegravir in vitro and in vivo. *Antimicrob. Agents Chemother.* **2010**, *54*, 491–501. [CrossRef]
31. Mbisa, J.L.; Martin, S.A.; Cane, P.A. Patterns of resistance development with integrase inhibitors in HIV. *Infect. Drug Resist.* **2011**, *4*, 65–76.

32. Mbisa, J.L.; Gupta, R.K.; Kabamba, D.; Mulenga, V.; Kalumbi, M.; Chintu, C.; Parry, C.M.; Gibb, D.M.; Walker, S.A.; Cane, P.A.; et al. The evolution of HIV-1 reverse transcriptase in route to acquisition of Q151M multi-drug resistance is complex and involves mutations in multiple domains. *Retrovirology* **2011**, *8*, 31. [CrossRef]
33. Malet, I.; Delelis, O.; Nguyen, T.; Leducq, V.; Abdi, B.; Morand-Joubert, L.; Calvez, V.; Marcelin, A.G. Variability of the HIV-1 3′ polypurine tract (3′PPT) region and implication in integrase inhibitor resistance. *J. Antimicrob. Chemother.* **2019**, *74*, 3440–3444. [CrossRef]
34. Hu, Z.; Kuritzkes, D.R. Altered viral fitness and drug susceptibility in HIV-1 carrying mutations that confer resistance to nonnucleoside reverse transcriptase and integrase strand transfer inhibitors. *J. Virol.* **2014**, *88*, 9268–9276. [CrossRef] [PubMed]
35. Gupta, S.F.; Frantzell, A.; Chappey, C.; Petropoulos, C.; Huang, W. Combinations of primary NNRTI- and integrase inhibitor-resistance mutations do not alter HIV-1 drug susceptibility but impair replication capacity. In Proceedings of the 16th Conference on Retroviruses and Opportunistic Infections, Montreal, QC, Canada, 8–11 February 2009.
36. Van Duyne, R.; Kuo, L.S.; Pham, P.; Fujii, K.; Freed, E.O. Mutations in the HIV-1 envelope glycoprotein can broadly rescue blocks at multiple steps in the virus replication cycle. *Proc. Natl. Acad. Sci. USA* **2019**, *116*, 9040–9049. [CrossRef]
37. Malet, I.; Subra, F.; Charpentier, C.; Collin, G.; Descamps, D.; Calvez, V.; Marcelin, A.G.; Delelis, O. Mutations Located outside the Integrase Gene Can Confer Resistance to HIV-1 Integrase Strand Transfer Inhibitors. *MBio* **2017**, *8*, e00922-17. [CrossRef]
38. Palmer, S.; Kearney, M.; Maldarelli, F.; Halvas, E.K.; Bixby, C.J.; Bazmi, H.; Rock, D.; Falloon, J.; Davey, R.T., Jr.; Dewar, R.L.; et al. Multiple, linked human immunodeficiency virus type 1 drug resistance mutations in treatment-experienced patients are missed by standard genotype analysis. *J. Clin. Microbiol.* **2005**, *43*, 406–413. [CrossRef] [PubMed]
39. Van Laethem, K.; Schrooten, Y.; Covens, K.; Dekeersmaeker, N.; De Munter, P.; Van Wijngaerden, E.; Van Ranst, M.; Vandamme, A.M. A genotypic assay for the amplification and sequencing of integrase from diverse HIV-1 group M subtypes. *J. Virol. Methods* **2008**, *153*, 176–181. [CrossRef]
40. Gupta, R.K.; Kohli, A.; McCormick, A.L.; Towers, G.J.; Pillay, D.; Parry, C.M. Full-length HIV-1 Gag determines protease inhibitor susceptibility within in vitro assays. *AIDS* **2010**, *24*, 1651–1655. [CrossRef] [PubMed]
41. Bainbridge, J.W.; Stephens, C.; Parsley, K.; Demaison, C.; Halfyard, A.; Thrasher, A.J.; Ali, R.R. In vivo gene transfer to the mouse eye using an HIV-based lentiviral vector; efficient long-term transduction of corneal endothelium and retinal pigment epithelium. *Gene Ther.* **2001**, *8*, 1665–1668. [CrossRef]
42. Wright, E.; Temperton, N.J.; Marston, D.A.; McElhinney, L.M.; Fooks, A.R.; Weiss, R.A. Investigating antibody neutralization of lyssaviruses using lentiviral pseudotypes: A cross-species comparison. *J. Gen. Virol.* **2008**, *89 Pt 9*, 2204–2213. [CrossRef]

pathogens MDPI

Article

Factors Associated with HIV Drug Resistance in Dar es Salaam, Tanzania: Analysis of a Complex Adaptive System

Anneleen Kiekens [1,*], Idda H. Mosha [2], Lara Zlatić [1,3], George M. Bwire [1,4], Ally Mangara [5], Bernadette Dierckx de Casterlé [6], Catherine Decouttere [7], Nico Vandaele [7], Raphael Z. Sangeda [4], Omary Swalehe [8], Paolo Cottone [3], Alessio Surian [3], Japhet Killewo [9] and Anne-Mieke Vandamme [1,10]

1 Department of Microbiology, Immunology and Transplantation, Rega Institute for Medical Research, Clinical and Epidemiological Virology, Institute for the Future, KU Leuven, 3000 Leuven, Belgium; lara.zlatic0508@gmail.com (L.Z.); georgemsema.bwire@kuleuven.be (G.M.B.); annemie.vandamme@kuleuven.be (A.-M.V.)
2 Department of Behavioural Sciences, Muhimbili University of Health and Allied Sciences, Dar es Salaam 65015, Tanzania; ihmosha@yahoo.co.uk
3 FISPPA Department, Università degli Studi di Padova, 35139 Padova, Italy; paolo.cottone@unipd.it (P.C.); alessio.surian@gmail.com (A.S.)
4 Department of Pharmaceutical Microbiology, Muhimbili University of Health and Allied Sciences, Dar es Salaam 65013, Tanzania; sangeda@gmail.com
5 Dar es Salaam Urban Cohort Study, Dar es Salaam 65013, Tanzania; mangaraalli@gmail.com
6 Department of Public Health and Primary Care, Academic Centre for Nursing and Midwifery, KU Leuven, 3000 Leuven, Belgium; bernadette.dierckxdecasterle@kuleuven.be
7 Faculty of Economics and Business, Access to Medicine Research Center, KU Leuven, 3000 Leuven, Belgium; catherine.decouttere@kuleuven.be (C.D.); nico.vandaele@kuleuven.be (N.V.)
8 Department of Business Studies, School of Business, Mzumbe University, Dar es Salaam 20266, Tanzania; oswalehe@mzumbe.ac.tz
9 Department of Epidemiology and Biostatistics, Muhimbili University of Health and Allied Sciences, Dar es Salaam 65001, Tanzania; jkillewo@yahoo.co.uk
10 Center for Global Health and Tropical Medicine, Unidade de Microbiologia, Instituto de Higiene e Medicina Tropical, Universidade Nova de Lisboa, 1349-008 Lisbon, Portugal
* Correspondence: anneleen.kiekens@kuleuven.be

Citation: Kiekens, A.; Mosha, I.H.; Zlatić, L.; Bwire, G.M.; Mangara, A.; Dierckx de Casterlé, B.; Decouttere, C.; Vandaele, N.; Sangeda, R.Z.; Swalehe, O.; et al. Factors Associated with HIV Drug Resistance in Dar es Salaam, Tanzania: Analysis of a Complex Adaptive System. *Pathogens* **2021**, *10*, 1535. https://doi.org/10.3390/pathogens10121535

Academic Editor: Hezhao Ji

Received: 28 September 2021
Accepted: 17 November 2021
Published: 24 November 2021

Abstract: HIV drug resistance (HIVDR) is a complex problem with multiple interconnected and context dependent causes. Although the factors influencing HIVDR are known and well-studied, HIVDR remains a threat to the effectiveness of antiretroviral therapy. To understand the complexity of HIVDR, a comprehensive, systems approach is needed. Therefore, a local systems map was developed integrating all reported factors influencing HIVDR in the Dar es Salaam Urban Cohort Study area in Tanzania. The map was designed based on semi-structured interviews and workshops with people living with HIV and local actors who encounter people living with HIV during their daily activities. We visualized the feedback loops driving HIVDR, compared the local map with a systems map for Sub-Saharan Africa, previously constructed from interviews with international HIVDR experts, and suggest potential interventions to prevent HIVDR. We found several interconnected balancing and reinforcing feedback loops related to poverty, stigmatization, status disclosure, self-esteem, knowledge about HIVDR and healthcare system workload, among others, and identified three potential leverage points. Insights from this local systems map were complementary to the insights from the Sub-Saharan systems map showing that both viewpoints are needed to fully understand the system. This study provides a strong baseline for quantitative modelling, and for the identification of context-dependent, complexity-informed leverage points.

Keywords: case study; complex adaptive system; HIV drug resistance; leverage points; systems mapping; Dar es Salaam; Tanzania

1. Introduction

Over the past years, Tanzania has made considerable progress towards reaching the global 95-95-95 goals [1]. In August 2020, an estimated 83% of people living with HIV (PLHIV) in Tanzania were aware of their HIV status, of which 90% were on HIV treatment. Of those on treatment, 92% were virally suppressed. In 2019, the HIV prevalence in Tanzania was estimated to be 4.8%. The Tanzanian epidemic consists entirely of the HIV-1 type as no HIV-2 infections have been reported so far [2,3]. In 2019 the WHO reported alarming increases in pre-treatment HIV drug resistance (PDR) with 12 out of 18 reporting countries exceeding the 10% non-nucleoside reverse transcriptase inhibitor (NNRTI) PDR threshold, triggering immediate national action [4]. A recently published study conducted between 2013 and 2019 found a prevalence of 11% PDR among the 801 antiretroviral therapy (ART)-naïve participants from Tanzania, Kenya, Uganda and Nigeria [5]. Among the ART-experienced participants with unsuppressed viral load (VL), resistance rates of 82.5%, 66.7% and 1.8% were reported for NNRTI, nucleoside reverse transcriptase inhibitor (NRTI) and protease inhibitor (PI) mutations, respectively. Another study in Dar es Salaam from 2010, although with a small sample size, found drug resistance mutations in 82.6% of the included therapy-experienced participants [6]. A systematic literature review published by the WHO showed that the prevalence of pre-treatment NNRTI resistance has been increasing the fastest in Eastern Africa, compared to other low- and middle-income regions [7]. These results underline the importance of addressing HIV drug resistance (HIVDR) in order to sustain the progress towards the goal of ending the epidemic by 2030.

HIVDR is influenced by a multitude of factors which transcend single disciplines and population levels, and which, together, form a complex, multi-layered and interconnected system [8]. Several individual, socio-economic, structural and health care system related factors influencing HIVDR in Tanzania have been described in a literature review by Msongole et al. [9]. Although the diverse factors influencing HIVDR are relatively well studied, preventing HIVDR (including acquired and transmitted drug resistance) in the real world remains difficult [4,10–12]. In order to understand and address the underlying challenges of HIVDR there is a need to shift away from the reductionist, linear cause-effect models towards a comprehensive systems approach and study the factors associated with HIVDR as a complex adaptive system (CAS) [13]. A core characteristic of such CAS lies in the understanding that successfully intervening on one element of a system does not guarantee resolving the central problem due to influences of other aspects of the system [14]. Interventions in a complex system ideally require a small shift in one place which has the potential to positively change the whole system. Such places to intervene on are called leverage points and can be divided into shallow and deep leverage points [15,16]. Shallow leverage points, such as parameters and feedbacks, are relatively easy to intervene on, but have a limited effect on the system, whereas interventions at deep leverage points are difficult to accomplish but can result in an extensive change of the system. Interventions at deep leverage points are aimed at changing the underlying structure, goal, or paradigm of the system. Achieving this requires a joint understanding of the system by scientists, stakeholders (including PLHIV) and societal actors, as well as a joint commitment towards supporting the envisioned change. With this study we took a first step in this direction and studied HIVDR in its totality as a CAS of interconnected and interacting factors. Concretely, we aimed to understand how these factors are interconnected with and embedded in the local context of our study area in the Ukonga and Gongolamboto areas of Dar es Salaam, Tanzania [14,17]. We compare this local systems map with one constructed from the knowledge of international experts, developed in a previous study, and discuss the differences and similarities [8]. We also provide a first assessment of potential intervention points.

2. Results

We interviewed 12 PLHIV and 10 local actors in the Dar es Salaam Urban Cohort Study (DUCS) located in the Ukonga and Gongolamboto areas of Dar es Salaam. Of the PLHIV, two were lost to follow-up and ten were engaged in care. Another 10 PLHIV and nine local actors engaged in the validation workshops. The sociodemographic and therapy data of the participants are described in Table 1. Not surprisingly, the majority of participating PLHIV were female, which can be explained by the higher HIV prevalence in women, as well as the lower linkage to care rates in men. Of the 22 PLHIV involved, 18 were on first line dolutegravir-based treatment. The other four were on first-line NVP or EFV-based regimens. Overall, we reached a diverse sample of participants which allowed us to study the factors influencing HIVDR from different angles. Data saturation for the factors influencing HIVDR (elements) was reached after 16 interviews and after about 19 interviews for the connections between those factors (Figures S1 and S2).

Table 1. Sociodemographic and therapy data of the participants of the interviews and validation workshops.

	PLHIV (N = 22)	Local Actors (N = 19)
Average age (year)	40 (21–56)	49 (33–73)
Gender		
Male	18% (4)	63% (12)
Female	82% (18)	37% (7)
Education		
No degree	14% (3)	16% (3)
Primary education	77% (17)	26% (5)
Secondary education	9% (2)	16% (3)
Higher education	0% (0)	42% (8)
Occupation		
Employed	64% (14)	100% (19)
Unemployed	36% (8)	0% (0)
Years of experience in local actor roll		
<5	/	16% (3)
5–10	/	21% (4)
≥10	/	58% (11)
Time since first positive HIV test		
≤1 year	14% (3)	/
2–5 years	36% (8)	/
>5 years	50% (11)	/
Time since start of treatment		
≤1 year	18% (4)	/
2–5 years	36% (8)	/
>5 years	45% (10)	/

Based on the collected data, we developed a systems map representing the factors influencing HIVDR in the Ukonga and Gongolamboto areas in Dar es Salaam as experienced by the local population. The map consists of several interconnected feedback loops which we will describe step by step. In Figures 1–5, parts of the system are shown, whereas the complete system is presented in Figure 6. The purple section of Figure 1 represents the biological mechanism of HIVDR selection. HIVDR is selected under selective pressure caused by incomplete VL suppression. A major cause of incomplete VL suppression is suboptimal adherence, here defined as the compliance of PLHIV with their therapy as well as the possibility for them to take their medication daily, thus including both factors that are within and out of their own control. Selection of HIVDR will lead to an increase in opportunistic infections and generally poorer health as a result of an unsuppressed VL. The interviewees described situations in which clients do not believe they are HIV-positive when they do not experience symptoms after testing or who believe they are cured when their health improves and therefore do not see the need to adhere anymore. These clients then re-start taking their ART when they develop symptoms. This may be fuelled by a lack of knowledge about HIV, by the influence of traditional healers or religious leaders who claim to cure HIV, or by the client not accepting their HIV status. A major barrier to adherence in the study site is poverty (Figure 1, green colour). Clients who cannot afford a meal each day, may skip their medication, out of fear of side effects. Clients living in poverty may also have difficulties picking up medication when they do not have money to pay for transportation or when they are offered an employment opportunity on the day of their refill and have to choose between income and medication. One participant described this as follows:

> "When I say that money is more important than health, it's not that health is not important but they depend on each other. It happens that you stayed hungry for three days and failed to take your medication because of the food insecurity. The fourth day someone calls you to go to work and get money, tell me if it were you, what would you do? Would you go to the clinic or to work?"—PLHIV (Female, 48 years old)

Clients migrating to other parts of Tanzania in search of an income or for other purposes may also experience difficulties remaining in care. The socio-economic aspects of HIVDR are very prominent in the study site as barriers to adherence but also as motivators. The knowledge that when adhering to therapy, one will be in good health, able to work and provide income for the family, drives clients to adhere well, a motivational strategy which is also used by the healthcare workers.

The yellow arrows in Figure 1 illustrate an issue caused by the stigmatized nature of HIV in the community. When joining social activities or travelling for work, some clients do not take their medication with them out of fear of involuntary status disclosure, subsequent stigmatization, and the possibility of losing employment opportunities.

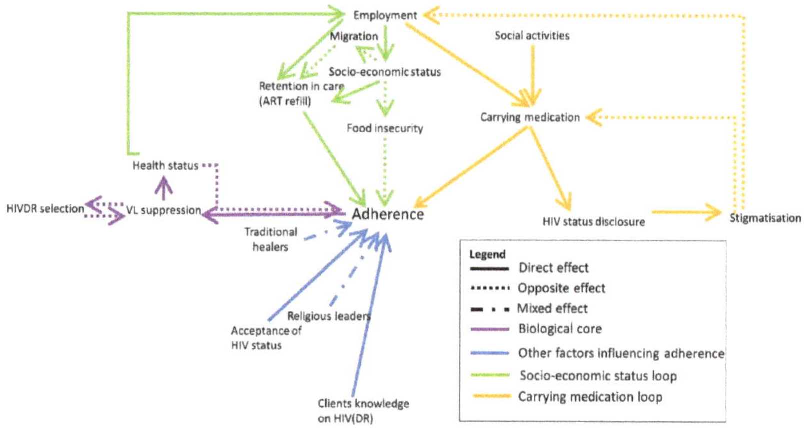

Figure 1. The participants' perspectives on HIV drug resistance in the study site, reflected in three core loops related to the health status (purple), socio-economic situation (green) and involuntary status disclosure when carrying medication (yellow). Some additional factors influencing HIVDR are indicated in blue. Full arrows indicate that both elements are evolving in the same direction (e.g., A->B: when A increases, B increases as well). Dotted arrows indicate an opposite effect (when A increases, B decreases). Mixed arrows indicate that the effect can be either direct or opposite.

Participants indicated that stigma and discrimination can have a profound effect on PLHIV's lives, reflected by the dark red and brown loop in Figure 2. Next to the risk of losing employment, the participants reported that stigma and discrimination can be the cause of marital or familial conflicts, discrimination at social gatherings and general discomfort due to gossip or being treated differently. Moreover, the impact on people's self-esteem can cause them to self-stigmatise. To avoid that, they often choose not to disclose their status, drop out of care, or become nonadherent. Some even go as far as to give fake contact details to the healthcare staff in order not to be traceable. Others prefer to go to a healthcare centre far from home in order not to be recognised. However, this may come with the challenge of sustainably accessing this healthcare centre for each refill and check-up due to for example financial constraints. The participants indicated that stigma and discrimination can be prevented by educating the community on HIV, its modes of transmission, prevention, treatment and required support. They also expressed the need to encourage the community to appreciate and support PLHIV who disclose their HIV health status. This can be achieved through the media, brochures, and seminars given by NGOs, or for example by religious leaders who have a wide reach.

Over time, the more PLHIV disclose their status and openly talk about HIV, the more the community will learn about HIV. This increased community education is expected to decrease the stigma surrounding HIV, encouraging more PLHIV to disclose their status and adhere to ART. This is a delayed reinforcing loop.

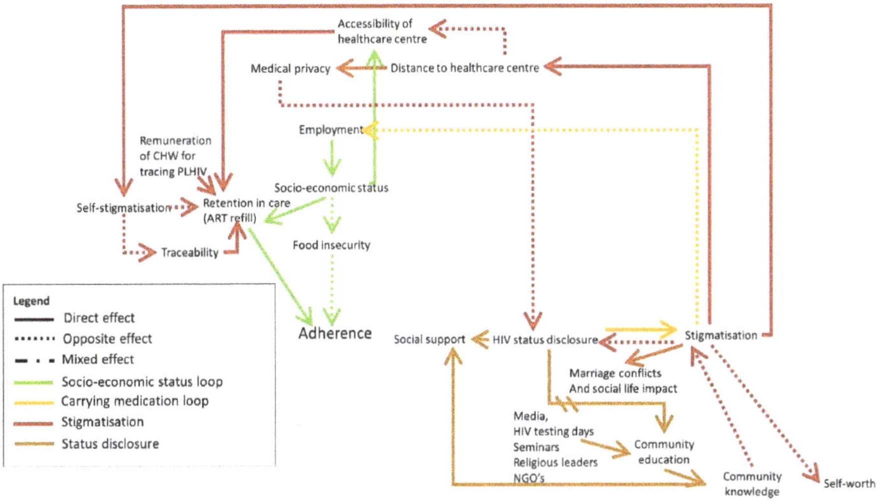

Figure 2. The causes and effects of stigmatisation and HIV status disclosure are indicated in dark red and brown. The arrow with double strikethrough indicates a relationship with a delayed effect. Full arrows indicate that both elements are evolving in the same direction (e.g., A->B: when A increases, B increases as well). Dotted arrows indicate an opposite effect (when A increases, B decreases). Mixed arrows indicate that the effect can be either direct or opposite.

HIV status disclosure can have positive and negative consequences: on the one hand, stigmatisation can have a profound effect on social life as discussed above. On the other hand, people may receive social support from their family who can help them to adhere and accept their status, or who can help them financially or by providing meals (Figure 3, beige arrows). A person living with HIV may experience both positive and negative consequences and may therefore choose to disclose their status only to a select group of people. Counselling can help to prepare PLHIV to disclose their status. Some participants reported not disclosing their status in order to spare their loved ones from worrying about them. However, the will to protect others may also motivate PLHIV to disclose their status in order to engage in safer sex and to adhere to their medication in order not to infect others.

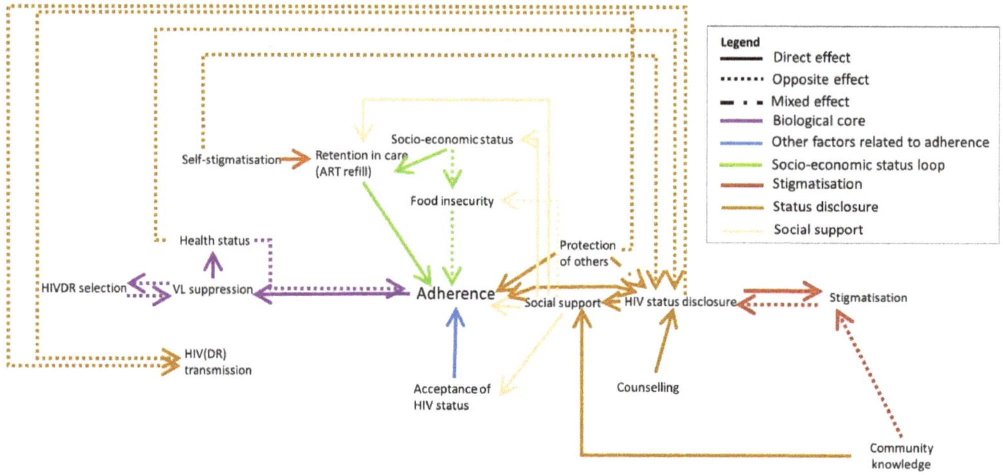

Figure 3. The influences of social support are indicated in beige. Full arrows indicate that both elements are evolving in the same direction (e.g., A->B: when A increases, B increases as well). Dotted arrows indicate an opposite effect (when A increases, B decreases). Mixed arrows indicate that the effect can be either direct or opposite.

Counselling can help PLHIV to accept their HIV status, gain a deeper understanding about HIV and ART and feel socially empowered to ask questions or demand VL tests for instance. In some cases, the health care provider gives very strict guidelines (such as dietary information or the guideline to take the medication strictly at a certain time) which may discourage the client to take the ART when they cannot meet these requirements.

> "... However, we shouldn't miss the nutrients they recommended in our foods. ... I don't know things like finger millet and others, we are missing them in our foods because we can't afford to get them, we are missing the nutrients. ... For instance, the ones with [financial] ability. Vegetables, small fried fishes aren't bad. They told us not to use beef, it isn't good that's what they said. For instance, they told me an old man like me what I should eat is like pig's meat, chicken and fishes. Now things I am able to get in most cases are green vegetables and stiff porridge. You see how it is hard. ... They told me so, but they didn't tell me the reasons. They told me that I shouldn't prefer using beef."—PLHIV (Male, 34 years old)

Elements important for good counselling sessions that arose from the interviews include: medical privacy (in some cases, there are multiple clients in the doctor's office or the door is left open), well-trained healthcare workers and community health workers (CHW) who are able to answer the clients' questions and who have a caring attitude, and a good client-provider relationship (Figure 4, dark blue). Participants also indicated that this could help clients to accept their HIV status.

Another important factor is the workload of the healthcare centre. Both PLHIV and local actors indicated that at times the healthcare centre is overburdened, and healthcare providers do not have enough time to provide thorough counselling for all clients, which may impact its efficiency.

The healthcare system workload increases when PLHIV have to visit the hospital more frequently because they have an unsuppressed VL or developed drug resistance, or when HIV(DR) is transmitted in the community and more people have to enrol in care. When healthcare staff are not sufficiently trained to handle certain cases or answer all questions of the client, they may have to refer the client to other colleagues, therefore also increasing their workload.

Next to decreased counselling efficiency, a high healthcare system workload also increases the waiting time at the healthcare centre which may lead to PLHIV not picking up their medication as they are afraid of being recognised by other people at the healthcare centre.

The healthcare system workload loop (Figure 4, dark green) is a reinforcing loop in which the consequences of high workload (decreased counselling quality and therefore a decreased adherence) will eventually lead to an even higher workload.

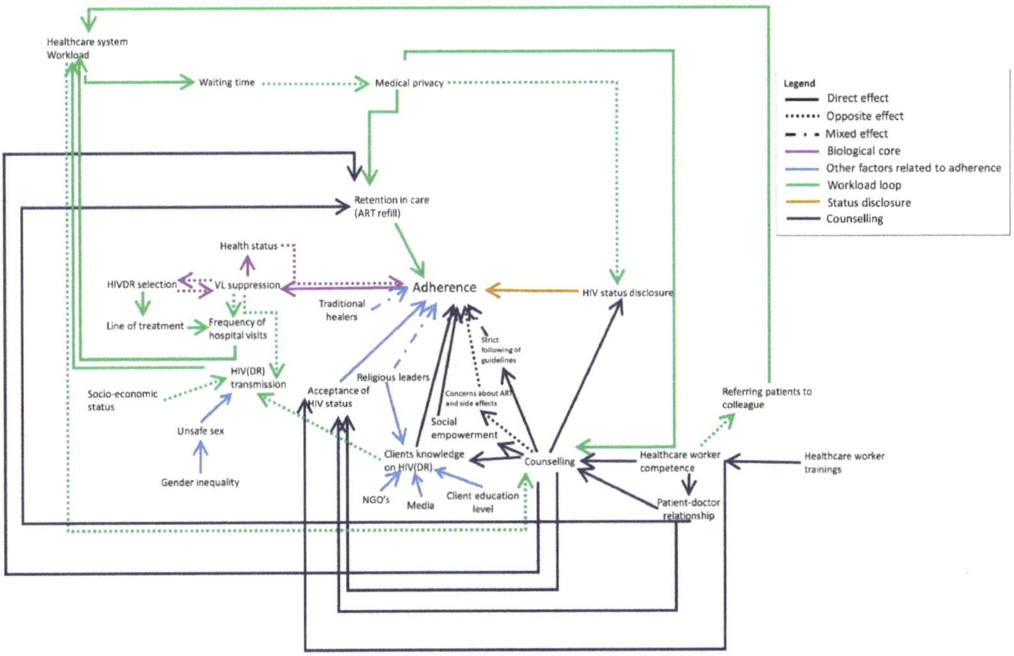

Figure 4. The reinforcing workload loop is indicated in dark green. Full arrows indicate that both elements are evolving in the same direction (e.g., A->B: when A increases, B increases as well). Dotted arrows indicate an opposite effect (when A increases, B decreases). Mixed arrows indicate that the effect can be either direct or opposite.

The following reinforcing loop is indicated in red in Figure 5. Having access to information about one's health status, such as VL and CD4 count information, especially when the client is doing well, contributes to the client's feeling of self-esteem. Clients are proud of their good health and are congratulated by healthcare staff, which motivates them to continue adhering. In black, we indicated the impact of the VL testing organization on the system. Test results sometimes arrive with a delay, or not at all because of which the test has to be repeated, further increasing workload. Possible causes of this are a lack of equipment for testing and a lack of uniform electronic data systems to facilitate sharing the results.

Figure 6 shows the full system of all identified factors influencing HIVDR in the study site. Additional to what is described above, other factors influencing adherence are substance abuse (possibly stemming from poor acceptance of one's HIV status), forgetfulness or pill fatigue as illustrated by the interview quote below. The burden of having to take medication each day for the rest of one's life may contribute to self-stigmatisation and may on its own be a reason to skip the medication from time to time. Although the first line ART in the study site consists of one pill per day, usually more medication needs to be taken such as medication for opportunistic infections.

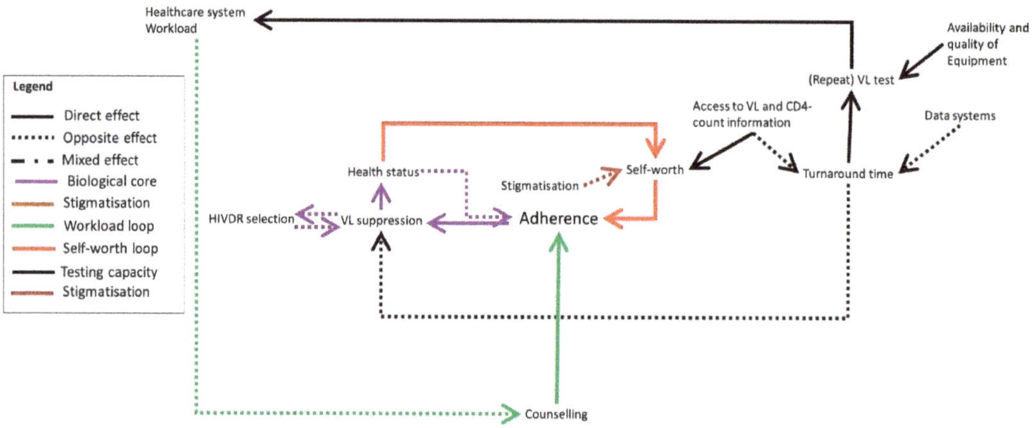

Figure 5. The importance of linking back testing results to the clients, and related practical requirements are indicated in red and black, respectively. Full arrows indicate that both elements are evolving in the same direction (e.g., A->B: when A increases, B increases as well). Dotted arrows indicate an opposite effect (when A increases, B decreases). Mixed arrows indicate that the effect can be either direct or opposite.

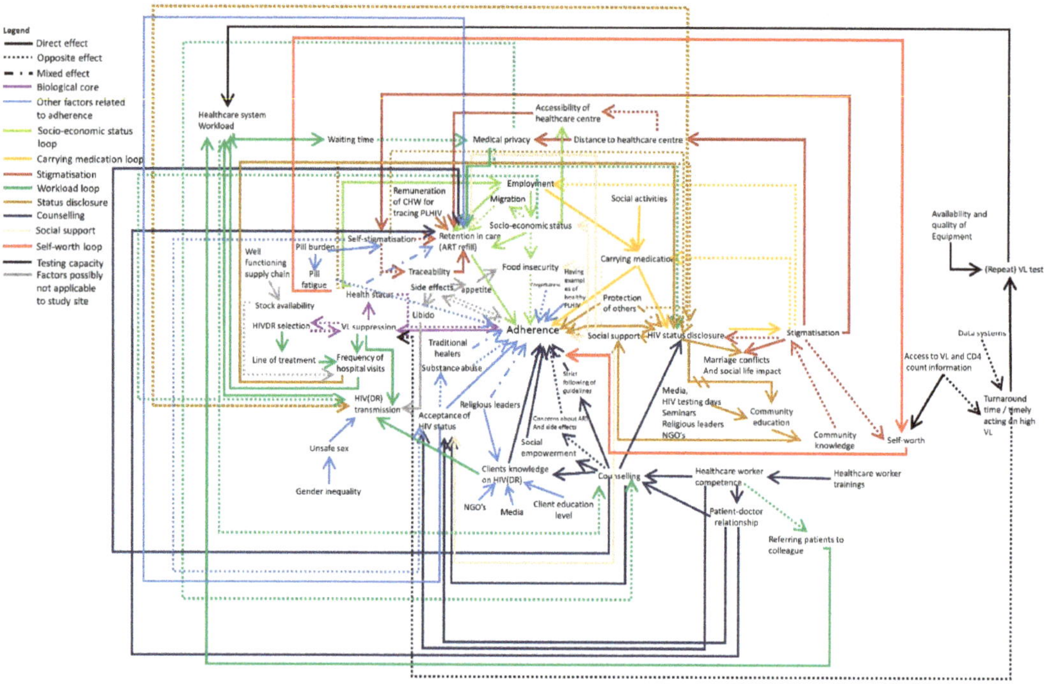

Figure 6. The full system of factors influencing HIVDR in the study site. Additional factors influencing adherence and some elements which are no longer applicable are indicated in blue and grey, respectively. Full arrows indicate that both elements are evolving in the same direction (e.g., A->B: when A increases, B increases as well). Dotted arrows indicate an opposite effect (when A increases, B decreases). Mixed arrows indicate that the effect can be either direct or opposite. See also Figure S3.

> "Truly, you can swallow the drugs and there are times you get tired of taking them and say let me skip them today. You can stop for a day; you just say today I am resting. ... Only one day, I am scared to skip them for two days because that's when you are told viruses increase in one day if you skip. ... Honestly, for instance for the drugs which I was given for three months. I can rest for one day. ... Ahh per three months I only rest once."—PLHIV (Female, 39 years old)

In light grey, two elements are added which are no longer applicable for the adult population in our study site. The participants reported relatively little supply issues in the study area and if needed the healthcare centres reorganize themselves and give half supplies to the clients so that everyone can be served until they have restocked. Additionally, the side effects are of lesser concern since first line treatment has been switched from tenofovir/lamivudine/efavirenz (TLE) to tenofovir/lamivudine/dolutegravir (TLD). It is important to note that side effects can demotivate clients from adhering to therapy directly, but clients can also experience being hungry after taking the medication and therefore skip the medication when they know they will not be able to satisfy their increased appetite. Some clients also report an increased libido after taking the medication and indicated that this increases the transmission risk.

While the above systems map represents the CAS in detail, Figure 7 summarizes the system into seven core loops representing the main mechanisms behind HIVDR in the study site. In the following paragraph the core loops and three identified leverage points are discussed. R1.1 is a reinforcing loop through which PLHIV are motivated to keep adhering to the ART because of their improved health status. The first, shallow level leverage point identified is the strengthening of this loop, for example through motivation by healthcare workers. Reinforcement of R1.1 will automatically weaken R2.1 and R2.2 which represent the effects of an increased healthcare system workload when adherence levels are not sufficient. The decreased time for counselling and other support for PLHIV will lead to a further decrease in adherence levels. Furthermore, R1.1 reinforcement would strengthen R1.2, which results in improved adherence through increased socio-economic opportunities. It would also decrease R1.3 as healthy looking PLHIV tend to be less stigmatized by others and by themselves. The second, also shallow leverage point is to weaken R2.3 and R2.4 which represent a decreased adherence through stigmatization and decreased socio-economic opportunities, respectively. This could be done by providing community education, potentially through religious leaders, community leaders or traditional healers, who have a wide range.

The third leverage point is identified at the design level and is therefore considered a deep leverage point. Based on the combined needs for economic support, education on HIV(DR) and improving the mental well-being of PLHIV, we propose the organization of microfinance groups specifically for PLHIV. Microfinance groups are informal financial support groups where members are educated on entrepreneurship, contribute a monthly amount of money and have the opportunity to request a loan from the group. These groups may be a platform for PLHIV to combine their economic support group with peer support-like activities such as education sessions on HIV(DR) and practical and psychological support [18]. Although the economics of microfinance groups for PLHIV have been described in the literature, more research remains to be conducted on the effect on health outcomes [19,20].

The summary system in Figure 7 is influenced by several other factors which are here considered external and therefore not represented. These are, for example, supply chain related factors, testing capacity and ART properties.

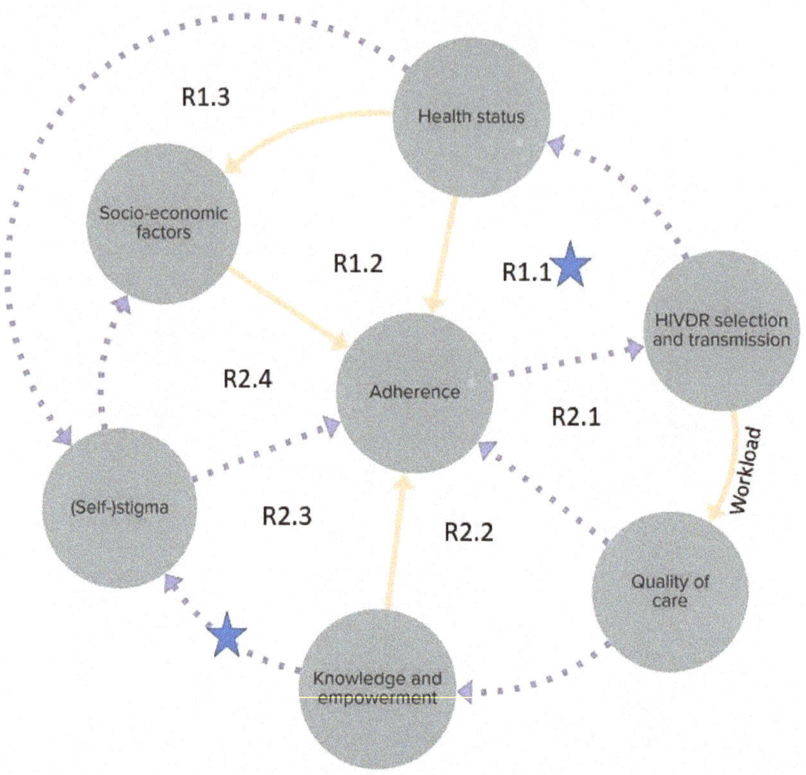

Figure 7. Summary figure of the CAS of factors associated with HIVDR in the study area. Seven reinforcing loops and two leverage points (blue stars) are indicated. The third leverage point is at the structural level and is therefore not visualised here. Individual reinforcing loops are indicated as R1.1 to R2.4. Full arrows indicate that both elements are evolving in the same direction (e.g., A->B: when A increases, B increases as well). Dotted arrows indicate an opposite effect (when A increases, B decreases).

3. Discussion

In this study, we gained insight into the complexity of HIVDR in the Ukonga and Gongolamboto areas of Dar es Salaam by developing a model representing the CAS of its interconnected factors, together with local actors and PLHIV. It is important to note that our aim was to understand the CAS of factors influencing HIVDR through the mental models of the people most affected by it. Therefore, the model does not represent one fixed reality but rather an interconnected network of elements influencing HIVDR, which are constantly evolving over time, and which are highly dependent on context.

Three leverage points were identified based on the insights provided by our systems map. The first, shallow, leverage point aims at reinforcing the motivation to adhere to therapy, for instance through the encouragement of positive health outcomes. The second also shallow one, aims at decreasing stigmatization by strengthening community education. The third identified leverage point is at a deeper level and requires the restructuring of certain aspects of care through combining microfinance and peer support groups for PLHIV. Our work provides valuable insights at the systems level which, after strengthening of the healthcare system viewpoint, can be used to design and test interventions at these leverage points.

In addition to the identified leverage points, we obtained some other system-level insights. First, our data clearly showed the impact of psychological wellbeing on the dynamics of the HIVDR system as also described extensively by Zlatić et al. [21]. In particular, stigmatization was found to be the driver of several important feedback loops. Second, at the healthcare system level, we found that some counsellors give very strict guidelines to their clients which are ill-adapted to their life circumstances. These are failing to convey their purpose, and therefore sometimes work counterproductively. Clients may refrain from taking their medication if they do not find the advised type of food or if they come home one hour late. Future seminars on HIVDR for healthcare workers may need to be revised to refocus on the objective of the counselling sessions (preventing HIVDR and ensuring good health of PLHIV) rather than on the individual rules they have to follow. Third, at the community level, we found a delayed reinforcing feedback loop, indicating that PLHIV openly disclosing and discussing their HIV status are conducting a type of community education. This can reduce community stigmatization over time, encouraging more PLHIV to disclose their status. Previous studies have shown the correlation between knowledge and HIV related stigma [22,23]. One study in South Africa found that a decrease in stigma was associated with an increase in knowledge over a period of four years [22]. To identify the tipping point at which this reinforcing loop is kicked into action additional research is needed.

To explore the contents of our systems map beyond the local level, we compared it with a systems map of factors influencing HIVDR for Sub-Saharan Africa, which was informed by experts and developed using the same methodology [8]. Overall, the content of the systems maps remains largely similar. As can be expected, however, the expert systems map contained more extensive information at the healthcare system level and the local map goes into more detail at the personal level. A notable difference is that, whereas in the expert map the economic factor food insecurity was considered to be important but external to the system, it became clear that at the local level those factors were at the very core of the system, forming daily barriers to adherence for PLHIV. This shows that in order to fully understand the CAS of HIVDR, the viewpoints of PLHIV, actors and experts, as well as those groups at the local and broader geographical level need to be integrated.

A shortcoming of this study is its timeframe as two important events happened: (1) at the time of data collection the healthcare centres in the study site had just switched their ART regimens from TLE to TLD, a therapy which evokes less side-effects and which has a lower chance of provoking mutations in the virus and (2) between the data collection and validation the world was hit by the COVID-19 pandemic which, for a period of time brought a number of changes to the system. From March until July 2020, all PLHIV in the study area were given ART for six months instead of the usual one or three months, wearing face masks was obligatory in the healthcare centre, which caused problems for clients who could not afford them and transportation fees increased due to strict rules for seat capacity of commuter buses. While further research is needed to clarify the impact of these interruptions on the HIVDR prevalence in the population, our systems map can help to understand how these measures may have impacted the adherence level of PLHIV. Moreover, the systems mapping method described can be used to study the impact of the COVID-19 pandemic on other aspects on the healthcare system, to study other public health problems, or to be transferred to study HIVDR in other study sites.

4. Materials and Methods

4.1. Study Design

An iterative systems mapping design was used to visualize and analyse the CAS of factors associated with HIVDR in our case study site in Dar es Salaam, Tanzania. Qualitative methods were used for data collection and analysis. The systems analysis and identification of leverage points were based on a systems thinking inspired analysis guide [24].

4.2. Study Site and Participants

The study was conducted at the DUCS site in the Ukonga and Gongolamboto administrative wards, Illala district, Dar es Salaam region, Tanzania. The DUCS follows more than 100,000 residents from more than 20,000 households and collects sociodemographic and other data on a six-monthly basis [17]. This study site was chosen because of the rich data available which may support future intervention designs. We included three types of stakeholders in this study, each representing a different perspective: local experts, local actors, and PLHIV. Local experts were people with professional expertise on HIVDR, based in Tanzania. For the purpose of this study, local actors are defined as people who have good insights in the daily lives of the local citizens and who, through their job, status or daily activities are able to make a positive impact in their society. The local actors were selected with the aim of including a range of people who could provide us with insights about HIV in the community from diverse angles in order to create an overview that is as comprehensive as possible. PLHIV in several stages of their treatment, on different therapy regimens and with varying treatment-adherence levels were selected purposefully and recruited by research assistants of the DUCS.

4.3. Data Collection Procedures

The systems map was developed in three phases (Table 2). During the preparation phase we organized a workshop with local experts to discuss factors influencing HIVDR in our study site. During this meeting we started from a Sub-Saharan systems map based on knowledge from international experts, developed in previous research and adapted this map to the local situation. This adapted map served as a basis to design the semi-structured interview guides and was not used further in data analysis. This way, the CAS of HIVDR in our study site was constructed anew from the interview data, truly allowing the perspectives and mental models of the local inhabitants to form the map, without the influence of previous research.

Table 2. Overview of the different activities and participants in the project.

Phase	Activity	Participants	Purpose
Preparation	Expert meeting + field visit (June 2019)	10 Tanzanian HIVDR experts	Discussion on factors influencing HIVDR in the Tanzanian context, informed by a systems map previously developed with Sub-Saharan African HIVDR experts. This meeting informed our semi-structured interview guide.
Data collection	Semi-Structured interviews (June 2019–February 2020)	12 PLHIV and 10 Local actors	Forming a detailed understanding of the perspectives of PLHIV and local actors on the CAS of factors influencing HIVDR in the study site.
Validation	Workshops (February–March 2021)	10 PLHIV and 9 Local actors	Validating the systems map developed based on the semi-structured interviews and brainstorming about possible interventions for preventing HIVDR.

4.4. Semi-Structured Interviews

The first draft of the systems map was designed based on semi-structured interviews with PLHIV and local actors at DUCS in the Ukonga and Gongolamboto areas in Dar es Salaam, Tanzania. Semi-structured interviews do not consist of a set of rigorous questions but rather use a set of common themes to be explored with all the participants. This type of interview allows new themes to come up and be explored, based on the interviewee's answers.

The participants were called on their cell-phone and invited for a face-to-face interview at the DUCS office in the local community centre located in the Ukonga area. This location is neutral and not linked to any activities involving PLHIV and was therefore chosen to avoid stigmatization of the participants. The interviews were held in Kiswahili by I.M., a local social scientist and participants were reimbursed for their transportation costs. Each interview session lasted for about forty-five minutes. The interviews were audio recorded after seeking consent from study participants, transcribed verbatim and translated into English.

The semi-structured interview guide was informed by the expert meeting and designed by A.K., A.V. and I.M. with the aim of capturing the deeper factors influencing

HIVDR in the DUCS area. After each interview day I.M., A.K. and A.V. met to debrief the interviews and the interview guide was adapted according to the insights gained. After a first analysis of the interviews, a selection bias was noted as only participants enrolled in care were interviewed. In order to have a more diverse perspective on the factors influencing HIVDR in the study area, two additional participants who had not been attending healthcare services regularly in the past months were recruited and interviewed during a phone conversation. Interviews were conducted until data saturation was reached. For the purpose of this study, data saturation was defined as the moment in which no new elements or connections are discovered in two consecutive interviews (Table S1).

4.5. Data Analysis

The analysis of the semi-structured interviews was conducted by two researchers (L.Z.) and (A.K.) with a combined background in psychology, biomedical science and systems thinking. The method used was inspired by the QUAGOL method [25]. After each interview, a technical report was written, containing all the specifics needed for a full comprehension of the data in their specific context. In order to ascertain a correct interpretation and cultural understanding of the transcripts, they were each individually discussed in a series of meetings between A.K., L.Z. and I.M.

For each transcript, a respective systems map was made, visualizing the factors influencing HIVDR mentioned in the interview and the connections between those factors. Seven interviews with PLHIV and five local actor interviews were schematized and coded by A.K. The other five interviews with PLHIV and five local actor interviews were schematized by both A.K. and L.Z. and the interviews were coded by L.Z. Possible differences were discussed until a consensus was found. In a next phase the separate schemes were merged together into one comprehensive systems map containing all the codes extracted from the interviews. The systems map was designed with the online mapping tool KUMU, which facilitates the visualization and analysis of the map, as different types of data can be stored behind the elements and connections [26]. Though here described linearly, the coding and mapping was an iterative process in which the interviews were re-read at several points in time, codes were revised throughout discussions between the researchers and findings were constantly compared with insights from previously analysed interviews.

4.6. Validation

A validation round of the systems map was held in two workshops, one with PLHIV and one with local actors, organized in February and March 2021. The discussion was organized around six central areas of the systems map. The participants discussed the model, changes in the model since the first data collection, and possible interventions. The workshops were organized in the form of a focus group discussion, conducted in Kiswahili. The workshops were recorded, transcribed, and translated into English and they were coded and analysed following the same method as for the semi-structured interviews above.

5. Conclusions

We successfully modelled the CAS of factors influencing HIVDR in the Ukonga and Gongolamboto areas of Dar es Salaam, Tanzania. The model provides a detailed understanding of the mechanisms that locally drive HIVDR, based on which we suggested three local leverage points. Together this forms a strong basis for the design of sustainable, complexity-informed interventions, tailored to the local context of the study site.

Supplementary Materials: The following are available online at https://www.mdpi.com/article/10.3390/pathogens10121535/s1, Figure S1: data saturation elements, Figure S2: data saturation connections, Figure S3: Systems map representing the CAS of factors related to HIVDR in the study site, Table S1: table containing all elements and connections.

Author Contributions: Conceptualization, A.K., A.-M.V., I.H.M., G.M.B., A.M., C.D., N.V., O.S., R.Z.S. and J.K.; Methodology, A.K., I.H.M., A.M., C.D. and B.D.d.C.; Validation, A.K., A.-M.V., B.D.d.C. and I.H.M.; Analysis, A.K., L.Z. and I.H.M.; Investigation, A.K., L.Z. and I.H.M.; Resources, A.M., I.H.M., G.M.B. and A.K.; Data Curation, A.K. and L.Z.; Writing—Original Draft Preparation, A.K.; Writing—Review and Editing, A.K., L.Z., I.H.M., G.M.B., B.D.d.C., A.M., N.V., C.D., O.S., R.Z.S., J.K., A.-M.V., A.S. and P.C.; Visualization, A.K.; Supervision, A.-M.V., J.K., R.Z.S., A.S. and P.C.; Project Administration, A.K.; Funding Acquisition, A.-M.V., A.K., R.Z.S. and J.K. All authors have read and agreed to the published version of the manuscript.

Funding: This research and the APC were funded by VLIR-UOS, grant number TZ2019SIN263.

Institutional Review Board Statement: The study was conducted according to the guidelines of the Declaration of Helsinki, and approved by the Institutional Review Board of MUHIMBILI UNIVERSITY FOR HEALTH AND ALLIED SCIENCES (protocol code No.DA.282/293/03/C/69, approved on 24 May 2019).

Informed Consent Statement: Informed consent was obtained from all subjects involved in the study.

Data Availability Statement: All data generated or analyzed during this study is included in this published article and its supplementary information files.

Acknowledgments: The authors thank the study participants and experts for sharing their insights. We also thank Winfrida Onesmo and Mwasiti Sadala for their help with translations and the DUCS field workers for accommodating the study and recruiting study participants.

Conflicts of Interest: The funders had no role in the design of the study; in the collection, analyses, or interpretation of data; in the writing of the manuscript, or in the decision to publish the results. AV declares consultancy fee from Gilead.

References

1. UNAIDS Country Factsheet United Republic of Tanzania. Available online: https://www.unaids.org/en/regionscountries/countries/unitedrepublicoftanzania (accessed on 1 October 2021).
2. UNICEF. *AIDS HIV and AIDS–Fact Sheet*; UNICEF: New York, NY, USA, 2020.
3. National AIDS Control Programme. *National Guidelines for the Management of HIV and AIDS*; Ministry of Health, Community Development, Gender, Elderly, and Children: Dar es Salaam, Tanzania, 2019; Volume 7.
4. World Health Organization (WHO). *HIV Drug Resistance Report 2019*; World Health Organization: Geneva, Switzerland, 2019.
5. Mayer, M.E.; Kong, G.; Barrington-trimis, J.L.; Mcconnell, R.; Leventhal, A.M.; Krishnan-sarin, S. Pre-Treatment and Acquired Antiretroviral Drug Resistance among Persons Living with HIV in Four African Countries. *Clin. Infect. Dis.* **2020**, *73*, e2311–e2322.
6. Sangeda, R.Z.; Gómes, P.; Rhee, S.-Y.; Mosha, F.; Camacho, R.J.; Van Wijngaerden, E.; Lyamuya, E.F.; Vandamme, A.-M. Development of HIV Drug Resistance in a Cohort of Adults on First-Line Antiretroviral Therapy in Tanzania during the Stavudine Era. *Microbiol. Res.* **2021**, *12*, 847–861. [CrossRef]
7. World Health Organization. *Global Action Plan on HIV Drug Resistance 2017–2021*; World Health Organization: Geneva, Switzerland, 2017; ISBN 9789241512848.
8. Kiekens, A.; Dierckx de Casterlé, B.; Pellizzer, G.; Mosha, I.; Mosha, F.; Rinke de Wit, T.; Sangeda, R.; Surian, A.; Vandaele, N.; Vranken, L.; et al. Identifying mechanisms behind HIV drug resistance in Sub-Saharan Africa: A systems approach. *BMC Public Health* **2021**. under peer review.
9. Msongole, B.A. HIV Drug Resistance in Tanzania: A Literature Review of Socio-Cultural, Economic and Health Systems Determinants. Master's Thesis, Vrije Universiteit Amsterdam, Amsterdam, The Netherlands, 2015.
10. Rusconi, S. The impact of adherence to HIV/AIDS antiretroviral therapy on the development of drug resistance. *Future Virol.* **2017**, *12*, 239–241. [CrossRef]
11. Shubber, Z.; Mills, E.J.; Nachega, J.B.; Vreeman, R.; Freitas, M.; Bock, P.; Nsanzimana, S.; Penazzato, M.; Appolo, T.; Doherty, M.; et al. Patient-Reported Barriers to Adherence to Antiretroviral Therapy: A Systematic Review and Meta-Analysis. *PLoS Med.* **2016**, *13*, e1002183. [CrossRef] [PubMed]
12. Eshun-Wilson, I.; Rohwer, A.; Hendricks, L.; Oliver, S.; Garner, P. Being HIV positive and staying on antiretroviral therapy in Africa: A qualitative systematic review and theoretical model. *PLoS ONE* **2019**, *14*, e0210408. [CrossRef]
13. Rutter, H.; Savona, N.; Glonti, K.; Bibby, J.; Cummins, S.; Finegood, D.T.; Greaves, F.; Harper, L.; Hawe, P.; Moore, L.; et al. The need for a complex systems model of evidence for public health. *Lancet* **2017**, *390*, 2602–2604. [CrossRef]
14. Plsek, P.E.; Greenhalgh, T. Complexity science: The challenge of complexity in health care. *BMJ* **2001**, *323*, 625–628. [CrossRef] [PubMed]
15. Abson, D.J.; Fischer, J.; Leventon, J.; Newig, J.; Schomerus, T.; Vilsmaier, U.; von Wehrden, H.; Abernethy, P.; Ives, C.D.; Jager, N.W.; et al. Leverage points for sustainability transformation. *Ambio* **2017**, *46*, 30–39. [CrossRef] [PubMed]

16. Meadows, D. Places to Intervene in a System. *Whole Earth* **1997**, *91*, 78–84.
17. Leyna, G.H.; Berkman, L.F.; Njelekela, M.A.; Kazonda, P.; Irema, K.; Fawzi, W.; Killewo, J. Profile: The Dar Es Salaam health and demographic surveillance system (Dar es Salaam HDSS). *Int. J. Epidemiol.* **2017**, *46*, 801–808. [CrossRef] [PubMed]
18. Kiekens, A.; Dehens, J.; Hemptinne, D.; Galouchka, M.; Van Otzel, R.P.; Wyszkowska, M.; Baert, S.; Bernard, J.; Ricardo, J.; Blanco, N.; et al. HIV-related peer support in dar es salaam: A pilot questionnaire inquiry. *Transdiscipl. Insights* **2019**, *3*, 1–18. [CrossRef]
19. Linnemayr, S.; Buzaalirwa, L.; Balya, J.; Wagner, G. A Microfinance Program Targeting People Living with HIV in Uganda: Client Characteristics and Program Impact. *J. Int. Assoc. Provid. AIDS Care* **2017**, *16*, 254–260. [CrossRef] [PubMed]
20. Wagner, G.; Rana, Y.; Linnemayr, S.; Balya, J.; Buzaalirwa, L. A qualitative exploration of the economic and social effects of microcredit among people living with HIV/AIDS in Uganda. *AIDS Res. Treat.* **2012**. [CrossRef] [PubMed]
21. Zlatic, L. A Systems Approach to Uncover Causes of HIV Drug Resistance in Dar es Salaam. Master's Thesis, University of Padua, Padova, Italy, 2020.
22. Mall, S.; Middelkoop, K.; Mark, D.; Wood, R. Changing patterns in HIV/AIDS stigma and uptake of voluntary counselling and testing services: The results of two consecutive community surveys conducted in the Western Cape, South Africa. *AIDS Care* **2013**, *25*, 194–201. [CrossRef] [PubMed]
23. Letshwenyo-maruatona, S.B.; Madisa, M.; George-kefilwe, B.; Kingori, C.; Ice, G.; Joseph, A.; Marape, M.; Haile, Z.T.; George-kefilwe, B.; Kingori, C.; et al. Association between HIV/AIDS knowledge and stigma towards people living with HIV/AIDS in Botswana Association between HIV/AIDS knowledge and stigma towards people. *Afr. J. AIDS Res.* **2019**, *18*, 58–64. [CrossRef] [PubMed]
24. Kiekens, A.; Dierckx de Casterlé, B.; Vandamme, A.-M. Qualitative systems mapping for complex public health problems: A practical guide. *PLoS ONE* **2021**. submitted.
25. Dierckx de Casterle, B.; Gastmans, C.; Bryon, E.; Denier, Y. QUAGOL: A guide for qualitative data analysis. *Int. J. Nurs. Stud.* **2012**, *49*, 360–371. [CrossRef]
26. Mohr, J.; Mohr, R. KUMU Inc. 2011. Available online: https://kumu.io/ (accessed on 1 October 2021).

pathogens

MDPI

Article

Retention in Care, Mortality, Loss-to-Follow-Up, and Viral Suppression among Antiretroviral Treatment-Naïve and Experienced Persons Participating in a Nationally Representative HIV Pre-Treatment Drug Resistance Survey in Mexico

Yanink Caro-Vega [1], Fernando Alarid-Escudero [2], Eva A. Enns [3], Sandra Sosa-Rubí [4], Carlos Chivardi [4], Alicia Piñeirúa-Menendez [5], Claudia García-Morales [6], Gustavo Reyes-Terán [6], Juan G. Sierra-Madero [1] and Santiago Ávila-Ríos [6,*]

1 Departamento de Infectología, Instituto Nacional de Ciencias Médicas y Nutrición Salvador Zubirán, Mexico City 14000, Mexico; yanink.caro@infecto.mx (Y.C.-V.); jsmadero@gmail.com (J.G.S.-M.)
2 Centro de Investigación y Docencia Económicas, Aguascalientes 20313, Mexico; fernando.alarid@cide.edu
3 Division of Health Policy and Management, School of Public Health, University of Minnesota, Minneapolis, MN 55455, USA; eens@umn.edu
4 Center for Health Systems Research, Instituto Nacional de Salud Pública, Cuernavaca 62100, Mexico; sandra.sosa.rubi@gmail.com (S.S.-R.); krloschivardi@gmail.com (C.C.)
5 Dirección de Atención Integral CENSIDA, Mexico City 14080, Mexico; aliciapina@yahoo.co.uk
6 Centro de Investigación en Enfermedades Infecciosas, Instituto Nacional de Enfermedades Respiratorias, Mexico City 14080, Mexico; claudia.garcia@cieni.org.mx (C.G.-M.); gustavo.reyesteran@gmail.com (G.R.-T.)
* Correspondence: santiago.avila@cieni.org.mx; Tel.: +52-(55)-5666-7985 (ext. 133)

Citation: Caro-Vega, Y.; Alarid-Escudero, F.; Enns, E.A.; Sosa-Rubí, S.; Chivardi, C.; Piñeirúa-Menendez, A.; García-Morales, C.; Reyes-Terán, G.; Sierra-Madero, J.G.; Ávila-Ríos, S. Retention in Care, Mortality, Loss-to-Follow-Up, and Viral Suppression among Antiretroviral Treatment-Naïve and Experienced Persons Participating in a Nationally Representative HIV Pre-Treatment Drug Resistance Survey in Mexico. *Pathogens* **2021**, *10*, 1569. https://doi.org/10.3390/pathogens10121569

Academic Editor: Nicola Coppola

Received: 29 October 2021
Accepted: 26 November 2021
Published: 1 December 2021

Abstract: We describe associations of pretreatment drug resistance (PDR) with clinical outcomes such as remaining in care, loss to follow-up (LTFU), viral suppression, and death in Mexico, in real-life clinical settings. We analyzed clinical outcomes after a two-year follow up period in participants of a large 2017–2018 nationally representative PDR survey cross-referenced with information of the national ministry of health HIV database. Participants were stratified according to prior ART exposure and presence of efavirenz/nevirapine PDR. Using a Fine-Gray model, we evaluated virological suppression among resistant patients, in a context of competing risk with lost to follow-up and death. A total of 1823 participants were followed-up by a median of 1.88 years (Interquartile Range (IQR): 1.59–2.02): 20 (1%) were classified as experienced + resistant; 165 (9%) naïve + resistant; 211 (11%) experienced + non-resistant; and 1427 (78%) as naïve + non-resistant. Being ART-experienced was associated with a lower probability of remaining in care (adjusted Hazard Ratio(aHR) = 0.68, 0.53–0.86, for the non-resistant group and aHR = 0.37, 0.17–0.84, for the resistant group, compared to the naïve + non-resistant group). Heterosexual cisgender women compared to men who have sex with men [MSM], had a lower viral suppression (aHR = 0.84, 0.70–1.01, $p = 0.06$) ART-experienced persons with NNRTI-PDR showed the worst clinical outcomes. This group was enriched with women and persons with lower education and unemployed, which suggests higher levels of social vulnerability.

Keywords: HIV; drug resistance; surveillance; public health; Mexico

1. Introduction

HIV pretreatment drug resistance (PDR), particularly to non-nucleoside reverse transcriptase inhibitors (NNRTI) is associated with lower viral suppression (VS) in persons that initiate NNRTI-based antiretroviral treatment (ART) regimens [1,2]. Solid evidence suggests that NNRTI PDR levels have been consistently increasing in low-/middle-income countries (LMICs) worldwide during the last decade [3], posing a significant threat for the achievement of UNAIDS 95–95–95 goals for ending the AIDS epidemic [4]. Mexico is not an exception to this trend, with recent studies showing increasing NNRTI PDR trends in three focal points of the HIV epidemic in the country [5]. A large nationally representative survey performed in Mexico in 2017–2018 showed a PDR level to NNRTI in all ART initiators of 9.9% (95% CI: 8.7–11.2%), ranging from 8.6% (7.4–9.9%) in ART-naïve individuals to 26.2% (19.5–34.3%) in previously antiretroviral-exposed individuals that re-start ART [6,7]. Up until late 2019, Mexican HIV treatment guidelines recommended NNRTI-based first-line ART options and did not recommend the use of routine drug resistance testing before ART initiation, which was instead reserved for cases of documented virological failure [6,7]. However, in 2019, the preferred first line ART options were modified, favoring the use of bictegravir and dolutegravir over efavirenz as the preferred third drug [8]. Since 2014, several LMICs have implemented nationally representative PDR surveys following WHO recommendations [6]. Among 18 countries reporting nationally representative PDR data, 12 showed NNRTI PDR levels over the 10% WHO-recommended threshold to urgently shift to a first-line non-NNRTI-based ART option [6]. Overall, NNRTI PDR levels were observed to be three-times higher among persons with previous exposure to antiretrovirals and two-times higher among women compared to men [6]. On the other hand, recent data on viral suppression at 12 months of ART initiation (defined as a viral load below 1000 copies/mL) in nine countries reporting nationally representative data on acquired drug resistance surveys designed according to WHO recommendations [6–9], ranged from 72% to 96% [6]. However, considering people not retained in care as virological failures, the prevalence of viral load suppression dropped by 12–22 points [6].

In Mexico, a significantly lower viral suppression among ART-naïve persons with documented PDR has been reported compared to those without PDR [10], but little is known about the association of HIV drug resistance and other outcomes such as retention in care or probability of death. Describing the sociodemographic characteristics, HIV drug resistance prevalence, pre-exposure levels to antiretroviral drugs, retention in care, and virological outcomes of persons initiating ART, could help strengthen HIV programs and support policy making. In this work, using nationally representative data on HIV drug resistance from a previously reported PDR survey [7], together with data from the National HIV Database SALVAR (Mexican System of Distribution, Logistics, and ART Surveillance), we explored longitudinal associations of PDR in persons entering to care and different outcomes such as retention in care, loss to follow-up (LTFU), viral suppression, and death in Mexico.

2. Results

2.1. Study Population Description

Of 2006 participants with an HIV drug resistance test in the published Mexico PDR survey [7], a total of 1823 (91%), were found in SALVAR and followed for a median of 1.88 years (IQR: 1.59–2.02) and are our study population. Among those, 231 (13%) were classified as ART-experienced and 185 (11%) were resistant to NNRTI. Considering prior exposure to ART and presence of NNRTI PDR, we classified 20 (1%) participants as experienced + resistant; 211 (11%) as experienced + non-resistant; 165 (9%) as naïve + resistant; and 1427 (78%) as naïve + non-resistant. Briefly, 333 (18%) of the study population were females and 1490 (72%) male. The median age was 30 years (IQR: 25–38). Regarding transmission risk, 304 (17%) were heterosexual cisgender women, 1008 (55%) were men who have sex with men (MSM), 326 (18%) were heterosexual cisgender men, 43 (2%) were persons who inject drugs (PWID), and 142 (8%) participants had missing information on transmission risk. Among heterosexual persons, 326 (52%) were cisgender men. The median CD4+ T cell count at the time of HIV drug resistance testing was 229 cells/mm^3 (IQR: 84–411). Regarding education level, 318 (17%) participants had elementary level or lower, and 1440 (79%) had high school level or higher. Additionally, 888 (51%) participants were employed, 680 (39%) were unemployed, and 160 (9%) were students. A total of 1728 (95%) participants had first ART regimen information, 1136 (66%) of them based on EFV. Clinical and sociodemographic characteristics of patients by group are shown in Table 1.

Table 1. Clinical and sociodemographic characteristics according to prior exposure to antiretroviral treatment and presence of efavirenz/nevirapine pretreatment drug resistance in Mexican individuals living with HIV, 2017–2019, N = 1823.

	Experienced -Resistant N = 20	Experienced -Non-Resistant N = 211	Naïve -Resistant N = 165	Naïve -Non-Resistant N = 1427	p-Value [1]
Female; n (%)	9 (45%)	69 (33%)	32 (19%)	223 (16%)	<0.01
Median age (years); (IQR)	34 (28–39)	34 (27–42)	30 (25–41)	29 (25–38)	<0.01
Transmission risk *; n					
Heterosexual cisgender women	8 (40%)	62 (29%)	30 (18%)	204 (14%)	
MSM	5 (20%)	83 (39%)	82 (49%)	838 (59%)	< 0.01
Heterosexual cisgender men	5 (20%)	34 (16%)	35 (21%)	252 (18%)	
PWID	1 (0.5%)	13 (6%)	3 (1.8%)	26 (1.8%)	
Mean CD4+ T cell count; cells/mm^3 (IQR)	223 (58–410)	143 (53–343)	244 (94–459)	237 (91–413)	0.31
Education; n (%)					
Elementary or lower	8 (40%)	62 (29%)	31 (19%)	217 (15%)	
High school or higher	12 (60%)	141 (67%)	128 (77%)	1159 (81%)	<0.01
Unknown	0 (0%)	8 (4%)	6 (4%)	51 (3.5%)	
Occupation; n (%)					
Employed	4 (20%)	81 (40%)	88 (51%)	824 (54%)	
Unemployed	16 (80%)	107 (53%)	63 (37%)	532 (35%)	<0.01
Student	0 (0%)	15 (7%)	21 (12%)	154 (10%)	
Median time of follow-up (years); (IQR)	1.93 (0.85–2.08)	1.91 (1.51–2.04)	1.86 (1.66–2.05)	1.87 (1.60–2.01)	0.74
First ART regimen group; n (%)					
Based on EFV	9 (45%)	120 (58%)	100 (64%)	907 (67%)	
Integrase Inhibitors	3 (15%)	15 (7%)	50 (33%)	366 (27%)	<0.01
Protease Inhibitors	7 (35%)	68 (33%)	4 (2%)	70 (5%)	
Other	1 (5%)	4 (2%)	1 (1%)	3 (0.2%)	

[1] The p-value compares the distribution of variables in each group, from Kruskal–Wallis, chi-squares, or fisher test according with the type of variable. * PWID: people who inject drugs includes 43 participants, 39 of them men and 4 women; 26 in the naïve + non-resistant group; 13 in the experienced + non-resistant; 1 in the experienced + resistant; and 3 in the naïve resistant. The missing information for risk of transmission was 1 for experienced + resistant, 19 in the experienced +non-resistant, 107 in the naive-resistant and 15 in the naïve + non-resistant (n = 142).

The percentage of ART-experienced individuals was higher among women and heterosexual men (70/333; 21% and 39/326, 12%, respectively) compared to MSM (88/1008, 9%; $p < 0.01$). Considering both persons with prior ART exposure and ART-naïve persons, the prevalence of resistance to NNRTI among women (41/333; 12%) and among heterosexual men (40/326, 12%) was higher than among MSM (87/1008, 8.6%; $p = 0.05$).

2.2. Characteristics of Participants without Information in the National HIV Database

A total of 184 (9.2%) persons were not included in the study because they were not found in the SALVAR dataset. Of them, 182 (99%) were naïve to ART, and 18 (10%) had NNRTI resistance, all of them belonging to the naïve group. When compared to those with available information in the SALVAR dataset, 17 (9.4%) were cisgender women ($p < 0.01$), the median age was 28 years (IQR: 24–37; $p = 0.21$), the median CD4 cell count was 287 cells/mm3 (IQR: 124–419; $p = 0.11$), 87% had high school level or higher education ($p = 0.02$), and 61% were employed ($p < 0.01$).

2.3. Final Outcomes

Considering 1823 persons with an HIV drug resistance test and information available in SALVAR, the present study represented 3034.3 person-years of follow-up. At the end of follow-up, 1276 (70%) of participants were reported as "in care" in SALVAR, 102 (6%) were reported as dead, and 435 (24%) were reported as LTFU. Among participants classified as LTFU, no specific reason was registered for 206 (46%), while 147 (33%) reported a change to a different health system (mainly due to employment status change and acquisition of social security), 82 (18%) left care for other reasons, and 10 (2%) discontinued ART. The distribution of final outcomes by group was non-significantly different ($p = 0.06$); however, we observed a higher proportion of participants retained in care among ART naïve persons (71%), compared to ART-experienced persons (63%, $p = 0.002$). Importantly, a trend toward higher mortality was observed in the experienced + resistant group (15%) compared to the experienced + non-resistant (8%), the naïve + non-resistant (5%), and the naïve + resistant (4%; $p = 0.08$) groups (Figure 1).

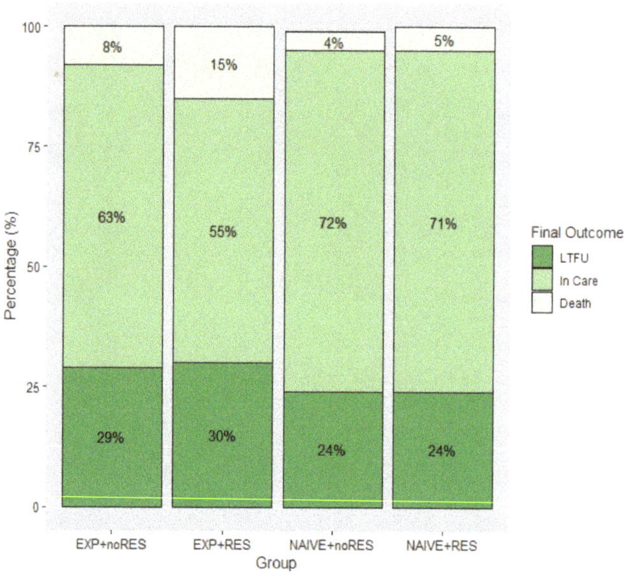

Figure 1. Final outcome by presence of efavirenz/nevirapine pre-treatment drug resistance and prior exposure to antiretroviral drugs in a cohort of Mexican persons living with HIV, 2017–2019. Note: Groups according to prior ART exposure and presence of NNRTI-PDR: EXP + noRES: experienced + non-resistant, EXP + RES: experienced + resistant, NAÏVE + noRES: naïve + non-resistant and NAÏVE + RES: naïve + resistant LTFU, lost to follow-up: defined as persons with a non-active status due to ART abandonment, migration to other healthcare systems, unknown status, as well as lack of viral load follow-up for more than 6 months at the dataset closure date.

2.3.1. Viral Suppression

Viral load data in the last six months of follow-up was available for 1637 (89%) participants, among whom 1126 (68%) had achieved viral suppression. When comparing across groups, 51% (92/179) among experienced + non-resistant; 36% (5/14) among experienced + resistant; 72% (929/1294) among naïve + non-resistant; and 67% (100/150) among naïve + resistant, achieved viral suppression ($p < 0.001$). Of the 1637 individuals with viral load follow up data available, 1259 (77%) were recorded as still in care at the end of follow-up, with 1021 (81%) of them achieving viral suppression; 330 (26%) classified as LTFU; and 48 (3%) as dead. After multivariable adjustment, experienced + non-resistant participants (aOR = 0.46, 95% CI: 0.32–0.66) and experienced + resistant (aOR = 0.28, 95% CI: 0.09–0.87) had lower odds of viral suppression compared to the naïve + non-resistant group. (Table 2, Model 1). Note that, in this analysis, 30% of the experienced + resistant group was not included due to lack of follow-up viral load data (Supplementary Material, Table S1). In the analysis using multiple imputation we observed significantly lower odds of viral suppression in experienced + non-resistant (aOR = 0.49, CI95%: 0.34–0.70), but not in experienced + resistant (aOR = 0.39, 95% CI: 0.13–1.15), and naïve + resistant (aOR = 0.79, 95% CI: 0.53–1.17) compared to naïve + non-resistant participants (Table 2, Model 2). Moreover, older participants had higher odds of viral suppression (aOR = 1.45,

95% CI: 1.04–2.04, for 50 years old vs. 30 years old) in the first model, but not in second with the imputed data set (aOR = 1.29, 95% CI: 0.93–1.79) (Table 2, Model 2).

Table 2. Factors associated with viral suppression in a cohort of Mexican persons living with HIV, 2017–2019.

	Model 1		Model 2		Model 3	
Characteristics	**OR; IC95%**	***p*-Value**	**OR; IC95%**	***p*-Value**	**OR; IC95%**	***p*-Value**
Group						
Naïve + non-resistant	1		1		1	
Naïve + resistant	0.74; 0.50–1.09	0.14	0.79; 0.53–1.17	0.25	0.71; 0.47–1.07	0.10
Experienced + non-resistant	0.46; 0.32–0.66	<0.001	0.49; 0.34–0.70	<0.001	0.37; 0.24–0.53	<0.001
Experienced + resistant	0.28; 0.09–0.87	0.02	0.39; 0.13–1.15	0.09	0.26; 0.08–0.83	0.02
CD4+ T cell count at the time of HIV drug resistance test (cells/mm^3)		0.16		0.27		0.04
100	1		1		1	
200	1.04; 0.89–1.21		1.04; 0.90–1.21		0.99; 0.85–1.16	
300	1.03; 0.82–1.31		1.05; 0.84–1.32		0.95; 0.74–1.22	
400	0.98; 0.77–1.25		1.00; 0.78–1.28		0.88; 0.67–1.14	
Age at the time of HIV drug resistance test (years) [1]		0.17		0.77		
30	1		1		1	0.03
40	1.25; 0.89–1.48		1.09; 0.97–1.24		1.10; 0.84–1.44	
50	1.45; 1.04–2.04		1.29; 0.93–1.79		1.52; 1.05–2.19	
Transmission Risk						
MSM	1		1		1	
Heterosexual cisgender men	0.77: 0.56–1.06	0.11	0.80; 0.58–1.07	0.13	0.75; 0.54–1.05	0.09
Heterosexual cisgender women	0.74; 0.53–1.03	0.82	0.73; 0.53–1.00	0.69	0.76; 0.53–1.08	0.97
Education level		0.56		0.73		
Elementary or lower	0.90; 0.64–1.27		0.94; 0.68–0.30		0.89; 0.62–1.28	0.55
High school or higher	1		1		1	
Employment status		0.73		0.99		
Unemployed	0.96; 0.75–1.22		1.00; 0.79–1.27		0.76; 0.59–0.99	0.004
Employed	1		1		1	
Change in ART regimen	NA	NA	NA	NA	1.78; 1.15–2.75	0.009

Model 1 was fitted by sex, antiretroviral treatment + exposure drug resistance group, CD4+ T cell count, age, transmission risk, education level and employment status, n = 1454; Model 2 includes the same variables of Model 1 using imputation of missing data to improve dataset completeness, n = 1780; and Model 3 includes the variable change in the ART regimen, n = 1445. [1] Age was modelled using splines with 3 nodes, the reference age selected for the results was 30 years old. MSM: Men who have sex with men, NA: not available.

2.3.2. Change in Antiretroviral Treatment Regimen

Of the 1136 (66%) participants who started ART with EFV-based regimens, 907 (80%) of them belonged to the naïve + non-resistant group, 9 (<1%) to the experienced + resistant, 100 (9%) to the naïve + resistant, and 120 (10%) to the experienced + non-resistant group. ART-experienced participants were more likely to switch to NNRTI-sparing regimens, with 40% of the non-resistant and 20% of the resistant. By contrast, within the ART naïve participants, 6% of the non-resistant, and 5% of the resistant changed ART regimen. When including information regarding change in ART regimen in the logistic model, the odds of viral suppression was significantly higher in persons who changed versus those who did not change regimen (aOR = 1.78, 95% CI: 1.15–2.75; $p < 0.01$). The odds of viral suppression for experienced + non-resistant (aOR = 0.37, 95% CI: 0.24–0.53) and experienced + resistant (aOR = 0.26, 95% CI: 0.08–0.83) compared to naïve + non-resistant persons including data on change in ART regimen, remained similar to those of the previous model (Table 2, Model 3).

2.3.3. Viral Suppression Outcome with Lost to Follow-Up and Death as Competing Events

Among the 1637 participants with viral load data available, we found that 1021 persons (62%) ended the study follow-up in care and virally suppressed, 238 (14%) were in care but without viral suppression, 330 (20%) were LTFU, and 48 (3%) were reported as dead. By group, the highest proportion of participants classified as in care and suppressed was observed among ART-naïve participants (84% among non-resistant and 77% among resistant), compared with ART-experienced participants (64% among non-resistant and 50% among resistant) (Supplementary Table S1). Using a Fine-Gray model, we found that being ART-experienced was associated with a lower probability of remaining in care with viral suppression over time (aHR = 0.68, 95% CI: 0.53–0.86, for the non-resistant group and aHR = 0.37, 0.17–0.84, for the resistant group, compared to the naïve + non-resistant group). Older age and higher education level did not show a significant association with viral suppression. Heterosexual cisgender women compared to MSM, had a lower hazard of viral suppression (aHR = 0.84, 95% CI: 0.70–1.01, $p = 0.06$) (Table 3). The estimated probability of remaining in care and virally suppressed, being LTFU and death, over time, for each group is shown in the Supplementary Material; Figure S1.

Table 3. Variables associated to the probability of viral suppression at the end of follow-up in a competing risk context. (Fine-Gray model).

	HR [1]	95% CI	*p*-Value
Group			
Naïve + non-resistant	1		
Naïve + resistant	0.97	(0.78–1.22)	0.81
Experienced + non-resistant	0.68	(0.53–0.86)	<0.001
Experienced + resistant	0.37	(0.17–0.84)	0.01
CD4+ T cell count at the time of HIV drug resistance test (per 100 cells/mm^3)	0.99	(0.96–1.03)	0.78
Age at the time of HIV drug resistance test	1.03	(0.97–1.10)	0.40
Transmission risk			
MSM	1		
Heterosexual cisgender women	0.84	(0.70–1.01)	0.06
Heterosexual cisgender men	0.91	(0.76–1.09)	0.29
Education level			
Elementary or lower	1		
High school or higher	1.14	(0.99–1.31)	0.07

[1] HR: hazard ratio, 95% CI: 95% confidence interval, MSM: men who have sex with men.

3. Discussion

The present study provides evidence that ART re-starters, as well as persons with pre-treatment NNRTI resistance, in general have worse clinical outcomes than persons without previous exposure to ART and persons without NNRTI resistance in a cohort of Mexican individuals followed for two years. In the adjusted model with ART-regimen change variable, prior exposure to ART was strongly associated with poor clinical outcomes, and with ART-experienced participants, having nearly 40% lower probability of remaining in care with viral suppression. Previous exposure to ART was more common in women with low education arriving late to clinical care. From a total of 1823 Mexican persons living with HIV with baseline drug resistance testing and followed by a median of almost 2 years of follow-up time, we classified 1% as experienced + resistant, 9% as naïve + resistant, 11% as experienced + non-resistant, and 78% as naïve + non-resistant. At the end of follow-up, the experienced + resistant group had the lowest proportion of participants remaining in care compared to other groups. Participants in the experienced + resistant group also showed higher mortality and LTFU, as well as lower levels of viral suppression, even after switching to NNRTI-sparing ART regimens.

Participants in the experienced + resistant group were more frequently women, with lower education level and more frequently unemployed, compared to other groups. Higher social and economic vulnerability among women living with HIV in Mexico has been observed in previous studies [10–15], including in circumstances associated with HIV diagnosis during pregnancy [15]. Additionally, a higher risk for ART discontinuation has been observed among Mexican women living with HIV compared to men [16], with a recent study reporting as high as 20% ART interruption rate [16], with reasons including access to care, depression, and ART adverse effects. Other common reasons observed for ART interruption, and higher viral failure rate in women include a general lower education level, economic dependence on other members of the household, responsibility to provide care and sustenance for children, long distance to clinics and difficulty to pay for transport [12,15]. In general, we found that MSM had better outcomes than heterosexual participants. This could reflect both significant structural differences in the MSM population compared to the heterosexual population living with HIV in Mexico [12], as well as a traditional focus on MSM as a priority group for HIV care and focus of most national HIV prevention efforts.

Changes in ART regimen were more commonly observed among ART-experienced than naïve patients, regardless of their resistance status. However, from this study, we cannot deduce whether clinicians were more proactive in changing ART regimens for ART-experienced and/or NNRTI resistant patients. We also do not know which information clinicians had available to them at the time of ART-regimen decision-making, as resistance test results. Thus, it is not possible to assess whether the results influenced selection of first-line ART regimens.

In Mexico, as of 2019, bictegravir, an integrase inhibitor drug with high genetic barrier to resistance [8], is recommended as the basis for first line ART-regimens. However, the use of bictegravir is contraindicated in patients using rifampicin or rifabutin; and in pregnant women. In 2020, 30% of patients were still on EFV-based regimens in Mexico [16]. Thus, the implementation of measures to improve adherence and prevent failures due to resistance are important and still needed. HIV drug resistance testing is recommended to guide the choice of second-line ART line, and adherence issues and potential drug interactions need to be addressed.

Our study provides an evaluation of clinical outcomes in real-life setting evaluating clinical outcomes among ART-naive and experienced persons with and without resistance to NNRTI, using surveillance data cross-referenced with the official ministry of health database analyzed with robust statistical techniques. We evaluated virological success among resistant patients, in a context of competing risk with lost to follow-up and death; including the effect of ART change and multiple imputation analyses to address possible bias due to missing data. However, our study also has limitations. First, the original surveillance study was not designed to follow-up participants or to evaluate their clinical outcomes in longer periods, which may reduce availability of information. Using the national database SALVAR allowed us to improve completeness of the data, but we acknowledge that some quality issues could exist with a possible impact on our results. The SALVAR database was designed to record viral load and CD4 T cell count studies, as well as antiretroviral drug dispensation practices for administrative purposes, and record of visits to the clinic or vital status are not among its main objectives. We used the information available as a proxy to inform retention in care, lost to follow-up and viral suppression. Second, not all participants of the original surveillance study were included due to lack of follow-up information, representing a possible selection bias. This situation is frequent in the Mexican setting due to the fragmentation of the health system, obligating persons with formal employment to seek clinical care and ART in social security clinics and persons without formal employment in ministry of health clinics. The lack of a unified national database and migration of persons between health systems, due to changes in employment status has been previously reported as an important reason for ART defaulting and LTFU [17]. The percentage of participants in our study in this situation was 9%, and we found some sociodemographic differences between the persons excluded due to missing data and the persons with data available in the SALVAR database, and thus included in the current study, raising representativeness issues. Nevertheless, these participants with missing data were mainly men, with a slightly higher median CD4+ count, with higher education, higher employment rates, and lower prevalence of re-starters. Interestingly, a Mexican study including outpatients of a large Ministry of Health clinic in Mexico City observed that persons arriving to care with CD4+ T cell counts < 100 cells/mm^3 were more frequently classified as intermittent ART users and 43% came from social security clinics [18], possibly suggesting a return to care in Ministry of Health clinics, in a worse condition after employment loss, ART defaulting, and LTFU. A program linking the different health care systems in Mexico and a unified HIV database are urgently needed to improve follow-up and care of patients repeatedly changing employment status. Finally, although our study leverages access to SALVAR, we recognize that the information available in this national database is limited. The variables collected for sociodemographic description of the study cohort only describe education level and employment, which may also be variable over time. Inclusion of more adequate variables to describe economic class or poverty level could help to better define socioeconomic status and risk associations with the evaluated outcomes.

Our study provides evidence on associations between pretreatment drug resistance and prior exposure to antiretrovirals in persons starting ART and deleterious clinical outcomes in the Mexican context. However, these observations may also be generally true elsewhere, mainly in other LMICs, and help in public health decision making.

4. Materials and Methods

4.1. Data Source

We analyzed PDR and sociodemographic data from 1823 persons that participated in a large nationally representative HIV PDR survey carried out in Mexico from 09/2017 to 03/2018 who entered to care in Ministry of Health clinics [7], and had follow-up data in Mexico's national Ministry of Health ART database (SALVAR). The SALVAR database comprises information regarding mortality, retention in HIV care, ART regimen history, and CD4+ T cell count, and viral load follow-up for persons without social security in Mexico. The administrative closure date for the dataset used in this study was 12/2019. The last status reported in the database was used to classify the final outcome of the participants.

4.2. Sample Selection

Persons recorded as alive and in follow-up in the SALVAR database were classified as remaining in care. Persons with a non-active status due to ART abandonment, migration to other healthcare systems [18], unknown status, as well as lack of viral load follow-up for more than 6 months at the dataset closure date, were classified as LTFU. Persons who died were not included in the LTFU group. Participants were stratified into four groups according to prior ART exposure and presence of NNRTI-PDR: experienced + resistant, experienced + non-resistant, naïve + resistant, and naïve + non-resistant. Retention in care, LTFU and death were compared between groups as final outcomes.

4.3. Statistical Analysis

We estimated the percentage of persons with viral suppression (last viral load < 200 copies/mL) at the end of follow-up by group, among those persons with viral load information available (within 6 months prior to the last database entry for each participant). A logistic regression model was developed to assess the relationship between ART exposure, NNRTI resistance, and viral suppression, adjusting for sociodemographic characteristics in the main analysis. A model including change in ART status after an HIV drug resistance test was performed to see the potential impact of this variable on the probability of reaching viral suppression. A Fine-Gray model was used to compare retention in care and viral suppression at the end of follow-up, with LTFU and death as final outcomes and competing events. In this model, we censored persons who ended in care but did not achieve viral suppression or did not have viral load information available. We included ART exposure drug resistance status groups, age, sex, mode of transmission, and educational level as co-variables. Due to the small size of groups, we combined sex and mode of HIV transmission to include them in the models. The variable "sex and mode of transmission" was categorized as: MSM, heterosexual cisgender men and heterosexual cisgender women. People who inject drugs were excluded from the models. Additional analyses using multiple imputations with 10 replications were conducted for viral suppression since we observed that 10% of the records had missing information for the last viral load. In particular, 30% (6/20) of the experienced + resistant group had missing viral load data. Additionally, to evaluate potential biases and the possible generalization of our results, we described and compared the characteristics of HIV drug resistance testing between persons with and without information in SALVAR. All the analyses were performed using R Version 1.2.5019.

Supplementary Materials: The following are available online at https://www.mdpi.com/article/10.3390/pathogens10121569/s1, Figure S1: Estimated probability for remaining in care under viral suppression in competing risk with death and LTFU. Table S1: Clinical outcomes according to availability of viral load information in Mexican persons living with HIV, 2017–2019.

Author Contributions: Conceptualization, Y.C.-V., C.G.-M., G.R.-T., J.G.S.-M. and S.Á.-R.; data curation, C.C., C.G.-M. and S.Á.-R.; formal analysis, Y.C.-V., F.A.-E., S.S.-R. and C.C.; funding acquisition, F.A.-E. and E.A.E.; investigation, A.P.-M. and C.G.-M.; methodology, Y.C.-V., F.A.-E., E.A.E., S.S.-R. and C.C.; resources, A.P.-M., C.G.-M. and S.Á.-R.; supervision, G.R.-T., J.G.S.-M. and S.Á.-R.; validation, C.G.-M. and S.Á.-R.; writing—original draft, Y.C.-V., A.P.-M. and S.Á.-R.; writing—review and editing, Y.C.-V., F.A.-E., E.A.E., C.C., A.P.-M., C.G.-M., G.R.-T., J.G.S.-M. and S.Á.-R. All authors have read and agreed to the published version of the manuscript.

Funding: This work was supported by Consejo Nacional de Ciencia y Tecnología (CONACyT SALUD-2017-01-289725), the Mexican Government (Programa Presupuestal P016; Anexo 13 del Decreto del Presupuesto de Egresos de la Federación), and the Canadian Institutes of Health Research (grants PJT-148621 and PJT-159625). E.A.E., F.A.-E. and C.C. had funding provided by the Center for Global Health and Social Responsibility at the University of Minnesota. August 2018–July 2019.

Institutional Review Board Statement: The study was conducted according to the guidelines of the Declaration of Helsinki, and approved by the Ethics Committee of Instituto Nacional de Ciencias Médicas y Nutrición Salvador Zubirán (protocol code INF-2795-18-19-1, date of approval 19 October 2018).

Informed Consent Statement: Patient consent was waived because we are using secondary information from datasets previously recorded; the written informed consent was obtained from the patient(s) to analyze the original information.

Data Availability Statement: The data presented in this study are available on request from the corresponding author. Databases with patient sequences and follow up data are not public due to national regulations.

Conflicts of Interest: The authors declare no conflict of interest. The funders had no role in the design of the study; in the collection, analyses, or interpretation of data; in the writing of the manuscript, or in the decision to publish the results.

References

1. Guidelines on the Public Health Response to Pretreatment HIV Drug Resistance. July 2017. Available online: https://apps.who.int/iris/bitstream/handle/10665/255880/9789241550055-eng.pdf;jsessionid=1FA5DAAEDF96CC18BAB5E3AAD2DCA704?sequence=1 (accessed on 28 November 2021).
2. Bertagnolio, S.; Hermans, L.; Jordan, M.R.; Avila-Rios, S.; Iwuji, C.; Derache, A.; Delaporte, E.; Wensing, A.; Aves, T.; Borhan, A.S.M.; et al. Clinical Impact of Pretreatment Human Immunodeficiency Virus Drug Resistance in People Initiating Nonnucleoside Reverse Transcriptase Inhibitor-Containing Antiretroviral Therapy: A Systematic Review and Meta-analysis. *J. Infect. Dis.* **2021**, *224*, 377–388. [CrossRef] [PubMed]
3. Gupta, R.K.; Gregson, J.; Parkin, N.; Haile-Selassie, H.; Tanuri, A.; Andrade Forero, L.; Kaleebu, P.; Watera, C.; Aghokeng, A.; Mutenda, N.; et al. HIV-1 drug resistance before initiation or re-initiation of first-line antiretroviral therapy in low-income and middle-income countries: A systematic review and meta-regression analysis. *Lancet Infect. Dis.* **2018**, *18*, 346–355. [CrossRef]
4. UNAIDS. 90-90-90 An Ambitious Treatment Target to Help End the AIDS Epidemic. 2014. Available online: https://www.unaids.org/sites/default/files/media_asset/90-90-90_en.pdf (accessed on 15 July 2018).

5. García-Morales, C.; Tapia-Trejo, D.; Quiroz-Morales, V.S.; Navarro-Álvarez, S.; Barrera-Arellano, C.A.; Casillas-Rodríguez, J.; Romero-Mora, K.A.; Gómez-Palacio-Schjetnan, M.; Murakami-Ogasawara, A.; Ávila-Ríos, S.; et al. HIVDR MexNet Group. HIV pretreatment drug resistance trends in three geographic areas of Mexico. *J. Antimicrob. Chemother.* **2017**, *72*, 3149–3158. [CrossRef] [PubMed]
6. World Health Organization. *HIV Drug Resistance Report 2019*; (WHO/CDS/HIV/19.21). Licence: CC BY-NC-SA 3.0 IGO; World Health Organization: Geneva, Switzerland, 2019. Available online: https://www.who.int/hiv/pub/drugresistance/hivdr-report-2019/en/ (accessed on 28 November 2021).
7. Ávila-Ríos, S.; García-Morales, C.; Valenzuela-Lara, M.; Chaillon, A.; Tapia-Trejo, D.; Pérez-García, M.; López-Sánchez, D.M.; Maza-Sánchez, L.; del Arenal-Sánchez, S.J.; Paz-Juárez, H.E.; et al. HIV-1 drug resistance before initiation or re-initiation of first-line ART in eight regions of Mexico: A sub-nationally representative survey. *J. Antimicrob. Chemother.* **2019**, *74*, 1044–1055. [CrossRef] [PubMed]
8. Guía de Manejo Antirretroviral de las Personas con VIH. México: Censida/Secretaría de Salud Décima Edición. 2019. Available online: https://www.gob.mx/cms/uploads/attachment/file/569287/GUIA_DE_MANEJO_ANTIRRETROVIRAL_DE_LAS_PERSONAS_CON_VIH_2019_-_VERSI_N_COMPLETA1.pdf (accessed on 28 November 2021).
9. WHO. HIV Drug Resistance Surveillance Concept Notes. Available online: https://www.who.int/hiv/topics/drugresistance/protocols/en/ (accessed on 28 November 2021).
10. Ávila-Ríos, S.; García-Morales, C.; Matías-Florentino, M.; Romero-Mora, K.A.; Tapia-Trejo, D.; Quiroz-Morales, V.S.; Reyes-Gopar, H.; Ji, H.; Sandstrom, P.; Casillas-Rodríguez, J.; et al. HIVDR MexNet Group. Pretreatment HIV-drug resistance in Mexico and its impact on the effectiveness of first-line antiretroviral therapy: A nationally representative 2015 WHO survey. *Lancet HIV* **2016**, *12*, e579–e591. [CrossRef]
11. Avila-Rios, S.; Sued, O.; Rhee, S.Y.; Shafer, R.W.; Reyes-Teran, G.; Ravasi, G. Surveillance of HIV Transmitted Drug Resistance in Latin America and the Caribbean: A Systematic Review and Meta-Analysis. *PLoS ONE* **2016**, *11*, e0158560. [CrossRef] [PubMed]
12. Bautista-Arredondo, S.; Servan-Mori, E.; Beynon, F.; González, A.; Volkow, P. A tale of two epidemics: Gender differences in socio-demographic characteristics and sexual behaviors among HIV positive individuals in Mexico City. *Int. J. Equity Health* **2015**, *14*, 147. [CrossRef] [PubMed]
13. Boender, T.S.; Hoenderboom, B.M.; Sigaloff, K.C.; Hamers, R.F.; Wellington, M.; Shamu, T.; Siwale, M.; Labib Maksimos, E.E.F.; Nankya, I.; Kityo, C.M.; et al. Pretreatment HIV drug resistance increases regimen switches in sub-Saharan Africa. *Clin. Infect. Dis.* **2015**, *61*, 1749–1758. [CrossRef] [PubMed]
14. Aguilar-Zapata, D.; Piñeirúa-Menéndez, A.; Volkow-Fernández, P.; Rodríguez-Zulueta, P.; Ramos-Alamillo, U.; Cabrera-López, T.; Martin-Onraet, A. Sociodemographic differences among HIV-positive and HIV-negative recently pregnant women in Mexico City. *Medicine* **2017**, *96*, e7305. [CrossRef] [PubMed]
15. Ramírez, R. HIV/HEP 2019. P012. Barriers to access HIV-healthcare services for women living with HIV in Mexico. *J. Int. AIDS Soc.* **2019**, *22*, e25263.
16. De la Torre-Rosas, A. Estado Actual de la Epidemia en México ¿Cómo van las Metas? 2021. Available online: https://simposiovih-sida.mx/assets/pdf/PROGRAMA_SIMPOSIO_VIH_SIDA2021.pdf (accessed on 28 November 2021).
17. Sierra-Madero, J.G.; Belaunzaran-Zamudio, P.F.; Crabtree-Ramírez, B.; Magis-Rodriguez, C. Mexico's fragmented health system as a barrier to HIV care. *Lancet HIV* **2019**, *2*, e74–e75. [CrossRef]
18. Piñeirúa-Menendez, A.; Del Hoyo, M.; Osorno González de León, F.; Badial Hernández, F.; Niño-Vargas, R. (Mexico City, Mexico). P035. HIV/HEP2018. The Continuum of Care among Very Immunosuppressed (Less Than 100 CD4+ Cells) Patients in an Outpatient Clinic in Mexico City: Gaps in Diagnosis, Linkage and Retention in Care. Available online: http://www.hivhepamericas.org/wp-content/uploads/2018/05/P035.pdf (accessed on 28 November 2021).

pathogens

MDPI

Article

HIV Pretreatment Drug Resistance Trends in Mexico City, 2017–2020

Claudia García-Morales [1], Daniela Tapia-Trejo [1], Margarita Matías-Florentino [1], Verónica Sonia Quiroz-Morales [1], Vanessa Dávila-Conn [1], Ángeles Beristain-Barreda [1], Miroslava Cárdenas-Sandoval [1], Manuel Becerril-Rodríguez [1], Patricia Iracheta-Hernández [2], Israel Macías-González [2], Rebecca García-Mendiola [3], Alejandro Guzmán-Carmona [3], Eduardo Zarza-Sánchez [1], Raúl Adrián Cruz [3], Andrea González-Rodríguez [2], Gustavo Reyes-Terán [4] and Santiago Ávila-Ríos [1,*]

[1] Centre for Research in Infectious Diseases, National Institute of Respiratory Diseases, Calzada de Tlalpan 4502, Colonia Sección XVI, Mexico City 14080, Mexico; claudia.garcia@cieni.org.mx (C.G.-M.); daniela.tapia@cieni.org.mx (D.T.-T.); margarita.matias@cieni.org.mx (M.M.-F.); veronica.quiroz@cieni.org.mx (V.S.Q.-M.); vanessa.davila@cieni.org.mx (V.D.-C.); angeles.beristain@gmail.com (Á.B.-B.); sandovalmiroslava14@gmail.com (M.C.-S.); manuel.becerril@cieni.org.mx (M.B.-R.); eduardo.zarza@cieni.org.mx (E.Z.-S.)

[2] Condesa Specialised Clinic, General Benjamín Hill 24, Colonia Condesa, Mexico City 06140, Mexico; patricia.iracheta.hedz@gmail.com (P.I.-H.); maglezis@gmail.com (I.M.-G.); andrea.gonzalez.condesa@gmail.com (A.G.-R.)

[3] Condesa Iztapalapa Specialised Clinic, Combate de Celaya s/n, Colonia Unidad Habitacional Vicente Guerrero, Mexico City 09730, Mexico; rebe_ime@yahoo.com.mx (R.G.-M.); alex.guzman75@gmail.com (A.G.-C.); acruzf@gmail.com (R.A.C.)

[4] Coordinating Commission of the National Institutes of Health and High Specialty Hospitals, Periférico Sur 4809, Colonia Arenal de Tepepan, Mexico City 14610, Mexico; gustavo.reyesteran@gmail.com

* Correspondence: santiago.avila@cieni.org.mx; Tel.: +52-55-5666-7985 (ext. 133)

Citation: García-Morales, C.; Tapia-Trejo, D.; Matías-Florentino, M.; Quiroz-Morales, V.S.; Dávila-Conn, V.; Beristain-Barreda, Á.; Cárdenas-Sandoval, M.; Becerril-Rodríguez, M.; Iracheta-Hernández, P.; Macías-González, I.; et al. HIV Pretreatment Drug Resistance Trends in Mexico City, 2017–2020. *Pathogens* **2021**, *10*, 1587. https://doi.org/10.3390/pathogens10121587

Academic Editor: Alessandra Borsetti

Received: 1 November 2021
Accepted: 30 November 2021
Published: 8 December 2021

Abstract: In response to increasing pretreatment drug resistance (PDR), Mexico changed its national antiretroviral treatment (ART) policy, recommending and procuring second-generation integrase strand-transfer inhibitor (INSTI)-based regimens as preferred first-line options since 2019. We present a four-year observational study describing PDR trends across 2017–2020 at the largest HIV diagnosis and primary care center in Mexico City. A total of 6688 baseline protease-reverse transcriptase and 6709 integrase sequences were included. PDR to any drug class was 14.4% (95% CI, 13.6–15.3%). A significant increasing trend for efavirenz/nevirapine PDR was observed (10.3 to 13.6%, $p = 0.02$). No increase in PDR to second-generation INSTI was observed, remaining under 0.3% across the study period. PDR was strongly associated with prior exposure to ART (aOR: 2.9, 95% CI: 1.9–4.6, $p < 0.0001$). MSM had higher odds of PDR to efavirenz/nevirapine (aOR: 2.0, 95% CI: 1.0–3.7, $p = 0.04$), reflecting ongoing transmission of mutations such as K103NS and E138A. ART restarters showed higher representation of cisgender women and injectable drug users, higher age, and lower education level. PDR to dolutegravir/bictegravir remained low in Mexico City, although further surveillance is warranted given the short time of ART optimization. Our study identifies demographic characteristics of groups with higher risk of PDR and lost to follow-up, which may be useful to design differentiated interventions locally.

Keywords: HIV pretreatment drug resistance; HIV acquired drug resistance; Mexico City; Mexico

1. Introduction

Antiretroviral therapy (ART) has provided undeniable benefits at the individual and population levels, significantly reducing morbidity and mortality among people living with HIV (PLVIH) [1] and averting new infections [2]. An estimated 27.5 million PLHIV were on ART by the end of 2020 worldwide [3]. However, the widespread use of

ART has been associated with the rise and spread of HIV drug resistance (HIVDR) [4]. According to the World Health Organization (WHO) operational definition, pretreatment drug resistance (PDR) refers to HIVDR detected in ART-naïve persons or previously antiretroviral (ARV)-exposed persons reinitiating first-line ART [5]. Over the last decade, there is growing evidence that PDR to non-nucleoside reverse transcriptase inhibitors (NNRTIs), mainly efavirenz and nevirapine, has been increasing in low- and middle-income countries (LMICs) [6]. Additionally, nationally representative surveys have been performed in several LMICs evidencing efavirenz/nevirapine PDR levels over 10% [4]. The high NNRTI PDR levels observed have led to the WHO recommendation and advocacy of the use of dolutegravir-based first-line regimens as the preferred option in LMICs [7].

In the Mexican context, two nationally representative surveys have shown efavirenz/nevirapine PDR levels close to 10% [8,9]. In addition, a study by our group demonstrated significant increases in efavirenz/nevirapine PDR levels in different areas of the country from 2008 to 2016, including Mexico City [10]. These results, together with advocacy and stewardship efforts, led to a change in national policy to recommend and procure ART regimens containing second-generation integrase strand-transfer inhibitors (INSTI), mainly bictegravir, as preferred first-line options since 2019 [11]. In Mexico, as in other LMICs, baseline HIVDR testing is not standard of care according to national guidelines.

To date, no data have been published updating PDR trends and describing the impact of national ART policy changes in México. Here, we present a four-year observational study describing PDR trends in Mexico City from 2017 to 2020. The study leverages a scientific collaboration between the largest primary care HIV clinic in Mexico City and a reference HIVDR testing laboratory, performing baseline HIV sequencing in all persons receiving an HIV diagnosis locally. Mexico City encompasses 18% of persons on ART in the country, and its epidemic is highly concentrated in men who have sex with men (MSM), with a high rate of linkage to care and ART use compared with other areas in the country [12].

2. Results

2.1. Characteristics of the Study Participants

Between January 2017 and December 2020, 8128 blood specimens were collected at the Condesa Specialized Clinic, the largest HIV primary care center in Mexico City. From these, 6785 (83.5%) were successfully sequenced. After curation, removal of duplicates (the first sequence of each individual in this case was kept), and sequence quality filtering (see Methods), 6661 unique individuals with protease-reverse transcriptase (PR.RT) as well as integrase (IN) sequence available were included in the database. Taking into account different amounts of missing information for different variables across the data set (Table 1), 95.1% (6234/6555) of the participants were cisgender men, 4.1% (267/6555) cisgender women, 0.8% (51/6555) transgender women, and 0.05% (3/6555) transgender men; 80.0% (4223/5280) lived in Mexico City and 18.3% (967/5280) in the surrounding municipalities of the State of Mexico; and 39.7% (2323/5853) arrived with <200 CD4+ T cells/mm^3 to clinical care. Subtype B largely predominated in the study population with only 1.3% (84/6661) of participants having non-B subtypes. The most frequent non-B subtypes observed were circulating recombinant forms (CRF02_AG: 0.29%; CRF01_AE: 0.26%) and unique recombinant forms (BG: 0.20%; BF: 0.17%).

Considering a subgroup of 1348 participants enrolled from June to December 2020, for whom more detailed metadata were collected (Table 2), and accounting for missing data, an estimated 11.0% (141/1286) reported previous exposure to ART, 59.9% (717/1196) self-identified as belonging to the middle social class, 40.3% (484/1201) had at least an undergraduate degree, and 3.3% (40/1196) reported speaking any indigenous language. Regarding additional risk variables, 40.2% (426/1059) reported having a sexually transmitted infection in the previous 6 months, 78.1% (793/1016) reported a receptive role in anal sex, 77.1% (807/1047) were not circumcised, and 9.2% (93/1013) reported using venues for sex (Table 2).

Table 1. Baseline demographic and clinical characteristics of study participants, 2017–2020 [a].

	Total Number of Observations [b] n = 6661	With PDR to Any Drug [c,d] n = 957	p Value	With PDR to EFV/NVP [d] n = 690	p Value
Gender, n (%)					
Cisgender Women	267 (4.0)	32 (12.0)	0.14	24 (9.0)	0.26
Cisgender Men	6234 (93.6)	907 (14.5)	0.06	653 (10.5)	0.13
Transgender Women	51 (0.8)	6 (11.8)	0.39	4 (7.8)	0.38
Transgender Men	3 (0.0)	0 (0.0)	0.62	0 (0.0)	0.72
Missing	106 (1.6)	12 (11.3)	0.23	9 (8.5)	0.33
Age (years) [e]					
Median (IQR)	28 (24–35)	28 (24–34)	0.09	28 (24–34)	0.30
State of residence, n (%)					
Mexico City	4223 (63.4)	621 (14.7)	0.16	448 (10.6)	0.20
Mexico State	967 (14.5)	142 (14.7)	0.40	107 (11.1)	0.23
Other	90 (1.4)	9 (10.0)	0.15	5 (5.6)	0.08
Missing	1381 (20.7)	185 (13.4)	0.13	130 (9.4)	0.10
HIV subtype, n (%)					
B	6577 (98.7)	946 (14.4)	0.44	680 (11.6)	0.37
Non-B	84 (1.3)	11 (13.1)		10 (11.9)	
Viral load (log RNA copies/mL) [f]					
Median (range)	4.8 (4.25-5-31)	4.7 (4.2–5.3)	0.02 *	4.7 (4.2–5.3)	0.03 *
CD4+ T cell count (cells/mm^3), n [g]					
Median (IQR)	249 (120–395)	250 (123–407)	0.22	254 (129–405)	0.16
CD4+ T cell count category, n (%)					
<200 cells/mm^3	2323 (34.87)	334 (14.4)	0.51	240 (10.3)	0.50
200–500 cells/mm^3	2721 (40.8)	389 (14.3)	0.46	285 (10.5)	0.41
>500 cells/mm^3	809 (12.2)	129 (15.9)	0.10	94 (11.6)	0.12
Missing	808 (12.1)	105 (13.0)	0.13	71 (8.8)	0.06
CD4+ T cell %, n [h]					
Median (IQR)	15 (9–21)	15 (9–22)	0.27	15 (10–22)	0.14

[a] Data for 6661 participants enrolled from January 2017 to December 2020. [b] Column percentages are shown. [c] Using the WHO definition for PDR (see Methods). [d] Row percentages are shown. [e] Data missing for 114 participants (n = 6547). [f] Data missing for 557 participants (n = 6104). [g] Data missing for 808 participants (n = 5853). [h] Data missing for 2234 participants (n = 4427). * $p < 0.05$. PDR; pretreatment drug resistance; EFV, efavirenz; NVP, nevirapine; IQR, interquartile range.

Table 2. Baseline demographic, clinical, and risk characteristics of study participants, June–December 2020 [a].

	Total Number of Observations [b] n = 1348	With PDR to Any Drug [c,d] n = 215 (15.9%)	p Value	With PDR to EFV/NVP [d] n = 158 (11.7%)	p Value
Gender, n (%)					
Cisgender Women	85 (6.3)	13 (15.3)	0.50	9 (10.6)	0.45
Cisgender Men	1234 (91.5)	196 (15.9)	0.46	145 (11.8)	0.53
Transgender Women	28 (2.1)	6 (21.4)	0.28	4 (14.3)	0.42
Transgender Men	1 (0.1)	0 (0.0)	0.84	0 (0.0)	0.88
Age (years)					
Median (IQR)	29 (25–36)	29 (25–35)	0.54	30 (25–35)	0.81
Prior ARV exposure, n (%)					
No	1145 (84.9)	164 (14.3)	<0.01 *	115 (10.0)	<0.01 *
Yes	141 (10.5)	41 (29.1)	<0.01 *	35 (24.8)	<0.01 *
Missing	62 (4.6)	10 (16.4)	0.88	8 (13.1)	0.72

Table 2. *Cont.*

	Total Number of Observations [b] n = 1348	With PDR to Any Drug [c,d] n = 215 (15.9%)	p Value	With PDR to EFV/NVP [d] n = 158 (11.7%)	p Value
State of residence, n (%)					
Mexico City	1035 (76.8)	180 (17.4)	<0.01 *	134 (13.0)	<0.01 *
Mexico State	279 (20.7)	32 (11.5)	0.01 *	23 (8.2)	0.02 *
Other	33 (2.5)	3 (9.1)	0.20	1 (3.0)	0.08
HIV subtype, n (%)					
B	1330 (98.7)	211 (15.8)	0.51	155 (11.6)	0.35
Non-B	18 (1.3)	4 (22.1)		3 (16.8)	
Viral load (log RNA copies/mL)					
Median (range)	4.6 (4.1–5.2)	4.6 (4.0–5.1)	0.22	4.6 (3.9–5.1)	0.20
CD4+ T cell count (cells/mm^3)					
Median (IQR)	173 (78–291)	154 (71–281)	0.15	152 (84–284)	0.38
CD4+ T cell count category, n (%)					
<200 cells/mm^3	757 (56.2)	137 (18.1)	<0.01 *	102 (13.5)	0.01
200–500 cells/mm^3	529 (39.2)	70 (13.2)	0.02 *	51 (9.6)	0.03 *
>500 cells/mm^3	60 (4.4)	8 (13.3)	0.36	5 (8.3)	0.28
Missing	2 (0.2)	0 (0.0)	0.70	0 (0.0)	0.78
CD4+ T cell %					
Median (IQR)	13 (7–19)	12 (7–18)	041	14 (8–19)	0.48
Sexual risk category, n (%)					
Heterosexual cis women	78 (5.8)	11 (14.1)	0.39	8 (10.3)	0.42
Heterosexual cis men	172 (12.8)	20 (11.6)	0.06	12 (7.0)	0.02 *
Cisgender MSM	888 (65.9)	139 (15.6)	0.36	105 (11.8)	0.47
Transgender women	31 (2.3)	6 (19.3)	0.37	3 (9.7)	0.50
Missing	179 (13.3)	39 (21.8)	0.02 *	30 (16.8)	0.02 *
Marital status, n (%)					
Single	958 (71.1)	153 (16.0)	0.53	115 (12.0)	0.34
Married	46 (3.4)	7 (15.2)	0.54	3 (6.5)	0.19
Domestic partnership	173 (12.8)	20 (11.6)	0.05	13 (7.5)	0.04 *
Other	29 (2.2)	3 (10.3)	0.29	2 (6.9.6)	0.32
Missing	142 (10.5)	32 (22.5)	0.02 *	25 (17.6)	0.02 *
Education, n (%)					
Illiterate	7 (0.5)	1 (14.3)	0.69	1 (14.3)	0.58
Elementary	59 (4.4)	11 (18.6)	0.33	8 (13.6)	0.38
High School	587 (43.5)	86 (14.6)	0.14	56 (9.5)	0.02 *
Technician	64 (4.7)	10 (15.6)	0.55	9 (14.1)	0.33
Degree	440 (32.6)	69 (15.7)	0.46	54 (12.3)	0.36
Postgraduate	44 (3.26)	5 (11.4)	0.27	4 (9.1)	0.40
Missing	147 (10.91)	33 (22.4)	0.02 *	26 (17.7)	0.02 *
Self-identified social class, n (%)					
Low	477 (35.4)	74 (15.5)	0.40	50 (10.5)	0.17
Middle	717 (53.2)	108 (15.1)	0.19	83 (11.6)	0.46
High	2 (0.2)	1 (50.0)	0.29	0 (0.0)	0.77
Missing	152 (11.3)	32 (21.0)	0.05	25 (16.4)	0.04 *
Indigenous languages spoken, n (%)					
No	1156 (85.7)	177 (15.3)	0.07	130 (11.2)	0.11
Yes	40 (3.0)	6 (15.0)	0.54	3 (7.5)	0.29
Missing	152 (11.3)	32 (21.0)	0.05	25 (16.4)	0.04 *

Table 2. *Cont.*

	Total Number of Observations [b] n = 1348	With PDR to Any Drug [c,d] n = 215 (15.9%)	p Value	With PDR to EFV/NVP [d] n = 158 (11.7%)	p Value
Other sexually transmitted infections, n (%)					
No	633 (47.0)	91 (14.4)	0.08	72 (11.4)	0.38
Yes	426 (31.6)	72 (16.9)	0.28	48 (11.3)	0.40
Preferred not to answer	58 (4.3)	10 (17.2)	0.45	5 (8.6)	0.31
Missing	231 (17.1)	42 (18.2)	0.17	33 (14.3)	0.11
Role in anal sex, n (%)					
Receptive	319 (23.6)	49 (15.4)	0.41	35 (11.0)	0.36
Insertive/Receptive	474 (35.3)	76 (16.0)	0.50	64 (13.5)	0.08
Insertive	223 (16.5)	32 (14.4)	0.27	17 (7.7)	0.02 *
Missing	332 (24.6)	58 (17.5)	0.22	42 (12.6)	0.30
Circumcision, n (%)					
No	807 (59.9)	131 (16.2)	0.39	97 (12.0)	0.37
Yes	240 (17.8)	28 (11.7)	0.03 *	20 (8.3)	0.04 *
Missing	301 (22.3)	56 (18.6)	0.09	41 (13.6)	0.14
Injectable drug use, n (%)					
No	1143 (84.8)	170 (14.9)	<0.01 *	123 (10.8)	<0.01 *
Yes	49 (3.6)	13 (26.5)	0.04 *	10 (20.4)	0.05
Missing	156 (11.6)	32 (20.5)	0.06	25 (16.0)	0.05
Venues for sex, n (%)					
At home	519 (38.5)	82 (15.8)	0.48	62 (11.9)	0.45
At partner's home	290 (21.5)	48 (16.5)	0.40	36 (12.4)	0.37
Venues for sex	93 (6.9)	14 (15.0)	0.47	8 (8.6)	0.22
Multiple	111 (8.2)	12 (10.8)	0.07	8 (7.2)	0.07
Missing	335 (24.8)	59 (17.6)	0.19	44 (13.1)	0.20

[a] Data for 1348 participants enrolled from June to December 2020. [b] Column percentages are shown. [c] Using the WHO definition for PDR (see Methods). [d] Row percentages are shown. * $p < 0.05$. ARV, antiretroviral; EFV, efavirenz; NVP, nevirapine; IQR, interquartile range; MSM, men who have sex with men.

2.2. Overall Estimations of Pretreatment Drug Resistance

After removal of sequences with quality control issues, 6688 PR-RT and 6709 IN sequences were available for HIVDR analysis (a total of 6661 participants had both PR-RT and IN sequences available). Considering the complete study period, overall PDR to any drug class in Mexico City was 14.4% (95% CI: 13.6–15.3%) (Figure 1a). PDR to NNRTI was higher than to any other drug class (12.0%, 95% CI: 11.3–12.8%, $p < 0.0001$), and exceeded the 10% threshold recommended by the WHO for public health action. PDR to NRTI was 4.2% (3.7–4.7%), and to PI, 3.1% (2.7–3.6%). PDR to any INSTI was the lowest (1.0%, 0.8–1.3%, $p < 0.0001$). In agreement with the preferential use of efavirenz-based first-line regimens in Mexico during most of the analysis period, PDR to efavirenz/nevirapine was 10.4% (9.7–11.2%). Nevertheless, PDR to efavirenz/nevirapine + any NRTI remained low (1.1%, 0.9–1.7%). Importantly, given the current preferential use of INSTI-based first-line regimens, PDR to first-generation INSTI was 1.0% (0.8–1.3%) and to second-generation INSTI 0.3% (0.2–0.4%, $p < 0.0001$).

Considering individual drugs, PDR to nevirapine (10.4%, 9.7–11.6%) and to efavirenz (9.3%, 8.6–10.0%) was the highest across the study period, followed by PDR to rilpivirine (5.1%, 4.6–5.7%) (Figure 1b). Emtricitabine and tenofovir showed the lowest PDR among NRTIs (0.5%, 0.4–0.8%, and 1.1%, 0.9–1.4%, respectively). Among the currently used drugs as third component, PDR to boosted darunavir (0.3%, 0.2–0.5%), dolutegravir (0.2%, 0.1–0.4%) and bictegravir (0.1%, 0.0–0.2%) was low.

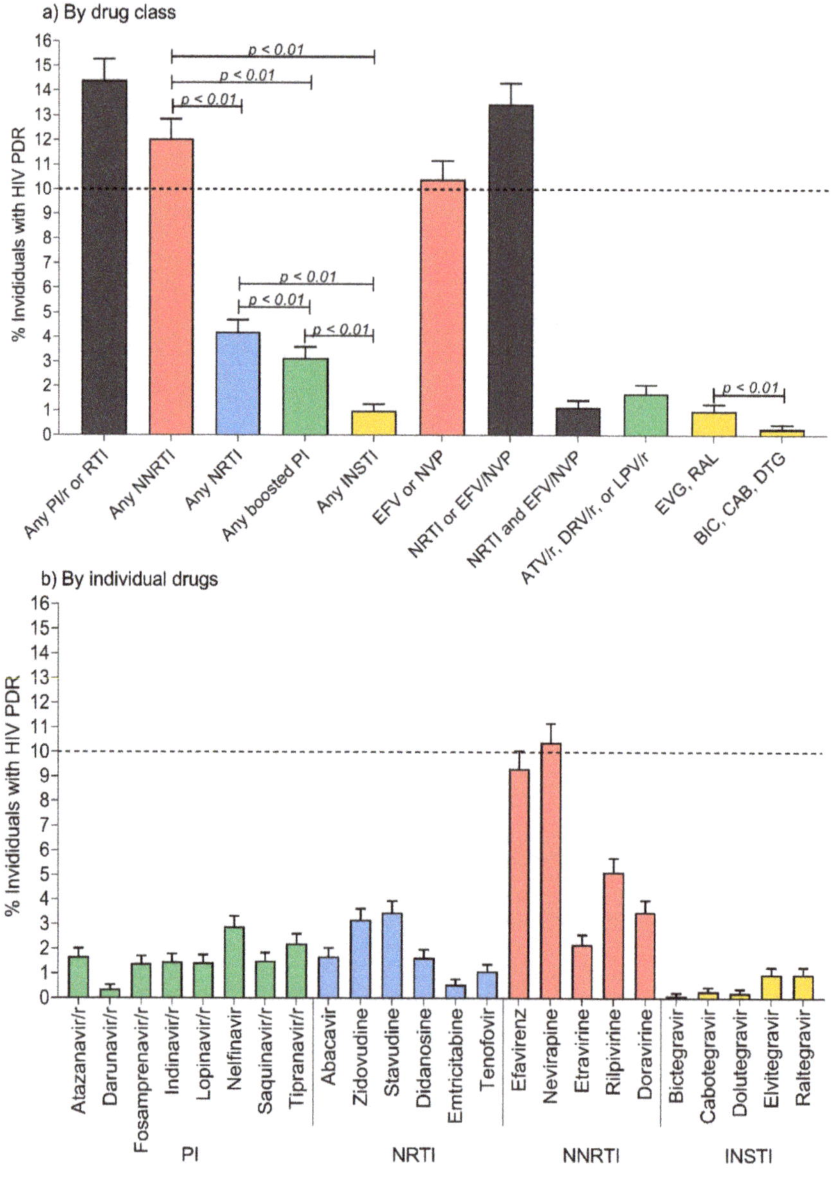

Figure 1. Overall pretreatment drug resistance levels in Mexico City, 2017–2020. Classified by (**a**) drug class, (**b**) individual drug. PDR was estimated from 6688 protease-reverse transcriptase and 6709 integrase sequences using the Stanford HIVdb tool (v9.0). Individuals with HIV PDR were defined as those having a score ≥15 to any of the drugs in the corresponding category, as defined in the Methods. Error bars represent 95% confidence intervals. Comparisons were made with Fisher's exact test. PDR, pretreatment drug resistance; PI, protease inhibitor; RTI, reverse transcriptase inhibitor; NRTI, nucleoside reverse transcriptase inhibitor; NNRTI, non-nucleoside reverse transcriptase inhibitor; INSTI, integrase strand-transfer inhibitor; EFV, efavirenz; NVP, nevirapine; ATV/r, atazanavir/ritonavir; DRV/r, darunavir/ritonavir; LPV/r, lopinavir/ritonavir; EVG, elvitegravir; RAL, raltegravir; BIC, bictegravir; CAB, cabotegravir; DTG, dolutegravir.

The most frequent surveillance drug resistance mutations (SDRMs) were K103NS (6.7%) to NNRTI; M41L (1.2%) and T215CDEF (2.1%) to NRTI; M46IL (1.7%) to PI; and E138AKT (0.2%), Q148HKR (0.1%), and S230R (0.1%) to INSTI (Figure 2a). However, other polymorphic non-SDRMs were also frequent (V106I (3.6%), V179DE (7.1%) in RT) (Figure 2b). Given the low prevalence of non-B subtypes in the study population, associations between specific viral subtypes and the presence of polymorphic mutations were not particularly relevant in the context of the study population, e.g., V106I was present in all F1 subtypes; however, only 6/6661 F1 viruses were observed, while V106IM (generally combined with other NNRTI mutations) was observed in 231/6577 (3.5%) subtype B viruses.

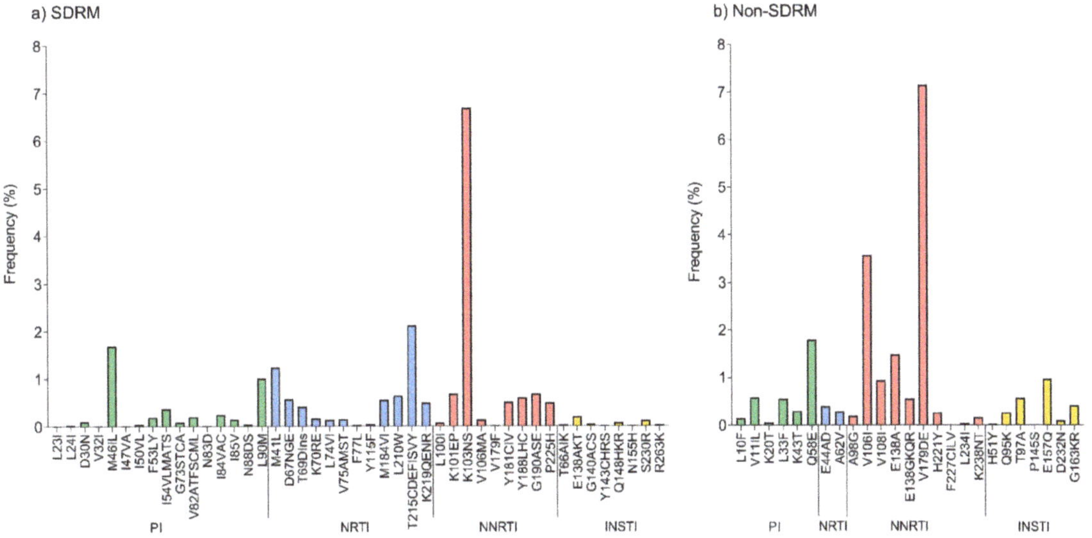

Figure 2. Drug resistance mutation frequency in Mexico City, 2017–2020. Frequencies of surveillance drug resistance mutations (SDRMs) (**a**) and non-SDRMs (**b**) for the complete study period are shown, including a total of 6688 protease-reverse transcriptase and 6709 integrase sequences from unique individuals. Only resistance-associated mutations observed in the sequences are shown. All SDRMs and non-SDRMs defined in the Stanford HIV drug resistance database were analyzed. PI, protease inhibitors; NRTI, nucleoside reverse transcriptase inhibitors; NNRTI, non-nucleoside reverse transcriptase inhibitors; INSTI, integrase strand-transfer inhibitors.

We explored associations of PDR with demographic, clinical, and risk variables collected for a subgroup of participants starting from June to December 2020. As expected, persons with prior exposure to ARV had overall significantly higher prevalence of PDR ($p < 0.01$) (Table 2, Figure 3). This was true for NNRTI and NRTI, but not for boosted PI or INSTI (Figure 3). Persons who inject drugs also showed higher PDR level ($p = 0.04$). Interestingly, persons with incomplete metadata collection in general (who failed to answer several questions of the questionnaire) showed higher PDR ($p < 0.05$). Additionally, persons living in a domestic partnership, with a high school level education, who identified as heterosexual cisgender men, who were circumcised, and who engaged more frequently in insertive sexual relations showed lower PDR to efavirenz/nevirapine (all $p < 0.05$) (Table 1). In general, persons with PDR had slightly lower viral load ($p < 0.05$) (Table 2).

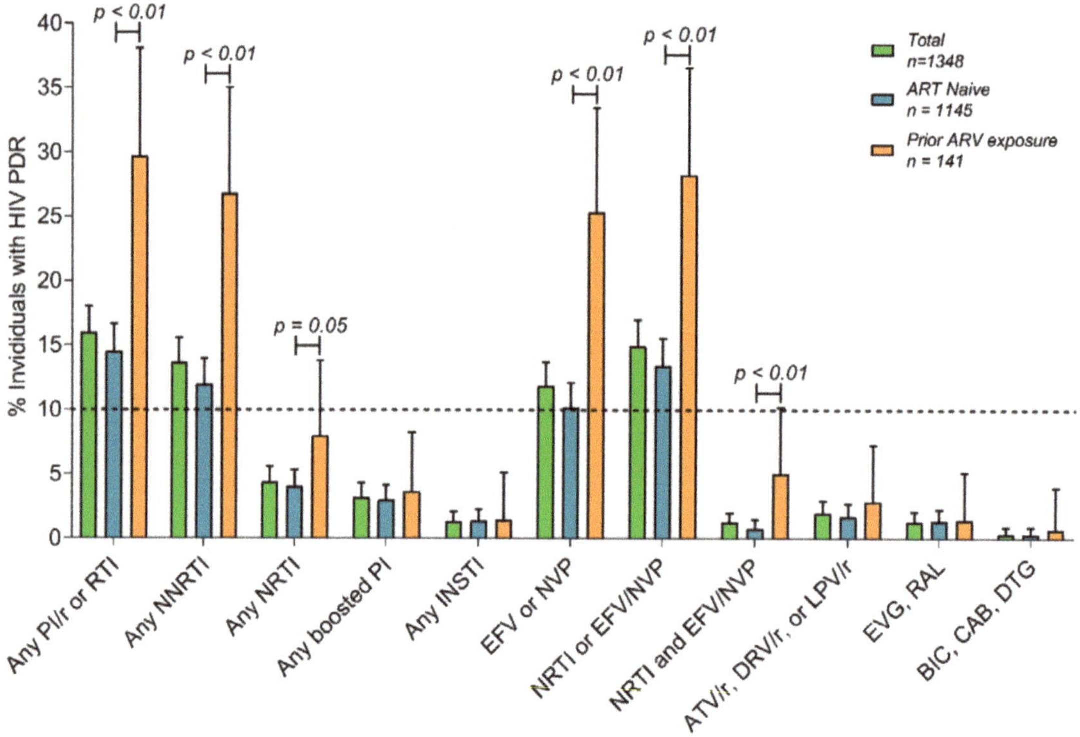

Figure 3. Pretreatment drug resistance in ART-naïve and prior ARV-exposed individuals in Mexico City, 2020. PDR levels are shown for a subset of 1348 participants enrolled from June to December 2020 (data on ARV exposure for 62 participants are missing), for whom data on prior exposure to antiretrovirals were available. Individuals with HIV PDR were defined as those having a score ≥ 15 to any of the drugs in the corresponding category, as defined in the Methods. Error bars represent 95% confidence intervals. Comparisons were made with Fisher's exact test. PDR; pretreatment drug resistance; PI, protease inhibitor; RTI, reverse transcriptase inhibitor; NRTI, nucleoside reverse transcriptase inhibitor; NNRTI, non-nucleoside reverse transcriptase inhibitor; INSTI, integrase strand-transfer inhibitor; EVG, elvitegravir; RAL, raltegravir; BIC, bictegravir; CAB, cabotegravir; DTG, dolutegravir.

The group of participants with prior exposure to ARVs showed significant differences in demographic, clinical, and risk characteristics in comparison to ART-naïve participants, including a higher frequency of cisgender women (12.8 vs. 5.6%), lower frequency of cisgender MSM (60.3 vs. 68.3%), higher age (median: 35 vs. 29 years), lower education (elementary or none: 12.2 vs. 4.8%), higher frequency of persons who inject drugs (8.5 vs. 3.1%), and lower use of apps for finding sexual partners (31.9 vs. 42.8%) ($p < 0.05$ in all cases; Supplementary Table S1). Considering only ART-naïve persons enrolled from June to December 2020, HIVDR reached 10.2% (CI 95%: 8.5–12.1%) to efavirenz/nevirapine, 4.0% (3.0–5.3%) to NRTI, 1.7% (1.1–2.7%) to boosted atazanavir, lopinavir or darunavir, and 1.4% (0.8–2.3%) to any INSTI (Figure 3). Of note, no cases of bictegravir or dolutegravir resistance were observed among prior ARV-exposed participants (only 1 participant (0.7%) showed cabotegravir resistance due to the N155H mutation).

2.3. Pretreatment Drug Resistance Trends across the Study Period

A significant increasing trend for NNRTI PDR was observed from 2017 to 2020 (10.3 to 13.6%, $p = 0.02$). PDR to all other drug classes remained stable: NRTI below 5%, PI below 3.5%, and INSTI below 1% (Figure 4a). Importantly, no increase in PDR to second-generation INSTI was observed, remaining under 0.3% across the complete study period.

The observed increase in NNRTI PDR was mainly attributable to increasing PDR to efavirenz (8.0 to 10.4%; $p = 0.05$), but also to rilpivirine (4.5 to 5.9%, $p = 0.03$) (Figure 4b). No other drugs showed significant trends (Figure S1).

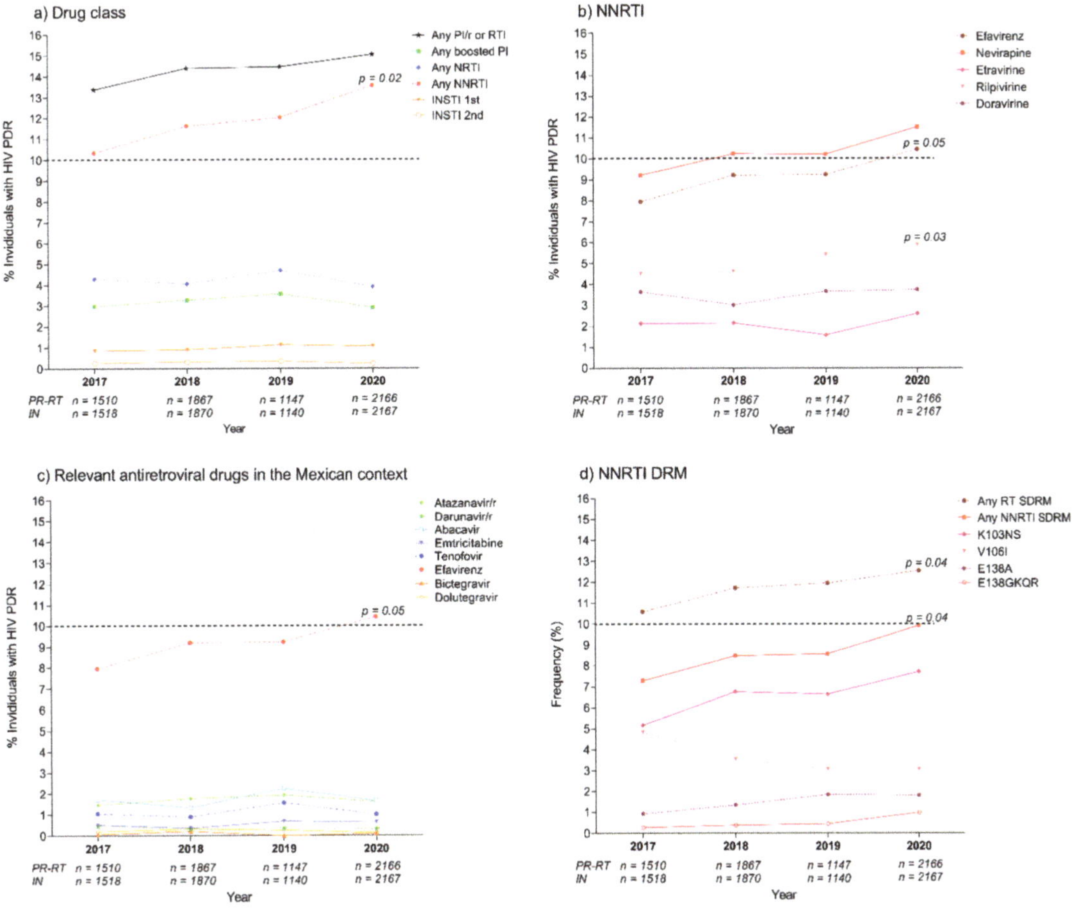

Figure 4. Pretreatment drug resistance trends in Mexico City, 2017–2020. (**a**) By drug class, (**b**) For NNRTI, (**c**) Including relevant antiretroviral drugs in the Mexican context, and (**d**) Including selected drug resistance mutations with relevance to NNRTI PDR. PDR was estimated from protease (PR), reverse transcriptase (RT) and integrase (IN) sequences using the Stanford HIVdb tool (v9.0). Individuals with HIV PDR were defined as those having a Stanford score ≥ 15 for any of the drugs in the corresponding category, as described in the Methods. DRMs included SDRM and non-SDRM. First-generation INSTIs include raltegravir and elvitegravir; second-generation INSTIs include dolutegravir, bictegravir and cabotegravir. Trends were tested using linear regression. PDR, pretreatment drug resistance; PI, protease inhibitors; RTI, reverse transcriptase inhibitors; NRTI, nucleoside reverse transcriptase inhibitors; NNRTI, non-nucleoside reverse transcriptase inhibitors; INSTI, integrase strand-transfer inhibitors; DRM, drug resistance mutation; SDRM, surveillance DRM.

In the Mexican context, PDR to all relevant drugs for currently recommended first-line ART regimens remained stable and below 2%, except for efavirenz (Figure 4c). Regarding possible NRTI backbones, PDR to abacavir, emtricitabine/lamivudine, and tenofovir, remained low (under 2%) and stable. The same was true for boosted darunavir (under 0.5%), and dolutegravir/bictegravir (under 0.3%).

A significant increasing trend was observed in the prevalence of any RT SDRM across the study period (10.6 to 12.5%, $p = 0.04$), particularly to any NNRTI SDRM (7.3 to 10.0%, $p = 0.04$). The prevalence of K103NS varied from 5.2 to 7.7%, but this increase was not significant ($p = 0.08$) (Figure 4d). No other DRM (including both SDRM and non-SDRM) showed significant prevalence changes during the period (Figure S2).

2.4. Associations of Pretreatment Drug Resistance with Epidemiological Variables

We analyzed possible associations between the presence of PDR and demographic and clinical variables. This analysis encompassed only individuals enrolled from June 2020 to December 2020, a period in which variables were collected through a computer-based questionnaire and the completeness of the metadata was acceptable. After multivariable adjustment, the presence of PDR to any drug remained strongly associated with prior exposure to ARV drugs (adjusted odds ratio, aOR: 2.7, 95% CI: 1.7–4.1, $p = 0.001$). The odds of PDR were higher in persons presenting to care with <200 CD4+ T cells/mm^3 compared to 200–499 CD4+ T cells/mm^3 (aOR: 1.6, 95% CI: 1.2–2.2, $p = 0.005$) (Table 3).

Table 3. Risk factors for HIV pretreatment drug resistance in Mexico City, June–December 2020.

	Resistance to Any ARV [a]			Resistance to NNRTI [a]		
	aOR	95% CI	*p* Value	aOR	95% CI	*p* Value
Age (years) [b]	1.0	1.0–1.0	0.07	1.0	1.0–1.0	0.1
Sexual risk category [c]						
Heterosexual cis men	Ref.			Ref.		
Heterosexual cis women	1.1	0.5–2.5	0.8	1.3	0.5–3.5	0.6
Cisgender MSM	1.5	0.9–2.4	0.2	1.9	1.0–3.5	0.1
Transgender women	1.9	0.7–5.4	0.2	1.5	0.4–5.7	0.6
Missing	2.8	1.1–7.0	0.03 *	3.2	1.1–9.3	0.03 *
Injectable drug use						
No	Ref.			Ref.		
Yes	1.7	0.9–3.7	0.07	1.8	0.8–3.8	0.1
Missing	0.9	0.4–2.0	0.7	1.0	0.4–2.6	1.0
CD4+ T cell count category						
200–499 cells/mm^3	Ref.			Ref.		
<200 cells/mm^3	1.6	1.2–2.2	0.005 *	1.6	1.1–2.4	0.01 *
≥500 cells/mm^3	1.0	0.4–2.1	0.9	0.8	0.3–2.1	0.6
Viral load (log copies/mL) [b]	0.9	0.7–1.1	0.2	0.9	0.7–1.1	0.2
Prior ARV exposure						
No	Ref.			Ref.		
Yes	2.7	1.7–4.1	0.001 *	3.4	2.1–5.3	0.001 *
Missing	0.9	0.4–1.8	0.7	1.0	0.4–2.2	0.9

[a] $n = 1348$; [b] Analyzed as a continuous variable; [c] Sexual risk category was assessed as a composite variable including sex at birth, gender identity and sexual practices. aOR, adjusted odds ratio; CI, confidence interval; ARV, antiretroviral; NNRTI, non-nucleoside reverse transcriptase inhibitors; MSM, men who have sex with men; Ref., reference category. * Statistically significant.

2.5. Analysis of HIV PDR Transmission within Mexico City's HIV Genetic Network

We identified clusters of individuals with PDR within Mexico City's HIV transmission network. The network was inferred from 6688 PR-RT sequences from individuals arriving to care from 2017 to 2020, from which 2960 (44.3%) were found to belong to 820 clusters, ranging in size from 2 to 41 nodes (Figure 5). No difference was observed between clustering and non-clustering individuals in the proportion of viruses with PDR to any drug (13.9 vs. 14.7%, p = 0.65) or to efavirenz/nevirapine (9.7 vs. 11.0%, p = 0.15). A total of 19.4% (159/820) of all clusters included at least one person with PDR and 14.8% (121/820) included at least one person with resistance to efavirenz/nevirapine. Resistance to efavirenz/nevirapine was associated with transmission of K103NS alone in 7.9% (65/820) of clusters, K103NS plus other NNRTI mutations in 3.4% (28/820) clusters and with other NNRTI mutations in 8.0% (66/820) of clusters (Figure 5). In 41.3% (50/121) of the clusters with efavirenz/nevirapine PDR, resistance was shared by 100% of the nodes, and in 32.4% (38/121) by 50 to 99% of the nodes. Some examples of the larger clusters evidencing NNRTI PDR transmission included cluster NNRTI-1, with 14 nodes, all men living in Mexico City with median age 28 years (IQR 23–31), all of them with K103NS; cluster NNRTI-2, with 27 nodes formed by men with median age 25 (23–30) enrolled across the complete study period, 11% (3/27) with K103NS and 74% (20/27) with other mutations; NNRTI-3, with 21 nodes, including men living in Mexico City and the State of Mexico and median age 24 (20–29), 62% (13/21) with K103NS; and cluster NNRTI-4, with 12 nodes, all men with median age 28 (25–32), all sharing E138A (Figure 5).

A total of 2.7% (22/820) of the clusters included at least one person with INSTI PDR and only 0.7% (6/820) with at least one person with bictegravir/dolutegravir resistance. The largest clusters with INSTI PDR transmission were cluster INSTI-1, with 5 nodes sharing the S230R mutation, formed by 4 cisgender men and 1 transgender woman, with median age 23 (20–32); and cluster INSTI-2, with 4 nodes, all men sharing the E157Q and G163K mutations and median age 28 (26–34).

Other interesting clusters evidencing PDR transmission within the network included cluster PI-1, with 29 nodes, all men with PI resistance and median age 24 (22–28) enrolled across all years; cluster NRTI-1, with 23 nodes, 22 cisgender men and 1 cisgender woman, with median age 22 (10–27) and constant growth across all years; cluster complex-1, with 10 nodes, all men enrolled from 2018 to 2020 and median age 23 (20–30), 60% (6/10) with PI + NRTI + NNRTI resistance and 40% (4/10) with PI + NRTI resistance; and complex-2, with 7 nodes, all men with median age 26 (21–31) sharing PR M46I, L90M, RT M41L, D67N, T69D, L210W, T215D and RT K103N, Y181C (Figure 5).

2.6. *Characteristics and Prevalence of Acquired Drug Resistance in Mexico City, 2020*

In order to describe acquired drug resistance in the context of ART optimization in Mexico City, starting in 2019, we analyzed all clinically indicated HIV genotypes for persons cared for at the Condesa clinics in 2020, who had two consecutive viral load estimations > 1000 copies/mL. A total of 143 individuals were eligible (see Methods). From these, we obtained 142 successful PR-RT sequences and 137 IN sequences. After quality filtering, 133 PR-RT and 128 IN sequences were used for the analysis. Overall, 39.8% (95% CI: 31.5–48.7%) individuals had ADR to any drug class (Figure 6a). Considering individual drug classes, 34.6% (26.6–43.3%) of individuals showed ADR to NNRTI, 26.3% (19.1–34.7%) to NRTI, 1.5% (0.2–5.3%) to boosted PI, and 2.3% (0.5–6.7%) to INSTI. A total of 21.1% (14.5–29.0%) showed resistance to NRTI and efavirenz/nevirapine. Considering individual drugs, 33.8% individuals were resistant to efavirenz, 23.3% to emtricitabine/lamivudine, and 8.3% to tenofovir. Resistance to dolutegravir/bictegravir was 2.3% and to darunavir 0%. Regarding other drugs commonly used in second or third line, ADR to etravirine was 14.3%, 18.8% to rilpivirine, 20.3% to doravirine, and 2.3% to zidovudine (Figure 6b). The most commonly observed DRMs were K103NS (24.1%) and M184VI (23.3%) in RT. Resistance in IN was mainly due to R263K (1.6%) and E138AKT, G140ACS, Q148HKR (0.8% each) (Figure 6c). The relatively high resistance to doravirine is noteworthy, and was mainly associated with mutations Y188L (4.5%, in most cases combined with V106I), L100IV (4.5%), K103EP (3.8%), P225H (3.0%).

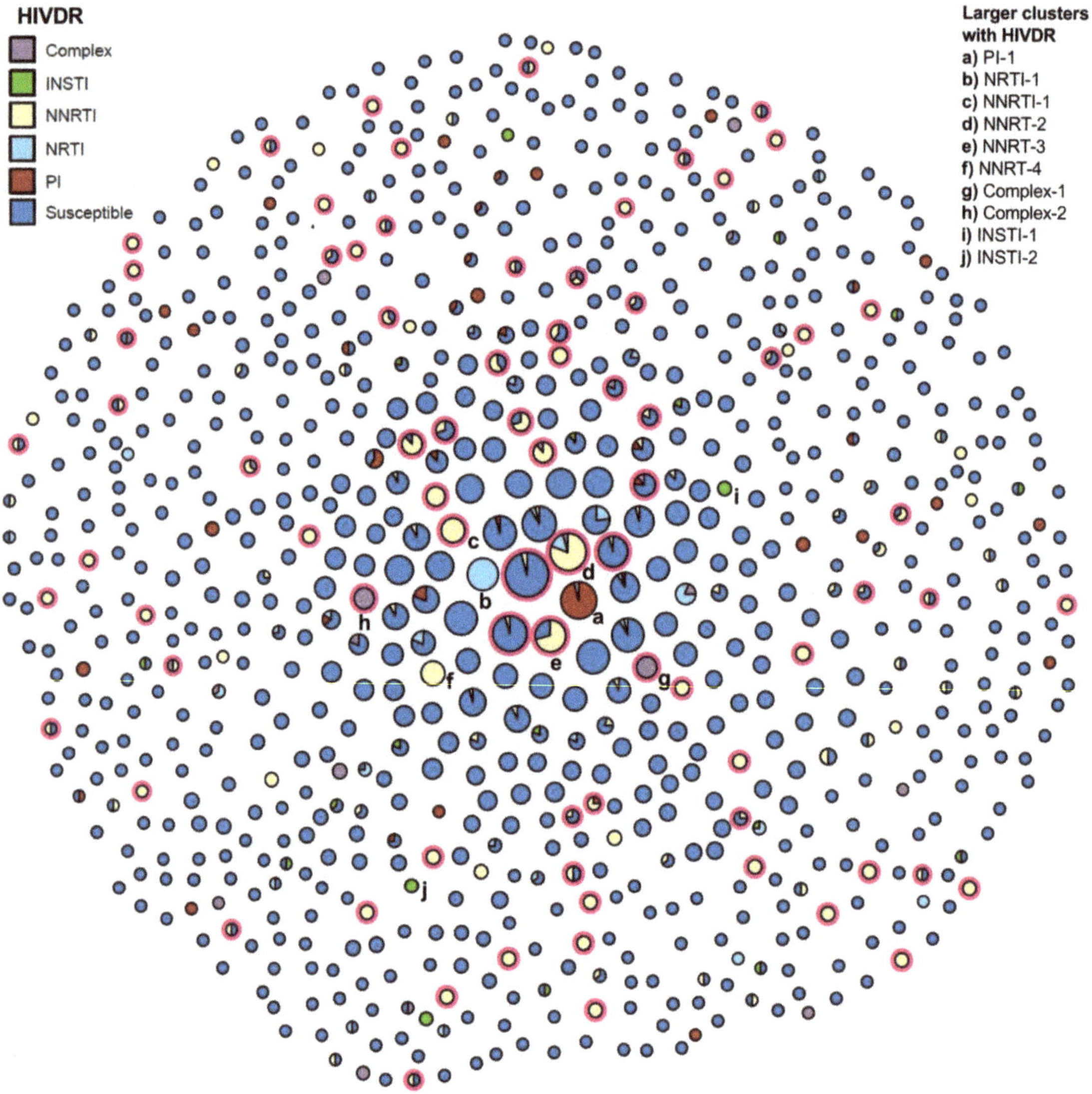

Figure 5. PDR transmission within Mexico City's HIV genetic network, 2017–2020. The network was inferred from 6688 protease-reverse transcriptase sequences from individuals arriving to care from 2017 to 2020, using a locally adapted version of the HIV-TRACE tool. Each circle represents a cluster. The size of the circle reflects the size of the cluster. Clusters are colored according to the presence of pretreatment drug resistance by drug class. Specific clusters mentioned in the text are identified with letters on the lower-right side. Red circles surrounding clusters show the presence of viruses with the K103NS mutation.

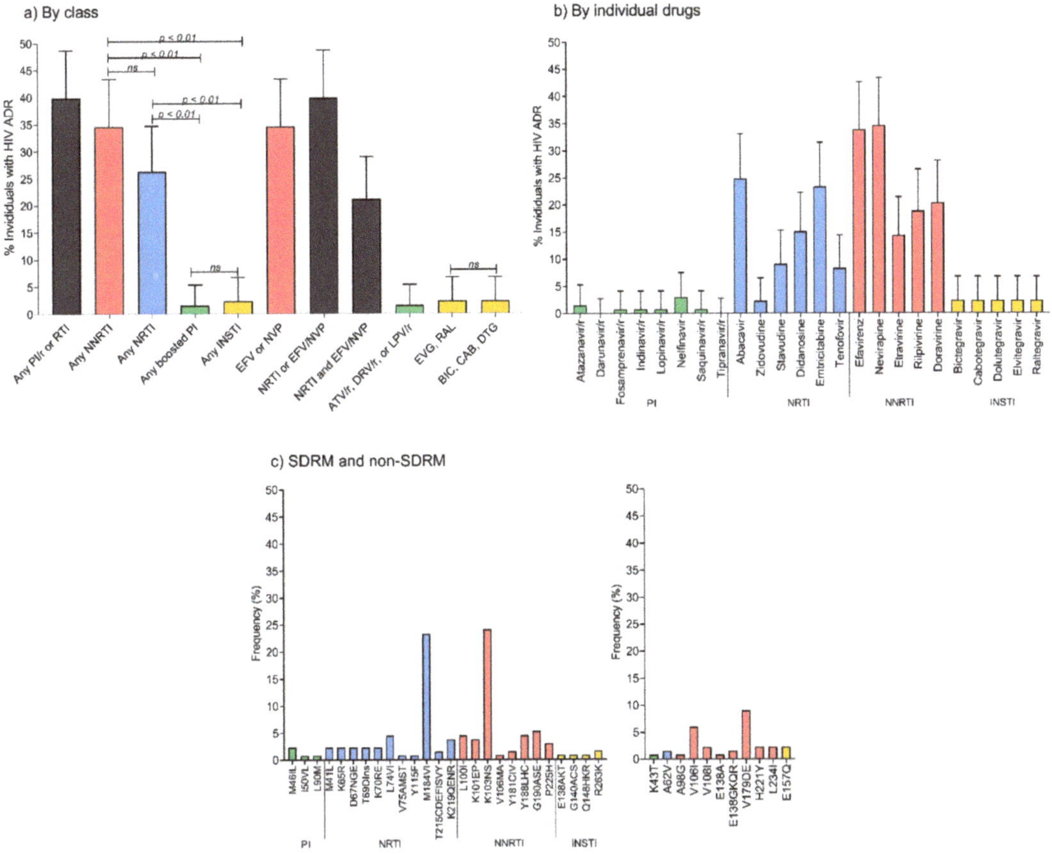

Figure 6. Acquired drug resistance in Mexico City, 2020. (**a**) By drug class, (**b**) by individual drugs, (**c**) SDRM and non-SDRM. ADR was estimated from protease (PR), reverse transcriptase (RT) and integrase (IN) sequences using the Stanford HIVdb tool (v9.0). Individuals with HIV ADR were defined as those having a Stanford score ≥ 15 for any of the drugs in the corresponding category, as described in the Methods. ADR, acquired drug resistance; PI, protease inhibitors; RTI, reverse transcriptase inhibitors; NRTI, nucleoside reverse transcriptase inhibitors; NNRTI, non-nucleoside reverse transcriptase inhibitors; INSTI, integrase strand-transfer inhibitors; EFV, efavirenz; NVP, nevirapine; ATV/r, atazanavir/ritonavir; DRV/r, darunavir/ritonavir; LPV/r, lopinavir/ritonavir; EVG, elvitegravir; RAL, raltegravir; BIC, bictegravir; CAB, cabotegravir; DTG, dolutegravir; DRM, drug resistance mutation; SDRM, surveillance DRM.

3. Discussion

The present study showed an increasing trend of PDR to efavirenz in Mexico City from 2017 to 2020, crossing the 10% threshold by the end of the study period, while PDR to dolutegravir and bictegravir remained low and under 0.5%. Given the high genetic barrier of second-generation INSTI-based ART regimens [13], as well as the low impact of baseline DRMs observed in the NRTI backbone in the effectiveness of these regimens [14], HIV PDR surveillance has become less of a priority in regions widely using dolutegravir and bictegravir. Nevertheless, given the historical rapid increase in NNRTI resistance in LMICs worldwide, it is important to maintain surveillance in order to detect increasing PDR trends in time and save important ART options for future management of HIV, strengthening HIV programs with focus on HIVDR-associated early warning indicators. Focused HIVDR surveillance to identify specific regions and populations with specific vulnerability issues and programmatic gaps is also important to improve the HIV care continuum with focused interventions and to optimize both first- and second-line ART regimens, as well as pre- (PrEP) and post-exposure prophylaxis (PEP) regimens.

As expected, PDR to efavirenz/nevirapine continued to grow in Mexico City across the study period, maintaining the previously observed trend [10]. Importantly, no changes in this trend were observed after the nationwide implementation and procurement of second-generation INSTI-based regimens as preferred first-line options since the second half of 2019, which suggests onward transmission of efavirenz resistance even in the context of a significantly reduced use of the drug. Indeed, when analyzing Mexico City's HIV transmission network for the study period, we observed 88 clusters for which at least 50% of the nodes shared NNRTI PDR mutations. These included large clusters formed mainly by young cisgender men sharing the K103NS mutation and other NNRTI PDR-associated mutations. It is also important to consider the possible impact of ongoing DRM transmission on the growing cross-resistance trend to rilpivirine observed in the present study for the future use of long-acting regimens as part of both first- and second-line ART as well as PrEP regimens.

As expected, efavirenz/nevirapine resistance and, in general, PDR to any ARV drug were strongly associated with prior exposure to ARVs. The group of persons with prior exposure to ARVs in Mexico City was mostly formed by persons that, after being lost to clinical follow-up, later returned to clinical care to restart ART, keeping in mind that PrEP is not yet widely available in Mexico. This group of ART restarters represents an important challenge and target for possible interventions, and it showed specific characteristics that were different from the rest of the study population, including higher representation of cisgender women and transgender women, higher age, lower education in general and higher representation of injectable drug users (Table S1). Some of these characteristics were described previously in a nationwide PDR study [9]. Unexpectedly, the odds of having PDR were not specifically higher in cisgender women, as observed in previous studies in Mexico and in other countries [5,9]. In the context of Mexico City, contrasted with other regions of Mexico, the epidemic is highly concentrated in MSM [15] who are generally younger, have a higher education level, and arrive earlier to clinical care than the heterosexual population [16,17]. In this context, MSM had significantly higher odds of efavirenz/nevirapine PDR compared to heterosexual cisgender men, possibly reflecting ongoing transmission of NNRTI resistance mutations such as K103NS and E138A. On the other hand, it is reassuring that both PDR and ADR to dolutegravir and bictegravir in 2020 remained low, although further surveillance is warranted given the short time of implementation of ART optimization nationwide. Taking this into consideration, most ADR cases observed in the present study could still be associated with failures to offer efavirenz-based first-line regimens in persons who had not yet switched to INSTI-based options, which is also consistent with the high frequency of K103NS and M184VI observed in persons with ADR. Also noteworthy is the fact that persons arriving to care with advanced infection had higher odds of PDR. This could be associated with ART defaulters who, years later, return to clinical care because of complications associated with opportunistic infections, but could also suggest a subpopulation of MSM characterized by late arrival to clinical care. Interestingly, this study identified a subset of individuals that did not answer several of the questions in the computer-based questionnaire and that were characterized overall by significantly higher PDR (Table 2). Further studies including in-depth interviews could be highly valuable for understanding this group, as it may present common vulnerability issues. Finally, although the level of ADR to dolutegravir/bictegravir observed in 2020 was low, it still warrants strengthening of strategies to improve adherence both at the clinic and community levels, especially in groups with a high risk of ART defaulting. This is especially relevant given that the overall level of ADR observed in this study was lower than that observed in other countries [5], possibly suggesting more frequent interruption of ART in persons without viral suppression. Also important is the high prevalence of cross-resistance to doravirine in persons with ADR. This drug is not yet available in Mexico, but the current level of cross-resistance observed could limit its use locally.

The present study has important limitations worth mentioning. First, all participants were enrolled at a single institution, which may cause selection bias. Even though the Condesa clinic encompasses an important proportion of new diagnoses in the metropolitan area of Mexico City, a fraction of the population living with HIV could be underrepresented, especially persons living in areas with local social security clinics that offer HIV testing within the city. Nevertheless, even though the Condesa clinics care for persons lacking health insurance, 42% of HIV diagnoses performed at the clinics are in persons with social security [15], from which approximately 20% are lost to follow-up and most probably later return to clinical care in subsequent years or die. This fact strengthens the representativeness of the study population, even when coming from a single center. Second, information bias could exist, especially given that metadata collection was poor, especially at the beginning of the study period. Still, given its role as the most important HIV diagnosis center in Mexico City and the size of the clinic, we expect the study population to be highly representative of the population of persons living with HIV locally. Third, the present study excludes important populations that warrant further studies in both their specific vulnerabilities and structural challenges and their contribution to HIV PDR, especially male adolescents who have sex with men.

4. Materials and Methods

4.1. Study Population

A cross-sectional, observational study was conducted at the Condesa Specialized Clinic, with two branches in Mexico City (located in the municipalities of Cuauhtémoc and Iztapalapa), between 2017–2020. The Condesa Specialized Clinic is the largest primary HIV care clinic and one of the main HIV diagnostic centers in Mexico, having diagnosed nearly 3500 individuals in 2020, approximately 70% of all the new infections in Mexico City's metropolitan zone [15]. All adults (>18 years) attending the Condesa Clinic for an HIV test, having received a positive result, including new diagnoses, referrals from other institutions, and persons returning to care after at least 3 months of ART defaulting, were invited to participate in the study between January 2017 and December 2020. These inclusion criteria were defined according to the WHO PDR definition [5]. Participants gave written informed consent to participate in the study. Since 2020, a computer-based self-administered questionnaire including demographic and clinical data was applied (a paper-based version of the questionnaire was available for participants preferring this option). Analysis of the variables included in the questionnaire was performed in a subset of the participants enrolled from June 2020 to December 2020. All participants donated a blood specimen for HIV sequencing and DR testing. HIV sequencing was performed at the Center for Research in Infectious Diseases of the National Institute of Respiratory Diseases (CIENI/INER), a reference center for HIV genotyping, following strict quality assurance processes. The study was reviewed and approved by the Institutional Review Board of the National Institute of Respiratory Diseases (project codes E12-17 and E02-20) and was conducted according to the principles of the Declaration of Helsinki.

Analysis of the characteristics and prevalence of acquired drug resistance was performed in an independent study group, including all clinically indicated HIV genotypes recorded at the National Ministry of Health HIV Database (SALVAR) from January 2020 to December 2020, as part of the national HIV program. HIV genotyping is recommended by the Mexican ART Guidelines for switching to second- and third-line regimens. All persons cared for at the Condesa clinic with two consecutive viral load values > 1000 copies/mL, whose second viral load test was performed in 2020, were included in the analysis. HIV sequencing was performed at CIENI/INER from the same blood specimen donated for the second viral load test, using internally validated Sanger sequencing methods, as explained below.

4.2. HIV Amplification and Sequencing

Sequences were obtained by next generation sequencing from a single amplicon including the complete protease (PR), reverse transcriptase (RT) and integrase (IN) genes (HXB2: PR 1-99, RT 1-560 and IN 1-288), using an in-house-validated method with Illumina sequencing technology on a MiSeq instrument (San Diego, CA, USA), as previously described [16,17]. A minority of the specimens in which amplification of this longer amplicon was not successful, as well as clinically indicated HIV genotypes for the ADR analysis, were amplified using a validated protocol developed by the US Centers for Disease Control and Prevention for the PR-RT region (HXB2 positions: PR 6-99, RT 1-251) [18] and an in-house developed and validated protocol for IN (HXB2: IN 1-288) [19]. These shorter amplicons were sequenced using NGS with standard Illumina protocols or by Sanger sequencing on a 3730xl Genetic Analyzer (ThermoFisher, Waltham, MA, USA) as previously described [10].

Next generation sequencing reads were filtered and assembled using HyDRA (Public Health Agency of Canada, Winnipeg, MB, Canada) [17,20]. Twenty percent consensus sequences (previously validated as Sanger-like sequences) were obtained and used for the HIVDR analyses [21]. Sanger sequences were assembled and edited using ReCall (BC Centre for Excellence in HIV/AIDS, Vancouver, BC, Canada) [22].

4.3. HIV Drug Resistance Assessment

Quality controls were applied to the sequences included in the database using the WHO HIVDR quality control tool [23,24]. Sequences not compliant with quality control were excluded from the study. Reasons for exclusion included inadequate sequence length, presence of stop codons, frameshift insertions/deletions, excess Apolipoprotein B mRNA-Editing Catalytic Polypeptide-like (APOBEC) or unusual mutations [23,24]. For participants with more than one sequence available, the first sequence was selected.

PDR was estimated using the Stanford HIVdb tool V.9.0 [24] and reported by drug class and individual drugs. Sequences with HIVDR were defined as those with a Stanford score $\geq$ 15 (at least low-level resistance) for efavirenz, nevirapine, any nucleoside reverse transcriptase inhibitor (NRTI), boosted darunavir, lopinavir, or atazanavir, raltegravir, elvitegravir, dolutegravir, or bictegravir, according to WHO standardized protocols [25]. PDR to INSTI was also reported referring to first-generation (raltegravir and elvitegravir) and second-generation INSTI (dolutegravir, bictegravir, and cabotegravir). HIVDR prevalence was estimated using a predefined Excel template developed for the WHO HIV ResNet Laboratory Network [26] (available by request from the corresponding author). HIV subtype was inferred using the REGAHIV-1 Subtyping Tool version 3.0 [27].

4.4. Associations between Pretreatment Drug Resistance and Epidemiological Variables

Exploratory analyses were performed comparing persons with and without PDR to any drug or with PDR to efavirenz/nevirapine, using Mann–Whitney U, chi square, or Fisher's exact tests, in accordance with the type of variable. Age and viral load were analyzed as continuous variables; gender, state of residence, marital status, education, social class, sexual risk, injectable drug use, use of venues for sex, and previous exposure to ARV were analyzed as categorical variables. CD4+ T cell count was stratified according to CDC clinical categories. Univariate associations between demographic, clinical and behavioral variables available and the presence of PDR to any ARV drug or PDR to efavirenz/nevirapine were explored with logistic regression, including only participants enrolled from June to December 2020, when completion of the metadata was best. Multivariable logistic regression models were constructed using all variables significantly associated with PDR in the univariate analyses. Additional variables were included a priori, owing to previous interest in HIVDR development. The best model was selected using Akaike information criterion, Bayesian information criterion, and Hosmer–Lemeshow goodness of fit test. Analyses were performed using STATA v16.

4.5. HIV Transmission Network Inference

The network was defined using a genetic matrix method based on PR-RT sequences, with Seguro HIV-TRAnsmission Cluster Engine (Seguro HIV-TRACE) [16], a locally adapted and secured version of the HIV-TRACE tool [28]. Clusters were defined when sequences showed pairwise Tamura–Nei 93 genetic distance < 1.5%. Although IN sequences were not used for network inference, the presence or absence of HIVDR to INSTI was considered as an additional attribute of each node.

5. Conclusions

The present study showed a continued increasing trend of NNRTI PDR in the context of Mexico City's HIV epidemic in 2017–2020, which was strongly associated with ongoing NNRTI DRM transmission, even with a much lower efavirenz use. It is reassuring that both PDR and ADR to dolutegravir and bictegravir have remained low locally after the widespread rollout of ART first-line regimens based on these drugs locally. Our study also identified demographic characteristics of groups with higher risk of PDR and higher probability of becoming lost to follow-up, in particular, ART restarters. The observations of the present study may be useful to guide clinical care algorithm design within the Condesa clinics in order to identify persons with these profiles who may need specific interventions differentiated from the rest of the population. In the same sense, our observations warrant further in-depth studies in the population of cisgender women, young MSM, and adolescents in order to design better strategies for retention in care and viral suppression.

Supplementary Materials: The following are available online at https://www.mdpi.com/article/10.3390/pathogens10121587/s1, Figure S1. Pretreatment drug resistance trends in Mexico City by antiretroviral drug, 2017–2020; Figure S2. Pretreatment antiretroviral drug resistance mutation frequency trends in Mexico City, 2017–2020; Table S1. Demographic, clinical, and behavioral characteristics of antiretroviral treatment restarters.

Author Contributions: Conceptualization, S.Á.-R. and C.G.-M.; methodology, D.T.-T., M.M.-F., V.S.Q.-M.; software, E.Z.-S.; formal analysis, C.G.-M. and V.D.-C.; investigation, S.Á.-R. and C.G.-M.; resources, S.Á.-R., G.R.-T. and A.G.-R.; local sampling, P.I.-H., R.G.-M., R.A.C. and A.G.-C.; data collection, Á.B.-B., M.C.-S. and M.B.-R.; participant recruitment, I.M.-G., Á.B.-B., M.C.-S. and M.B.-R.; data curation, C.G.-M. and D.T.-T.; writing—original draft preparation, S.Á.-R. and C.G.-M.; writing—review and editing, all authors; funding acquisition, G.R.-T., A.G.-R. and S.Á.-R. All authors have read and agreed to the published version of the manuscript.

Funding: This work was supported by Consejo Nacional de Ciencia y Tecnología (PRONAII Virología 303079 and CONACyT SALUD-2017-01-289725), the Mexican Government (Programa Presupuestal P016; Anexo 13 del Decreto del Presupuesto de Egresos de la Federación), the Canadian Institutes of Health Research (PJT-148621 and PJT-159625), the San Diego Center for AIDS Research International Pilot Grant (P30 AI036214, subaward no. 112605914). Á.B.-B. was supported by a scholarship from the AIDS Healthcare Foundation (AHF) Mexico.

Institutional Review Board Statement: The study was conducted according to the guidelines of the Declaration of Helsinki and approved by the Institutional Review Board of the National Institute of Respiratory Diseases (protocol code E02-17 approved on 1 October 2016 and E20-20 approved on 23 January 2020).

Informed Consent Statement: Written informed consent was obtained from all subjects involved in the study, except for individuals included in the acquired drug resistance analysis, for which national surveillance data were used, without the interaction of researchers and study participants.

Data Availability Statement: Data sets supporting the observations of the present study are available upon request from the corresponding author.

Acknowledgments: The authors would like to thank Edna Rodríguez-Aguirre for performing CD4+ T cell counts; Ramón Hernández-Juan for performing viral loads, Eduardo López-Ortiz for assistance in figure preparation, the laboratory staff at Condesa Specialised Clinic: Karina Nava-Memije, Maritza M. García-Lucas, Alieth A. Piña-Cruz, and the administrative staff at CIENI/INER: Guadalupe

Hernández-Reyes, Marisol Cruz, María de Jesús Espinosa, Omar Quevedo, Ofelia Gómez-Guerrero, Dania Pulido-Ravelo, Diana Ek-Reyes.

Conflicts of Interest: The authors declare no conflict of interest. The funders had no role in the design of the study; in the collection, analyses, or interpretation of data; in the writing of the manuscript; or in the decision to publish the results.

References

1. Palella, F.J.; Loveless, M.O.; Holmberg, S.D. Declining Morbidity and Mortality among Patients with Advanced Human Immunodeficiency Virus Infection. *N. Engl. J. Med.* **1998**, *338*, 853–860. [CrossRef]
2. Eaton, J.W.; Johnson, L.F.; Salomon, J.A.; Bärnighausen, T.; Bendavid, E.; Bershteyn, A.; Bloom, D.E.; Cambiano, V.; Fraser, C.; Hontelez, J.A.C.; et al. HIV Treatment as Prevention: Systematic Comparison of Mathematical Models of the Potential Impact of Antiretroviral Therapy on HIV Incidence in South Africa. *PLoS Med.* **2012**, *9*, e1001245. [CrossRef]
3. WHO. HIV Data and Statistics. Available online: https://www.who.int/teams/control-of-neglected-tropical-diseases/yaws/diagnosis-and-treatment/hiv (accessed on 28 October 2021).
4. WHO. HIV Drug Resistance Report. 2019. Available online: https://www.who.int/publications/i/item/WHO-CDS-HIV-19.21 (accessed on 28 October 2021).
5. WHO. Surveillance of HIV Drug Resistance in Adults Initiating Antiretroviral Therapy Pretreatment HIV Drug Resistance. Concept Note. 2014. Available online: https://www.who.int/publications/i/item/9789241507196 (accessed on 18 November 2021).
6. Gupta, R.K.; Gregson, J.; Parkin, N.; Haile-Selassie, H.; Tanuri, A.; Andrade Forero, L.; Kaleebu, P.; Watera, C.; Aghokeng, A.; Mutenda, N.; et al. HIV-1 Drug Resistance before Initiation or Re-Initiation of First-Line Antiretroviral Therapy in Low-Income and Middle-Income Countries: A Systematic Review and Meta-Regression Analysis. *Lancet Infect. Dis.* **2018**, *18*, 346–355. [CrossRef]
7. WHO. Consolidated Guidelines on HIV Prevention, Testing, Treatment, Service Delivery and Monitoring: Recommendations for a Public Health Approach. Available online: https://www.who.int/publications-detail-redirect/9789240031593 (accessed on 28 October 2021).
8. Ávila-Ríos, S.; García-Morales, C.; Matías-Florentino, M.; Romero-Mora, K.A.; Tapia-Trejo, D.; Quiroz-Morales, V.S.; Reyes-Gopar, H.; Ji, H.; Sandstrom, P.; Casillas-Rodríguez, J.; et al. Pretreatment HIV-Drug Resistance in Mexico and Its Impact on the Effectiveness of First-Line Antiretroviral Therapy: A Nationally Representative 2015 WHO Survey. *Lancet HIV* **2016**, *3*, e579–e591. [CrossRef]
9. Ávila-Ríos, S.; García-Morales, C.; Valenzuela-Lara, M.; Chaillon, A.; Tapia-Trejo, D.; Pérez-García, M.; López-Sánchez, D.M.; Maza-Sánchez, L.; del Arenal-Sánchez, S.J.; Paz-Juárez, H.E.; et al. HIV-1 Drug Resistance before Initiation or Re-Initiation of First-Line ART in Eight Regions of Mexico: A Sub-Nationally Representative Survey. *J. Antimicrob. Chemother.* **2019**, *74*, 1044–1055. [CrossRef]
10. García-Morales, C.; Tapia-Trejo, D.; Quiroz-Morales, V.S.; Navarro-Álvarez, S.; Barrera-Arellano, C.A.; Casillas-Rodríguez, J.; Romero-Mora, K.A.; Gómez-Palacio-Schjetnan, M.; Murakami-Ogasawara, A.; Ávila-Ríos, S.; et al. HIV Pretreatment Drug Resistance Trends in Three Geographic Areas of Mexico. *J. Antimicrob. Chemother.* **2017**, *72*, 3149–3158. [CrossRef]
11. Secretaría de Salud, Centro Nacional para la Prevencion y el Control del VIH y el SIDA. Guia de Manejo Antirretroviral de las Personas que Viven con el VIH/SIDA. CENSIDA: Mexico City, Mexico, 2021; ISBN 9789707210127.
12. Secretaría de Salud, Centro Nacional para la Prevención y el Control del VIH y el SIDA. *Boletín de Atención Integral de Personas que Viven con VIH*; CENSIDA: Mexico City, Mexico, 2021. Available online: https://www.gob.mx/censida/articulos/boletin-de-diagnostico-y-tratamiento-antirretroviral-censida?idiom=es (accessed on 28 October 2021).
13. Anstett, K.; Brenner, B.; Mesplede, T.; Wainberg, M.A. HIV Drug Resistance against Strand Transfer Integrase Inhibitors. *Retrovirology* **2017**, *14*, 36. [CrossRef] [PubMed]
14. Paton, N.I.; Musaazi, J.; Kityo, C.; Walimbwa, S.; Hoppe, A.; Balyegisawa, A.; Kaimal, A.; Mirembe, G.; Tukamushabe, P.; Ategeka, G.; et al. Dolutegravir or Darunavir in Combination with Zidovudine or Tenofovir to Treat HIV. *N. Engl. J. Med.* **2021**, *385*, 330–341. [CrossRef] [PubMed]
15. Gonzalez-Rodríguez, A. Clínicas Especializadas Condesa. Epidemiologic Response to HIV/AIDS and HCV in Mexico City, 2020. 2021. Available online: http://condesadf.mx/pdf/Respuesta2020_cdmx17feb21OK.pdf (accessed on 28 October 2021).
16. Dávila-Conn, V.; García-Morales, C.; Matías-Florentino, M.; López-Ortiz, E.; Paz-Juárez, H.E.; Beristain-Barreda, Á.; Cárdenas-Sandoval, M.; Tapia-Trejo, D.; López-Sánchez, D.; Becerril-Rodríguez, M.; et al. Characteristics and Growth of the Genetic HIV Transmission Network of Mexico City during 2020. *JIAS* **2021**, *24*, e25836. [CrossRef] [PubMed]
17. Matías-Florentino, M.; Chaillon, A.; Ávila-Ríos, S.; Mehta, S.R.; Paz-Juárez, H.E.; Becerril-Rodríguez, M.A.; del Arenal-Sánchez, S.J.; Piñeirúa-Menéndez, A.; Ruiz, V.; Iracheta-Hernández, P.; et al. Pretreatment HIV Drug Resistance Spread within Transmission Clusters in Mexico City. *J. Antimicrob. Chemother.* **2020**, *75*, 656–667. [CrossRef] [PubMed]
18. Zhou, Z.; Wagar, N.; DeVos, J.R.; Rottinghaus, E.; Diallo, K.; Nguyen, D.B.; Bassey, O.; Ugbena, R.; Wadonda-Kabondo, N.; McConnell, M.S.; et al. Optimization of a Low Cost and Broadly Sensitive Genotyping Assay for HIV-1 Drug Resistance Surveillance and Monitoring in Resource-Limited Settings. *PLoS ONE* **2011**, *6*, e28184. [CrossRef] [PubMed]

19. Van Laethem, K.; Schrooten, Y.; Covens, K.; Dekeersmaeker, N.; De Munter, P.; Van Wijngaerden, E.; Van Ranst, M.; Vandamme, A.-M. A Genotypic Assay for the Amplification and Sequencing of Integrase from Diverse HIV-1 Group M Subtypes. *J. Virol. Methods* **2008**, *153*, 176–181. [CrossRef] [PubMed]
20. Public Health Agency of Canada. HyDRA Web. Available online: https://hydra.canada.ca/ (accessed on 1 July 2021).
21. Parkin, N.T.; Avila-Rios, S.; Bibby, D.F.; Brumme, C.J.; Eshleman, S.H.; Harrigan, P.R.; Howison, M.; Hunt, G.; Ji, H.; Kantor, R.; et al. Multi-Laboratory Comparison of Next-Generation to Sanger-Based Sequencing for HIV-1 Drug Resistance Genotyping. *Viruses* **2020**, *12*, 694. [CrossRef] [PubMed]
22. BC Centre for Excellence in HIV/AIDS. Recall. Available online: https://recall.bccfe.ca/ (accessed on 28 October 2021).
23. WHO. WHO/HIV ResNet HIV Drug Resistance Quality Control Tool. Available online: https://sequenceqc-dev.bccfe.ca/who_qc (accessed on 28 October 2021).
24. Stanford University. HIV Drug Resistance Database. Available online: https://hivdb.stanford.edu/ (accessed on 28 October 2021).
25. WHO. WHO/HIV ResNet HIV Drug Resistance Laboratory Operational Framework. 2017. Available online: https://www.who.int/publications-detail-redirect/978-92-4-000987-5 (accessed on 28 October 2021).
26. WHO HIV ResNet. Available online: https://www.who.int/groups/who-hivresnet (accessed on 28 October 2021).
27. REGA HIV-1 Subtyping Tool. Available online: http://dbpartners.stanford.edu:8080/RegaSubtyping/stanford-hiv/typingtool/ (accessed on 19 November 2021).
28. Kosakovsky Pond, S.L.; Weaver, S.; Leigh Brown, A.J.; Wertheim, J.O. HIV-TRACE (TRAnsmission Cluster Engine): A Tool for Large Scale Molecular Epidemiology of HIV-1 and Other Rapidly Evolving Pathogens. *Mol. Biol. Evol.* **2018**, *35*, 1812–1819. [CrossRef] [PubMed]

pathogens

MDPI

Article

Spectrum of Atazanavir-Selected Protease Inhibitor-Resistance Mutations

Soo-Yon Rhee [1,*], Michael Boehm [2], Olga Tarasova [3], Giulia Di Teodoro [4], Ana B. Abecasis [5], Anders Sönnerborg [6], Alexander J. Bailey [1], Dmitry Kireev [7], Maurizio Zazzi [8], the EuResist Network Study Group † and Robert W. Shafer [1]

1 Department of Medicine, Stanford University, Stanford, CA 94305, USA; alexjamesbailey@gmail.com (A.J.B.); rshafer@stanford.edu (R.W.S.)
2 Institute of Virology, Faculty of Medicine and University Hospital of Cologne, University of Cologne, 50935 Cologne, Germany; michael.boehm@uk-koeln.de
3 Department of Bioinformatics, Institute of Biomedical Chemistry, 119121 Moscow, Russia; olga.a.tarasova@gmail.com
4 Department of Computer, Control and Management Engineering Antonio Ruberti, Sapienza University of Rome, 00185 Rome, Italy; giulia.diteodoro@uniroma1.it
5 Global Health and Tropical Medicine, Instituto de Higiene e Medicina Tropical, Universidade Nova de Lisboa, 1349-008 Lisboa, Portugal; ana.abecasis@ihmt.unl.pt
6 Division of Infectious Diseases, Department of Medicine Huddinge, Karolinska Institute, Huddinge, 14186 Stockholm, Sweden; anders.sonnerborg@ki.se
7 Central Research Institute of Epidemiology, 111123 Moscow, Russia; dmitkireev@yandex.ru
8 Department of Medical Biotechnologies, University of Siena, 53100 Siena, Italy; maurizio.zazzi@unisi.it
* Correspondence: syrhee@stanford.edu; Tel.: +1-(650)736-0911
† Collaborators/Membership of the EuResist Network Study Group is provided in the Supplementary Material.

Citation: Rhee, S.-Y.; Boehm, M.; Tarasova, O.; Di Teodoro, G.; Abecasis, A.B.; Sönnerborg, A.; Bailey, A.J.; Kireev, D.; Zazzi, M.; the EuResist Network Study Group; et al. Spectrum of Atazanavir-Selected Protease Inhibitor-Resistance Mutations. *Pathogens* **2022**, *11*, 546. https://doi.org/10.3390/pathogens11050546

Academic Editor: Richard Y. Zhao

Received: 23 March 2022
Accepted: 3 May 2022
Published: 5 May 2022

Abstract: Ritonavir-boosted atazanavir is an option for second-line therapy in low- and middle-income countries (LMICs). We analyzed publicly available HIV-1 protease sequences from previously PI-naïve patients with virological failure (VF) following treatment with atazanavir. Overall, 1497 patient sequences were identified, including 740 reported in 27 published studies and 757 from datasets assembled for this analysis. A total of 63% of patients received boosted atazanavir. A total of 38% had non-subtype B viruses. A total of 264 (18%) sequences had a PI drug-resistance mutation (DRM) defined as having a Stanford HIV Drug Resistance Database mutation penalty score. Among sequences with a DRM, nine major DRMs had a prevalence >5%: I50L (34%), M46I (33%), V82A (22%), L90M (19%), I54V (16%), N88S (10%), M46L (8%), V32I (6%), and I84V (6%). Common accessory DRMs were L33F (21%), Q58E (16%), K20T (14%), G73S (12%), L10F (10%), F53L (10%), K43T (9%), and L24I (6%). A novel nonpolymorphic mutation, L89T occurred in 8.4% of non-subtype B, but in only 0.4% of subtype B sequences. The 264 sequences included 3 (1.1%) interpreted as causing high-level, 14 (5.3%) as causing intermediate, and 27 (10.2%) as causing low-level darunavir resistance. Atazanavir selects for nine major and eight accessory DRMs, and one novel nonpolymorphic mutation occurring primarily in non-B sequences. Atazanavir-selected mutations confer low-levels of darunavir cross resistance. Clinical studies, however, are required to determine the optimal boosted PI to use for second-line and potentially later line therapy in LMICs.

Keywords: HIV-1; antiviral therapy; drug resistance; protease inhibitor; protease; mutation; atazanavir

1. Introduction

Ritonavir-boosted atazanavir has become increasingly important as an option for second-line therapy in low- and middle-income countries (LMICs) [1]. Although it appears to have comparable efficacy to ritonavir-boosted lopinavir (lopinavir/r) [2,3], there are few data on the mutations arising in patients receiving boosted or unboosted atazanavir compared with the extensive data available for lopinavir/r [4–12]. Characterizing the spectrum of mutations arising in patients receiving atazanavir, whether boosted or unboosted, provides an insight into the genetic barrier to atazanavir resistance and into the use of boosted darunavir (darunavir/r) for third line therapy in LMICs.

Therefore, in this paper, we analyze publicly available protease sequences from previously protease inhibitor (PI)-naïve patients with virological failure (VF) on a boosted or unboosted atazanavir-containing regimen. We compare the spectrum of protease mutations observed in patients with subtype B as opposed to non-B viruses, in patients receiving boosted as opposed to unboosted atazanavir, and in patients with early PI resistance (e.g., harboring few PI-associated drug-resistance mutations (DRMs)) with advanced PI resistance (e.g., harboring four or more PI-associated DRMs). We also examine the predicted susceptibility of the different patterns of atazanavir-selected mutations to lopinavir/r and darunavir/r.

2. Results

2.1. Studies

Overall, 1763 protease sequences from 1497 patients reported in 30 studies who received either boosted or unboosted atazanavir as their first PI were available for the analysis (Table 1). These sequences included 773 sequences from 740 patients in 27 studies from Stanford HIV Drug Resistance Database (HIVDB) [13], and previously unpublished sequences, including (i) 741 sequences from 562 patients from the EuResist Integrated Database (EIDB) [14]; (ii) 206 sequences from 152 patients from the Stanford University Hospital (SUH); and (iii) 43 sequences from 43 patients from the RHIVDB [15], a freely accessible database of HIV-1 sequences and clinical data of infected patients. Of the 184 patients with more than 1 sequence, 17 had sequences that differed from one another by one or more DRMs. For these patients, we selected the sequence containing the largest number of PI-associated DRMs. The complete set of 1497 one-per-person HIV-1 group M sequences from persons receiving atazanavir was provided in Table S1.

Table 1. Studies containing publicly available sequences from previously PI-naïve patients receiving boosted or unboosted atazanavir (ATV).

AuthorYr	Study Type	# Total ATV	# bATV	# ATV	% DRMs [1]	Median Year	Country	Subtypes (%) [2]
Large clinical trials and cohorts for which genotypic resistance testing was routinely available at virological failure								
EuResist Network [14]	Cohort	562	286	276	10.3	2012	Europe	B (57.8), G (16.2), 02_AG (12)
Stanford University Hospital	Cohort	152	142	10	9.2	2010	U.S.	B (96.7)
Mollan12 [16]	ACTG A5202	137	137	0	5.8	2006	U.S.	B (97.1)
Kantor15 [17]	ACTG A5175	117	19	98	14.5	2006	Multi-continents	C (55.6), B (41.9)
Lennox14 [18]	ACTG A5257	69	69	0	2.9	2010	U.S.	B (97.1)
Case series and cohorts for which genotypic resistance testing may not have been routinely available at virological failure								
Soldi19 [10]	Cohort	149	81	68	30.2	2015	Brazil	B (75.8), F (12.8)

Table 1. *Cont.*

AuthorYr	Study Type	# Total ATV	# bATV	# ATV	% DRMs [1]	Median Year	Country	Subtypes (%) [2]
Tarasova21 [15]	Cohort	43	16	27	37.2	2017	Russia	A (90.7)
Kouamou19 [19]	Cohort	40	40	0	12.5	2017	Zimbabwe	C (100)
de Carvalho Lima20 [20]	Cohort	37	28	9	54.1	2010	Brazil	B (81.1), F (16.2)
Acharya14 [21]	Cohort	35	35	0	48.6	2013	India	C (80), A (20)
Ndashimye18 [22]	Cohort	33	33	0	42.4	2016	Uganda	A (57.6), D (24.2), B (15.2)
Gulick04 [23]	ACTG A5095	24	1	23	8.3	2003	U.S.	B (100)
Colonno04 [24]	Case series from clinical trials [3]	21	0	21	100	2000	Multi-continents	B (71.4), C (28.6)
Chimukangara16 [25]	Cohort	17	17	0	29.4	2015	Zimbabwe	C (100)
Posada Cespedes21 [12]	Cohort	13	7	6	7.7	2015	South Africa	C (100)
Makwaga20 [26]	Cohort	11	11	0	36.4	2020	Kenya	A (63.6), B (18.2), D (18.2)
de Sa Filho08 [27]	Cohort	10	8	2	80	2006	Brazil	B (80), F (20)
Kolomeets14 [28]	Cohort	10	0	10	30	2012	Russia	A (70), 02_AG (30)
Alves19 [29]	Cohort	3	2	1	0	2017	Brazil	C (66.7), B (33.3)
Kim13 [30]	Cohort	3	1	2	33.3	2011	Korea	B (100)
Karkashadze19 [31]	Cohort	2	0	2	100	2015	Republic Of Georgia	A (50), B (50)
Armenia20 [32]	Cohort	1	1	0	0	2012	Italy	B (100)
El-Khatib10 [33]	Cohort	1	1	0	100	2008	South Africa	C (100)
Hoffmann13 [34]	Cohort	1	0	1	0	2010	South Africa	C (100)
Mziray20 [35]	Cohort	1	1	0	0	2018	Tanzania	C (100)
Neogi16 [36]	Cohort	1	0	1	0	2013	South Africa	C (100)
Riddler08 [37]	ACTG A5142	1	1	0	0	2004	U.S.	D (100)

Table 1. *Cont.*

AuthorYr	Study Type	# Total ATV	# bATV	# ATV	% DRMs [1]	Median Year	Country	Subtypes (%) [2]
Rosen-Zvi08 [38]	Cohort	1	1	0	0	2006	Germany	B (100)
Svard17 [39]	Cohort	1	1	0	0	2013	Tanzania	A (100)
Vergani08 [40]	Cohort	1	0	1	0	2006	Italy	B (100)

Footnotes: [1] DRMs were defined as those with a Stanford HIV drug resistance program penalty score for ≥1 PI. [2] Subtypes with ≥10% sequences were listed. [3] Colonno04 contained sequences from previously PI-naïve patients with virological failure with resistance on ATV-containing regimens in three clinical trial, AI424-007/041, AI424-008/044, and AI424-034. Additional notes: All studies used the Sanger dideoxynucleoside sequencing method, except for Alves19 in which next-generation sequencing was used; samples from peripheral blood mononuclear cells (PBMCs) were used in Alves19, Makwaga20, and Mziray20, and from both PBMC and plasma in Kim13. In the remaining studies, plasma was used. Abbreviation: b-ATV—boosted atazanavir.

The 30 studies were published between 2004 and 2021. The median number of patients per study was 12 (IQR: 1–39). The distribution of studies and patients by region included Africa (10 studies; 119 patients), North America (5 studies; 383 patients), Europe (4 studies; 565 patients), Latin America (4 studies; 199 patients), Eastern Europe (3 studies; 55 patients), and Asia (2 studies; 38 patients). Two studies included 138 patients from 1 or more regions.

The median sample year was 2011 (IQR: 2007–2015). Approximately 99% of sequences were obtained from plasma and 1% from peripheral blood mononuclear cells (PBMCs). Next-generation sequencing (NGS) was performed in 1 of the 30 studies. The most common subtypes were B (61.9%), C (13.6%), A (6.7%), G (6.1%), 02_AG (4.9%), F (3.1%) and D (1.1%). Of 1497 patients, 62.7% (n = 939) received boosted atazanavir and 37.3% (n = 558) received unboosted atazanavir. A higher proportion of patients with subtype B (70.4% of 927) compared with non-subtype B (50.2% of 570) viruses received boosted ($p < 0.001$). Table 2 summarizes the numbers of patients according to the administration of atazanavir (boosted vs. unboosted), subtype (B vs. non-subtype B), previous antiretroviral therapy (ART) (naïve vs. experienced), and year of ART initiation.

Table 2. Proportion of patients with PI-associated drug resistance mutations (DRMs) and median number of DRMs per patient according to ART history and HIV-1 subtype.

	# Patients, (% of Total; n = 1437)	# Patients with ≥1 DRMs [1], (% of Row Total)	Median # DRMs in Patients with ≥1 DRM (IQR)
Unboosted* vs. *boosted			
Unboosted	558 (37.3)	117 (21.0)	3.0 (1.0–4.0)
Boosted	939 (62.7)	147 (15.7)	2.0 (1.0–4.0)
Subtype B* vs. *non-subtype B			
Subtype B	570 (38.1)	150 (16.2)	3.0 (1.0–4.0)
Non-subtype B	927 (61.9)	114 (20.0)	3.0 (1.0–4.0)
ART-naïve* vs. *ART-experienced			
ART-naïve	907 (60.6)	136 (15.0)	3.0 (1.0–4.0)
ART-experienced	590 (39.4)	128 (21.7)	2.0 (1.0–4.0)
Year of ART initiation [2]			
1993–2004	134 (11.9)	24 (17.9)	2.0 (1.0–2.1)
2005–2006	362 (32.1)	44 (12.1)	1.0 (1.0–2.4)
2007–2009	316 (28.0)	26 (8.2)	2.0 (1.0–2.8)
2010–2018	315 (28.0)	29 (9.2)	2.0 (1.0–2.3)

Footnotes: [1] DRMs were defined as those with an HIVDB drug resistance program penalty score for ≥1 PI. [2] Patients with available year of ART initiation (n = 1127) were grouped into four time periods containing approximately equal numbers of patients.

2.2. Mutation Prevalence

Of the 1497 patients, 264 (17.6%) had 1 or more PI-associated DRMs. Of the 57 HIVDB PI-associated DRMs, 48 occurred in ≥1 patient, 38 in ≥2 patients, and 24 in ≥5 patients. The most commonly occurring major DRMs were I50L (34.1%), M46I (32.6%), V82A (22.3%), L90M (19.3%), I54V (16.3%), N88S (10.2%), M46L (7.6%), V32I (6.4%), and I84V (6.1%) (Table 3). The most common accessory DRMs were L33F (20.8%), Q58E (15.9%), K20T (14.4%), G73S (11.7%), L10F (9.8%), F53L (9.8%), K43T (8.7%), and L24I (6.1%).

Table 3. Drug resistance mutations (DRMs) occurring in ≥1 sequences from patients receiving boosted or unboosted atazanavir as their first PI.

DRM [1]	Classification [2]	% in the 264 Patients with a PI-Associated DRM	Median # Co-Occurring DRMs (IQR)
I50L	Major	34.1	2 (0.2–3)
M46I	Major	32.6	3 (2–5)
V82A	Major	22.3	4 (3–5)
L90M	Major	19.3	3 (2–4.5)
I54V	Major	16.3	4 (3–5)
N88S	Major	10.2	3 (2–4)
M46L	Major	7.6	3 (2–4)
V32I	Major	6.4	3 (2–5)
I84V	Major	6.1	3 (2–5)
I54L	Major	4.2	3 (3–4.5)
G48V	Major	3.4	3 (2–3)
I47V	Major	2.7	5 (4.5–7)
I50V	Major	2.3	4 (3–5)
L76V	Major	2.3	5.5 (4.2–6)
I47A	Major	1.5	3.5 (2–5)
V82M	Major	1.5	2 (1.7–3)
V82T	Major	1.5	4.5 (3.5–5.5)
D30N	Major	1.1	4 (3.5–7)
G48A	Major	1.1	6 (4.5–6.5)
V82F	Major	1.1	6 (5–6.5)
V82L	Major	1.1	3 (1.5–4.5)
I54A	Major	0.8	3.5 (3.2–3.7)
V82S	Major	0.8	3 (3–3)
G48M	Major	0.4	2 (2–2)
I54M	Major	0.4	5 (5–5)
I54S	Major	0.4	2 (2–2)
I54T	Major	0.4	2 (2–2)
V82C	Major	0.4	4 (4–4)
N88T	Major	0.4	3 (3–3)
L33F	Accessory	20.8	4 (2–5)
Q58E	Accessory	15.9	3 (1–5)
K20T	Accessory	14.4	2 (1–4)

Table 3. *Cont.*

DRM [1]	Classification [2]	% in the 264 Patients with a PI-Associated DRM	Median # Co-Occurring DRMs (IQR)
G73S	Accessory	11.7	3 (1–4)
L10F	Accessory	9.8	4 (2–5)
F53L	Accessory	9.8	3.5 (2–5)
K43T	Accessory	8.7	4 (2–5)
L24I	Accessory	6.1	4 (2–4.2)
L23I	Accessory	4.2	3 (1.5–4.5)
T74P	Accessory	3	3 (2–4)
G73T	Accessory	1.5	3.5 (2.7–4.5)
L89V	Accessory	1.5	3.5 (2–5.2)
N83D	Accessory	1.1	3 (3–4)
N88D	Accessory	1.1	3 (2.5–6.5)
G73C	Accessory	0.8	3.5 (2.2–4.7)
L24F	Accessory	0.4	0 (0–0)
M46V	Accessory	0.4	2 (2–2)
G73A	Accessory	0.4	6 (6–6)
G73V	Accessory	0.4	8 (8–8)

[1] DRMs were defined as those with a Stanford HIVDB drug resistance program penalty score for ≥1 PI. [2] See the method for DRM classification.

Of the 264 sequences with 1 or more PI-associated DRMs, the proportions of the sequences containing 1 DRM, 2–3 DRMs and ≥4 DRMs were 33.7%, 31.4% and 34.9%, respectively. The distribution of DRMs differed according to the total number of DRMs per sequence (Figure 1). Among sequences with a single DRM, the most common major DRMs were I50L, M46I/L, L90M, and N88S, while the most common accessory DRMs were Q58E, K20T, G73S, and L33F. In contrast, among sequences with ≥4 DRMs, the most common major DRMs were M46I/L, V82A, L90M, I54V, I50L, and N88S, while the most common accessory DRMs were unchanged. The major DRMs V32I and I84V occurred in approximately 5% to 6% of sequences regardless of the total number of DRMs.

An additional 197 mutations, previously classified as nonpolymorphic treatment selected mutations (NP-TSMs), occurred in 149 sequences, including in 109 of the 264 sequences containing a PI-associated DRM and 40 of the 1215 sequences without a PI-associated DRM. There were 33 different NP-TSMs of which the most common were L89T (34.9% of 149 sequences), K55R (15.4%), I85V (11.4%), A71I (9.4%), and E34Q (7.4%) (Table S2). These mutations were not classified as DRMs because they do not receive an HIVDB mutation penalty score.

2.3. *Unboosted versus Boosted Atazanavir*

PI-associated DRMs occurred in 21.0% of 558 patients receiving unboosted atazanavir and 15.7% of 939 patients receiving boosted atazanavir ($p = 0.01$) (Table 2). However, among patients with a DRM, the median number of DRMs was not significantly greater in those receiving unboosted atazanavir (3 DRMs; IQR: 1–4) compared with boosted atazanavir (2 DRMs; IQR: 1–4; $p = 0.1$). Of the 48 reported DRMs, I50L was the only DRM that occurred more commonly in patients receiving unboosted as compared with boosted atazanavir (10.4% vs. 3.4%; adjusted $p < 0.001$).

Sequences from patients receiving unboosted atazanavir were also slightly more likely to have one or more NP-TSMs compared with sequences from patients receiving boosted atazanavir (12.2% of 558 vs. 8.6% of 939; $p = 0.03$). Each of the 33 reported NP-TSMs occurred in similar proportions in patients receiving unboosted and boosted atazanavir.

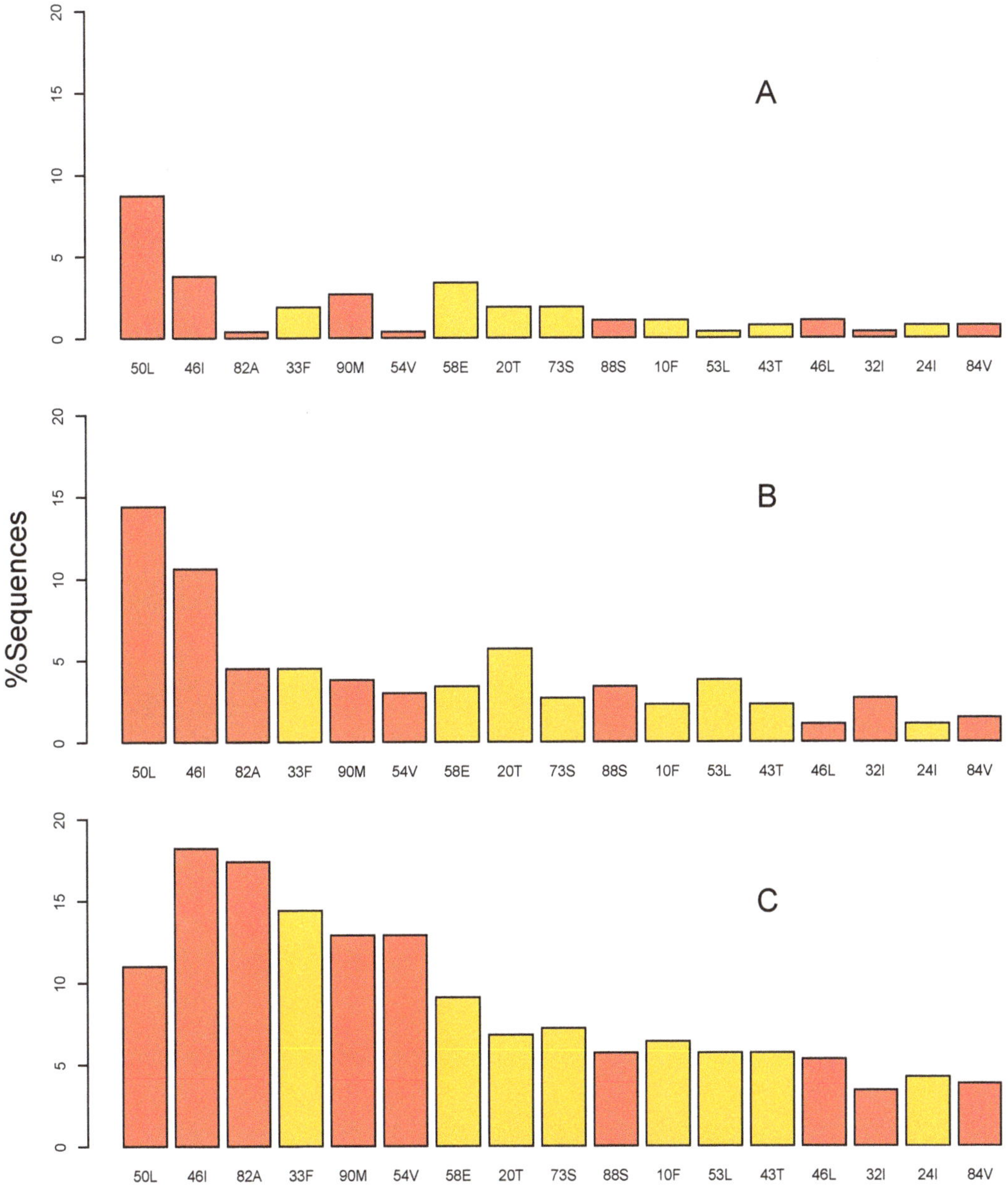

Figure 1. Prevalence of PI-associated drug-resistance mutations (DRMs) in 264 sequences containing 1 or more DRMs from previously PI-naïve patients receiving a boosted or unboosted atazanavir-containing regimen. The distribution of DRMs is plotted separately according to the number of PI-associated DRMs in the sequence: (**A**) 1 DRM, (**B**) 2 to 3 DRMs, and (**C**) ≥4 DRMs. The DRMs shown are those occurring in ≥5% of the sequences, including 9 major DRMs indicated in red and 8 accessory DRMs indicated in yellow.

2.4. Subtypes

The proportion of sequences containing one or more PI-associated DRMs was similar in subtype B (20.0% of 570) versus non-subtype B (16.2% of 927; $p = 0.07$) sequences (Table 2). Of the 48 reported PI-associated DRMs, G73S was significantly more common in subtype B (3.1% of 927) than non-subtype B (0.4% of 570; adjusted $p = 0.005$) sequences. Of the 33 reported NP-TSMs, only L/M89T was significantly more common in non-subtype B than in subtype B sequences (8.4% of 570 vs. 0.4% of 927; adjusted $p < 0.001$). In subtypes A, C, G, CRF01_AE, and CRF02_AG, the consensus amino acid at position 89 is methionine (M) [41] and 89T requires just a single transition in these subtypes (ATG => ACG). In contrast, changing to 89T requires a one transition plus one transversion change in subtype B (CTN or TTR => ACN).

2.5. ART Experience

Among the 1497 patients receiving atazanavir, 907 (60.6%) were previously ART-naïve and 590 (39.4%) were ART-experienced (Table 2). The proportion of sequences containing one or more PI-associated DRMs was 21.7% in previously ART-experienced patients and 15.0% in previously ART-naïve patients ($p = 0.001$). Among those with one or more PI-associated DRMs, the number of DRMs was not significantly different in previously ART-experienced patients (median 2 DRMs; IQR: 1–4 DRMs) compared with previously ART-naïve patients (median 3 DRMs; IQR: 1–4 DRMs; $p = 0.3$).

Among the 907 previously ART-naïve patients, atazanavir was administered with 2 nucleoside RT inhibitors (NRTIs) in 840 (92.6%) patients. Among the remaining 67 patients, the co-administered antiretroviral drugs (ARVs) were not provided for 44 (4.9%), while 23 (2.5%) received a variety of other ARVs.

Among the 590 previously ART-experienced patients, atazanavir was administered with 2 NRTIs in 345 (58.5%) patients. Among the remaining 245 patients, the co-administered ARVs were not provided for 163 (27.6%), while 82 (13.9%) received a variety of other ARVs. Only four patients received atazanavir plus one additional ARV.

The year of ART-initiation was available for 1127 (75.3%) of all patients. The patients could be pooled into four time periods containing approximately equal numbers spanning the years between 1993 and 2018 (Table 2). The proportion of patients with one or more PI-associated DRMs decreased over time (binomial coefficient = −0.26; 95% CI: −0.45 to −0.07; $p = 0.007$), but the number of DRMs in patients with one or more DRMs did not change.

Using just those patients for whom the year of ART initiation was available, a multivariate logistic regression analysis was performed to assess the association between four factors and the development of a PI-associated DRM. The four factors included the year of ART initiation, subtype (B vs. non-subtype B), the use boosted vs. unboosted atazanavir, and previous ART (naïve vs. experienced). The analysis found that a later year of ART initiation (OR: 0.62; 95%CI: 0.49–0.79; $p = 0.0001$) and the administration of boosted atazanavir (OR: 0.57; 95%CI: 0.35–0.93; $p = 0.02$) were associated with a decreased risk of developing a PI-associated DRM.

2.6. Bayesian Network Analysis of Correlated Mutations

We used the 1437 (96%) sequences containing 0 to 4 PI-associated DRMs (i.e., sequences with ≥5 PI-associated DRMs were excluded) to calculate Jaccard similarity coefficients and their standard Z scores for all pairs of DRMs and NP-TSMs. Eleven pairs of mutations comprising six major DRMs (M46I, I50L, I54V, V82A, N88S and L90M), three accessory DRMs (K20T, L33F and G73S), and the NP-TSM L89T participated in one or more significant pairwise correlations ($p < 0.01$). We then performed a Bayesian network analysis to determine the conditional dependency between the mutations in each of the pairwise correlations (Figure 2).

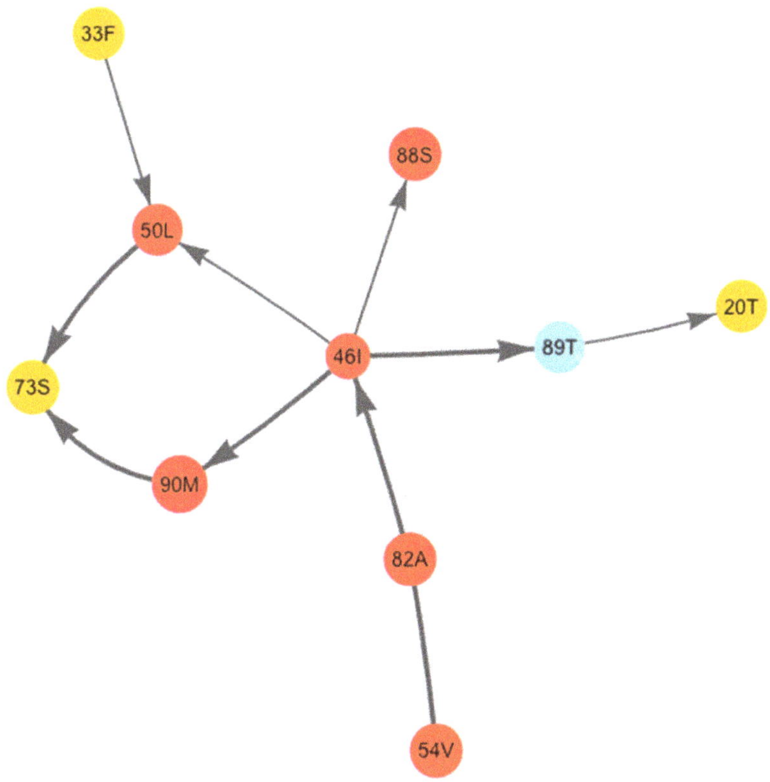

Figure 2. Bayesian network analysis of positively correlated mutation pairs with a hill-climbing search. The Bayesian network analysis yielded 11 mutation pairs, including 6 major DRMs (red), 3 accessory DRMs (yellow), and an additional nonpolymorphic treatment-selected mutation (light blue) with a significant Jaccard correlation coefficient ($p < 0.01$). The thickness of the arrows indicates the strength of the probabilistic relationship of the two mutations. The direction of the probabilistic causation is shown with an arrowhead. For the direction between V82A and I54V for which the probabilistic causation is not greater than the probabilistic causation of the opposite direction by 0.1, the arrowhead is not shown.

2.7. Estimated Cross Resistance to LPV/r and DRV/r

Among the 264 sequences with 1 or more PI-associated DRMs, there were 182 distinct DRM patterns, including 124 patterns (164 sequences; 62.1% of 264) interpreted by HIVDB as causing high-level atazanavir resistance, 19 patterns (20 sequences; 7.6% of 264) as causing intermediate atazanavir resistance, and 29 patterns (51 sequences; 19.3% of 264) as causing low- or potential low-level atazanavir resistance. The remaining 10 DRM patterns (n = 29 sequences patterns; 11.0% of 264) consisting primarily of singe accessory DRMs (e.g., K20T, Q58E) were not interpreted as causing reduced atazanavir susceptibility.

A total of 56 distinct DRM patterns (58 sequences; 22.0% of 264) were interpreted as causing high-level lopinavir resistance, 40 patterns (43 sequences; 16.3% of 264) as causing intermediate lopinavir resistance, and 44 patterns (62 sequences; 23.5% of 264) as causing low- or potential low-level lopinavir resistance. A total of 3 distinct DRM patterns (3 sequences; 1.1% of 264) were interpreted as causing high-level darunavir resistance, 14 patterns (14 sequences; 5.3% of 264) as causing intermediate darunavir resistance, and 32 patterns (34 sequences; 12.9% of 264) as causing low- or potential low-level darunavir resistance.

2.8. Virological Failure with Resistance

Five of the thirty studies included participants from three clinical trials and from two clinical cohorts for which genotypic resistance testing was routinely available (Table 1). Together, these five studies included 1037 (69.3%) of all 1497 patients from whom sequences were available. Of these 1037 patients, 63.0% and 37.0% received boosted and unboosted atazanavir, respectively. In these studies, the proportion of sequences containing one or more PI-associated DRMs ranged from 2.9% to 14.5% and the overall proportion of sequences containing one or more PI-associated DRMs in patients receiving boosted and unboosted atazanavir were 7.2% and 13.5%, respectively.

2.9. Studies Not Included in the Analysis

We identified 32 additional studies reporting sequences from 1089 previously PI-naïve patients receiving boosted or unboosted atazanavir-containing regimens (Table S3). Approximately 10% of the sequences in these studies were reported to contain one or more PI-associated DRMs. However, as the sequences were not available and as different mutations were reported in different studies, we did not include the data from these studies in our analysis.

3. Discussion

The spectrum of atazanavir-selected mutations has been largely influenced by data published in the earliest in vitro passage experiments and clinical trials. During in vitro passage experiments with three subtype B clones, the most commonly emerging DRMs were V32I, M46I, I50L, I84V, and N88S [42]. The initial reports of the in vivo selection of PI-associated DRMs, based on the use of unboosted atazanavir in ART-naïve patients, demonstrated that I50L and G73S were the most commonly occurring mutations in patients with VF [24,43]. A few cases of VF and emergent PI-associated DRMs have been reported in the clinical trials of ART-naïve patients receiving boosted atazanavir [16,44], consistent with the hypothesis that PI-resistance mutations develop only in viruses exposed to a narrow window of suboptimal drug concentrations that both exert selective pressure on the virus and allow virus replication [45]. Nonetheless, PI resistance in previously PI-naïve patients receiving lopinavir/r for second-line therapy has increasingly been reported, usually beginning after 12–18 months of therapy [46]. In addition, phenotypic studies have shown that DRMs selected by other PIs confer atazanavir cross resistance particularly when they occur in combination [47,48].

In the years since atazanavir has been introduced, there has been a gradual accumulation of data on the spectrum of mutations emerging in previously PI-naïve patients with VF on an ART-regimen containing boosted and less commonly unboosted atazanavir. In contrast to the earliest clinical trials of boosted atazanavir, these studies included cohorts of patients who were ART experienced at the time atazanavir was administered and who may not have been monitored as closely for VF thus enabling their viruses to evolve for longer period of time under atazanavir selection pressure. Moreover, these studies have included an increasing proportion of sequences from patients with non-subtype B viruses.

Our analysis confirmed that the five major DRMs selected in vitro by atazanavir (V32I, M46I, I50L, I84V, and N88S) were among the most commonly occurring major DRMs. Four additional DRMs also occurred commonly, including M46L, I54V, V82A, and L90M. I50L is a signature atazanavir-associated DRM because it has only been reported in patients receiving atazanavir and it increases susceptibility to PIs other than atazanavir [48,49]. N88S is also considered a signature atazanavir-associated DRM because it is rarely selected by other PIs and it does not significantly reduce susceptibility to other PIs, with the exception of nelfinavir and indinavir [48]. L/M89T may also be a signature atazanavir-associated mutation because it appears to occur more commonly in patients receiving atazanavir than in patients receiving any other PI; for example, it has only been reported in three previously PI-naïve patients receiving lopinavir/r (https://hivdb.stanford.edu/cgi-bin/Mutations.

cgi?Gene=PR; accessed on 1 November 2021). In contrast, each of the remaining atazanavir-selected mutations appear to be commonly selected by other PIs, in particular lopinavir/r.

With the exception of L10F and L33F, each of the above 17 most commonly selected major or accessory DRMs was significantly associated with reduced atazanavir susceptibility in a previously published weighted least squares regression analysis of 1644 sequences [48]. Few published phenotypic data are available on sequences containing L89T.

Some limitations of our review should be discussed. First, most of the sequences that we reviewed were obtained from retrospective cohort studies and case series. For these studies, the duration of therapy, accompanying ARVs, frequency of virological monitoring and genotypic resistance testing, and duration of virological failure were generally not available. Therefore, the extent to which these factors were associated with emergent PI-associated DRMs could not be explored. Second, the dataset contained an under-representation of subtypes other than subtype B. Third, we could not be sure that every sequence was obtained from a patient receiving atazanavir as his/her first PI as treatment histories are often incomplete. Nonetheless, we emailed the authors of those studies containing the largest numbers of DRMs and received confirmation that, to the authors' knowledge, the patients had just received atazanavir. Fourth, at least 32 studies in PubMed that contained sequences from 1000 patients receiving boosted or unboosted atazanavir could not be included in our analysis because the primary sequence data and complete list of protease mutations were not available.

In conclusion, to our knowledge, this is the only comprehensive analysis of atazanavir-selected mutations. Our analysis shows that the spectrum of atazanavir-selected mutations extends beyond those mutations observed in the earliest clinical trials in which patients received either boosted or unboosted atazanavir. The expanded spectrum is likely due to the large number of sequences in our analysis and the likelihood that many of the patients in the studies we reviewed had prolonged VF and ongoing replication while receiving atazanavir. The study also identified one novel nonpolymorphic atazanavir-selected mutation that predominantly occurred in non-subtype B sequences. The relatively low cross-resistance to darunavir/r combined with preliminary data suggests that boosted atazanavir can be an efficacious regimen for second-line therapy. However, comparative clinical trials are required to determine the optimal boosted PI to use for second-line and potentially later-line therapy in LMICs.

4. Materials and Methods

4.1. Study Selection Criteria

We analyzed publicly available HIV-1 group M protease nucleotide sequences obtained from previously PI-naïve patients receiving boosted or unboosted atazanavir. Sequences were obtained from HIVDB, which is populated with sequences from GenBank annotated with the ART history of the patients from whom the sequences were obtained [13]. The analysis was last updated 31 December 2021. We supplemented the data in HIVDB with previously unpublished sequences performed at SUH and with previously unpublished sequences from two collaborating research groups: the EIDB [14] and the RHIVDB [15]. Additionally, we performed a PubMed search to identify studies describing HIV-1 group M protease sequences that were not present either in HIVDB or GenBank.

Publications reporting eligible protease sequences were reviewed to determine the treatment history of the patient from whom each sequence was obtained to confirm that the patient had received no PI prior to atazanavir and to distinguish those patients receiving unboosted atazanavir from boosted atazanavir. Each sequence was annotated with the year and country of virus isolation, the type of sample (e.g., PBMCs), the sequencing method (Sanger dideoxynucleoside sequencing versus NGS), and the nature of the study population. HIV-1 subtype was determined using the HIVDB subtyping program [50].

We also characterized each study according to whether it included patients in a clinical trial or in a treatment cohort for whom genotypic resistance testing was routinely available for patients with VF as opposed to a case series or case reports for which the indications for genotypic resistance testing were not reported. Studies that performed routine genotypic resistance testing on all patients with VF provide information on how often PI resistance arises in patients receiving atazanavir. In contrast, the remaining studies were considered likely to be enriched for patients with acquired PI resistance.

4.2. Mutations

PI-associated DRMs were defined as those with an HIVDB drug resistance program penalty score for ≥1 PI as of December 31, 2021 [51]. The DRMs included 57 mutations at 24 positions: L10F, K20T, L23I, L24I/F/M, D30N, V32I, L33F, K43T, M46I/L/V, I47A/V, G48A/L/M/Q/S/T/V, I50I/L, F53L, I54A/L/M/S/T/V, Q58E, G73A/C/D/S/T/V, T74P, L76V, V82A/C/F/L/M/S/T, N83D, I84A/C/V, N88D/G/S/T, L89V, and L90M. Major mutations were defined as those with a greater effect on the susceptibility to one or more PIs, an increased occurrence in patients with VF on PI-containing regimens, and a low likelihood of occurring without selective drug pressure. Additional PI-associated NP-TSMs that are not classified as DRMs were also examined [52]. The NP-TSMs included 56 mutations at 31 positions: L10R/Y, V11L, K20A, A22V, L33M, E34D/N/Q/R/V, M36A, L38W, K43I/N/P/Q/S, K45I/Q/V, G48E, G51A, F53I/W/Y, K55R/N, I66F/L/V, C67F/L, A71I/L, I72K/L, G73I/N, T74E, P79N, V82G, N83S, I85V, L89P/T, T91C/S, Q92R, C95F/L/V, and T96S.

4.3. Analyses

The Fisher's Exact Test was used to compare the proportion of each mutation in sequences from patients receiving boosted versus unboosted atazanavir, from patients who were previously ART-naïve versus ART-experienced, and from patients according to whether they had subtype B versus non-subtype B sequences. The Wilcoxon Rank Sum Test was used to compare the median number of mutations between two groups. The Holm's method was used to control for the familywise error rate for multiple hypothesis testing [53].

A binomial regression model was used to examine the relationship between the year of ART initiation and the presence or absence of PI-associated DRMs. To assess the association of covariates with the presence or absence of PI-associated DRMs, a multivariate generalized linear mixed logistic regression analysis was performed using the R package lme4. To account for study heterogeneity, study was included in the model as a random effect.

To identify the patterns of covariation among DRMs and NP-TSMs, we calculated Jaccard similarity coefficients and their standard Z scores for all pair of mutations [54]. To capture conditional dependency among the significantly co-occurring mutation pairs, defined as those pairs that had Jaccard similarity coefficient $p < 0.01$, we constructed a Bayesian network with a hill-climbing search using the R package bnlearn [55] and created a directed edge network graph using the R package visNetwork [56]. To learn the structure of the Bayesian network of core mutations associated with atazanavir, we excluded sequences containing more than four DRMs in this analysis.

For each sequence containing one or more DRMs, we determined the level of predicted resistance to atazanavir and the levels of predicted cross resistance to lopinavir/r and darunavir/r using the HIVDB drug resistance interpretation system.

4.4. Accession Numbers

Sequences in this study had been submitted to GenBank (accession numbers ON058287-ON058987).

Supplementary Materials: The following supporting information can be downloaded at https://www.mdpi.com/article/10.3390/pathogens11050546/s1, Text S1: The EuResist Network Study Group; Table S1: The complete set of 1497 one-per-person HIV-1 group M protease sequences from persons receiving atazanavir; Table S2: Nonpolymorphic PI treatment-selected mutations (NP-TSMs) occurring in ≥1 sequences from patients receiving boosted or unboosted atazanavir (ATV) as their first PI; Table S3: Studies in PubMed containing sequences from previously PI-naïve patients receiving boosted or unboosted atazanavir (ATV) for which the sequences were not available.

Author Contributions: Conceptualization, R.W.S.; Methodology, S.-Y.R. and R.W.S.; Validation, S.-Y.R., R.W.S. and M.Z.; Formal Analysis, S.-Y.R.; Resources, M.B., O.T., A.B.A., A.S. and D.K.; Data Curation, G.D.T., A.J.B. and S.-Y.R.; Writing—Original Draft Preparation, S.-Y.R. and R.W.S.; Writing—Review and Editing, S.-Y.R., O.T., D.K., A.B.A., M.Z. and R.W.S.; Visualization, S.-Y.R.; Funding Acquisition, R.W.S. All authors have read and agreed to the published version of the manuscript.

Funding: S.-Y.R., A.J.B. and R.W.S. were supported in part by the National Institute of Allergy and Infectious Diseases (NIAID) of the National Institute of Health (NIH) (award number AI136618). The work of O.T. and D.K. was supported by the Russian Science Foundation Grant No. 19-75-10097. A.B.A. received funding from Fundação para a Ciência e Tecnologia through projects PTDC/SAU-INF/31990/2017 (INTEGRIV) and PTDC/SAU-PUB/4018/2021 (MARVEL). G.D.T. was supported by EuResist Network GEIE.

Institutional Review Board Statement: The Stanford University review board approved this study (IRB-13900; approved on 30 June 2021).

Informed Consent Statement: Patient consent was waived by the IRB because the study involved the analysis of anonymized data that had already been collected.

Data Availability Statement: Datasets used in the present study are available in Tables 1 and S1.

Conflicts of Interest: A.S. received research grants from Gilead Sciences, and personal fees for advisory boards from Gilead Sciences, MSD, and ViiV Healthcare, all outside the present work. M.Z. received research grants from Gilead Sciences, MSD, Theratechnologies and ViiV Healthcare and personal fees for advisory boards from Gilead Sciences, Janssen-Cilag, MSD, Theratechnologies and ViiV Healthcare, all outside the present work. The funder had no role in the design of the study; in the collection, analyses, or interpretation of data; in the writing of the manuscript, or in the decision to publish the results.

References

1. WHO Consolidated Guidelines on the Use of Antiretroviral Drugs for Treating and Preventing HIV Infection. 2016. Available online: https://www.who.int/publications-detail-redirect/9789241549684 (accessed on 10 February 2022).
2. Laker, E.A.O.; Nabaggala, M.S.; Kaimal, A.; Nalwanga, D.; Castelnuovo, B.; Musubire, A.; Kiragga, A.; Lamorde, M.; Ratanshi, R.P. An Observational Study in an Urban Ugandan Clinic Comparing Virological Outcomes of Patients Switched from First-Line Antiretroviral Regimens to Second-Line Regimens Containing Ritonavir-Boosted Atazanavir or Ritonavir-Boosted Lopinavir. *BMC Infect. Dis.* **2019**, *19*, 280. [CrossRef] [PubMed]
3. Engamba, D.C.; Wester, C.W.; Mutinta, M.M.; Kumar, A.P.; Chirwa, B.; Phiri, G.; Sinkala, E.; Kampamba, D.; Mpanji, S.; Mbewe, N.; et al. Predictors of Viral Suppression Following Enhanced Adherence Counseling: VISEND Trial. In Proceedings of the Conference on Retroviruses and Opportunistic Infections, Virtual, 12–16 February 2022; p. 490.
4. Barber, T.J.; Harrison, L.; Asboe, D.; Williams, I.; Kirk, S.; Gilson, R.; Bansi, L.; Pillay, D.; Dunn, D.; UK HIV Drug Resistance Database and UK Collaborative HIV Cohort (UK CHIC) Study Steering Committees. Frequency and Patterns of Protease Gene Resistance Mutations in HIV-Infected Patients Treated with Lopinavir/Ritonavir as Their First Protease Inhibitor. *J. Antimicrob. Chemother.* **2012**, *67*, 995–1000. [CrossRef] [PubMed]
5. Van Zyl, G.U.; Liu, T.F.; Claassen, M.; Engelbrecht, S.; de Oliveira, T.; Preiser, W.; Wood, N.T.; Travers, S.; Shafer, R.W. Trends in Genotypic HIV-1 Antiretroviral Resistance between 2006 and 2012 in South African Patients Receiving First- and Second-Line Antiretroviral Treatment Regimens. *PLoS ONE* **2013**, *8*, e67188. [CrossRef] [PubMed]
6. Rawizza, H.E.; Chaplin, B.; Meloni, S.T.; Darin, K.M.; Olaitan, O.; Scarsi, K.K.; Onwuamah, C.K.; Audu, R.A.; Chebu, P.R.; Imade, G.E.; et al. Accumulation of Protease Mutations among Patients Failing Second-Line Antiretroviral Therapy and Response to Salvage Therapy in Nigeria. *PLoS ONE* **2013**, *8*, e73582. [CrossRef] [PubMed]
7. Nerrienet, E. HIV-1 Protease Inhibitors Resistance Profiles in Patients with Virological Failure on LPV/r-Based 2nd Line Regimen in Cambodia. *J. AIDS Clin. Res.* **2013**, *1*. [CrossRef]
8. Grossman, Z.; Schapiro, J.M.; Levy, I.; Elbirt, D.; Chowers, M.; Riesenberg, K.; Olstein-Pops, K.; Shahar, E.; Istomin, V.; Asher, I.; et al. Comparable Long-Term Efficacy of Lopinavir/Ritonavir and Similar Drug-Resistance Profiles in Different HIV-1 Subtypes. *PLoS ONE* **2014**, *9*, e86239. [CrossRef]
9. Steegen, K.; Bronze, M.; Papathanasopoulos, M.A.; van Zyl, G.; Goedhals, D.; Van Vuuren, C.; Macleod, W.; Sanne, I.; Stevens, W.S.; Carmona, S.C. Prevalence of Antiretroviral Drug Resistance in Patients Who Are Not Responding to Protease Inhibitor-Based Treatment: Results From the First National Survey in South Africa. *J. Infect. Dis.* **2016**, *214*, 1826–1830. [CrossRef]
10. De Faria Romero Soldi, G.; Ribeiro, I.C.; Ahagon, C.M.; Coelho, L.P.O.; Cabral, G.B.; Lopes, G.I.S.L.; de Paula Ferreira, J.L.; de Macedo Brígido, L.F.; Salvage Therapy Working Group. Major Drug Resistance Mutations to HIV-1 Protease Inhibitors (PI) among Patients Exposed to PI Class Failing Antiretroviral Therapy in São Paulo State, Brazil. *PLoS ONE* **2019**, *14*, e0223210. [CrossRef]

11. Thompson, J.A.; Kityo, C.; Dunn, D.; Hoppe, A.; Ndashimye, E.; Hakim, J.; Kambugu, A.; van Oosterhout, J.J.; Arribas, J.; Mugyenyi, P.; et al. Evolution of Protease Inhibitor Resistance in Human Immunodeficiency Virus Type 1 Infected Patients Failing Protease Inhibitor Monotherapy as Second-Line Therapy in Low-Income Countries: An Observational Analysis Within the EARNEST Randomized Trial. *Clin. Infect. Dis.* **2019**, *68*, 1184–1192. [CrossRef]
12. Posada-Céspedes, S.; Van Zyl, G.; Montazeri, H.; Kuipers, J.; Rhee, S.-Y.; Kouyos, R.; Günthard, H.F.; Beerenwinkel, N. Comparing Mutational Pathways to Lopinavir Resistance in HIV-1 Subtypes B versus C. *PLoS Comput. Biol.* **2021**, *17*, e1008363. [CrossRef]
13. Rhee, S.-Y.; Gonzales, M.J.; Kantor, R.; Betts, B.J.; Ravela, J.; Shafer, R.W. Human Immunodeficiency Virus Reverse Transcriptase and Protease Sequence Database. *Nucleic Acids Res.* **2003**, *31*, 298–303. [CrossRef]
14. EuResist Network | Research in HIV | HIV Resistance Database. Available online: https://www.euresist.org (accessed on 1 March 2022).
15. Tarasova, O.; Rudik, A.; Kireev, D.; Poroikov, V. RHIVDB: A Freely Accessible Database of HIV Amino Acid Sequences and Clinical Data of Infected Patients. *Front. Genet.* **2021**, *12*, 679029. [CrossRef] [PubMed]
16. Mollan, K.; Daar, E.S.; Sax, P.E.; Balamane, M.; Collier, A.C.; Fischl, M.A.; Lalama, C.M.; Bosch, R.J.; Tierney, C.; Katzenstein, D.; et al. HIV-1 Amino Acid Changes among Participants with Virologic Failure: Associations with First-Line Efavirenz or Atazanavir plus Ritonavir and Disease Status. *J. Infect. Dis.* **2012**, *206*, 1920–1930. [CrossRef] [PubMed]
17. Kantor, R.; Smeaton, L.; Vardhanabhuti, S.; Hudelson, S.E.; Wallis, C.L.; Tripathy, S.; Morgado, M.G.; Saravanan, S.; Balakrishnan, P.; Reitsma, M.; et al. Pretreatment HIV Drug Resistance and HIV-1 Subtype C Are Independently Associated with Virologic Failure: Results from the Multinational PEARLS (ACTG A5175) Clinical Trial. *Clin. Infect. Dis.* **2015**, *60*, 1541–1549. [CrossRef]
18. Lennox, J.L.; Landovitz, R.J.; Ribaudo, H.J.; Ofotokun, I.; Na, L.H.; Godfrey, C.; Kuritzkes, D.R.; Sagar, M.; Brown, T.T.; Cohn, S.E.; et al. Efficacy and Tolerability of 3 Nonnucleoside Reverse Transcriptase Inhibitor-Sparing Antiretroviral Regimens for Treatment-Naive Volunteers Infected with HIV-1: A Randomized, Controlled Equivalence Trial. *Ann. Intern. Med.* **2014**, *161*, 461–471. [CrossRef] [PubMed]
19. Kouamou, V.; Manasa, J.; Katzenstein, D.; McGregor, A.M.; Ndhlovu, C.E.; Makadzange, A.T. Drug Resistance and Optimizing Dolutegravir Regimens for Adolescents and Young Adults Failing Antiretroviral Therapy. *AIDS* **2019**, *33*, 1729–1737. [CrossRef] [PubMed]
20. De Carvalho Lima, E.N.; Lima, R.S.A.; Piqueira, J.R.C.; Sucupira, M.C.; Camargo, M.; Galinskas, J.; Diaz, R.S. Evidence of Genomic Information and Structural Restrictions of HIV-1 PR and RT Gene Regions from Individuals Experiencing Antiretroviral Virologic Failure. *Infect. Genet. Evol.* **2020**, *78*, 104134. [CrossRef] [PubMed]
21. Acharya, A.; Vaniawala, S.; Shah, P.; Misra, R.N.; Wani, M.; Mukhopadhyaya, P.N. Development, Validation and Clinical Evaluation of a Low Cost in-House HIV-1 Drug Resistance Genotyping Assay for Indian Patients. *PLoS ONE* **2014**, *9*, e105790. [CrossRef]
22. Ndashimye, E.; Avino, M.; Kyeyune, F.; Nankya, I.; Gibson, R.M.; Nabulime, E.; Poon, A.F.Y.; Kityo, C.; Mugyenyi, P.; Quiñones-Mateu, M.E.; et al. Absence of HIV-1 Drug Resistance Mutations Supports the Use of Dolutegravir in Uganda. *AIDS Res. Hum. Retrovir.* **2018**, *34*, 404–414. [CrossRef]
23. Gulick, R.M.; Ribaudo, H.J.; Shikuma, C.M.; Lustgarten, S.; Squires, K.E.; Meyer, W.A.; Acosta, E.P.; Schackman, B.R.; Pilcher, C.D.; Murphy, R.L.; et al. Triple-Nucleoside Regimens versus Efavirenz-Containing Regimens for the Initial Treatment of HIV-1 Infection. *N. Engl. J. Med.* **2004**, *350*, 1850–1861. [CrossRef]
24. Colonno, R.; Rose, R.; McLaren, C.; Thiry, A.; Parkin, N.; Friborg, J. Identification of I50L as the Signature Atazanavir (ATV)-Resistance Mutation in Treatment-Naive HIV-1-Infected Patients Receiving ATV-Containing Regimens. *J. Infect. Dis.* **2004**, *189*, 1802–1810. [CrossRef] [PubMed]
25. Chimukangara, B.; Varyani, B.; Shamu, T.; Mutsvangwa, J.; Manasa, J.; White, E.; Chimbetete, C.; Luethy, R.; Katzenstein, D. HIV Drug Resistance Testing among Patients Failing Second Line Antiretroviral Therapy. Comparison of in-House and Commercial Sequencing. *J. Virol. Methods* **2017**, *243*, 151–157. [CrossRef] [PubMed]
26. Makwaga, O.; Adhiambo, M.; Mulama, D.H.; Muoma, J.; Adungo, F.; Wanjiku, H.; Ongaya, A.; Maitha, G.M.; Mwau, M. Prevalence of Human Immunodeficiency Virus-1 Drug-Resistant Mutations among Adults on First- and Second-Line Antiretroviral Therapy in a Resource-Limited Health Facility in Busia County, Kenya. *Pan Afr. Med. J.* **2020**, *37*, 311. [CrossRef] [PubMed]
27. De Sa-Filho, D.J.; da Silva Soares, M.; Candido, V.; Gagliani, L.H.; Cavaliere, E.; Diaz, R.S.; Caseiro, M.M. HIV Type 1 Pol Gene Diversity and Antiretroviral Drug Resistance Mutations in Santos, Brazil. *AIDS Res. Hum. Retrovir.* **2008**, *24*, 347–353. [CrossRef] [PubMed]
28. Kolomeets, A.N.; Varghese, V.; Lemey, P.; Bobkova, M.R.; Shafer, R.W. A Uniquely Prevalent Nonnucleoside Reverse Transcriptase Inhibitor Resistance Mutation in Russian Subtype A HIV-1 Viruses. *AIDS* **2014**, *28*, F1–F8. [CrossRef]
29. Alves, B.M.; Siqueira, J.D.; Prellwitz, I.M.; Botelho, O.M.; Da Hora, V.P.; Sanabani, S.; Recordon-Pinson, P.; Fleury, H.; Soares, E.A.; Soares, M.A. Estimating HIV-1 Genetic Diversity in Brazil through Next-Generation Sequencing. *Front. Microbiol.* **2019**, *10*, 749. [CrossRef]
30. Kim, M.H.; Song, J.E.; Ahn, J.Y.; Kim, Y.C.; Oh, D.H.; Choi, H.; Ann, H.W.; Kim, J.K.; Kim, S.B.; Jeong, S.J.; et al. HIV Antiretroviral Resistance Mutations among Antiretroviral Treatment-Naive and -Experienced Patients in South Korea. *AIDS Res. Hum. Retrovir.* **2013**, *29*, 1617–1620. [CrossRef]

31. Karkashadze, E.; Dvali, N.; Bolokadze, N.; Sharvadze, L.; Gabunia, P.; Karchava, M.; Tchelidze, T.; Tsertsvadze, T.; DeHovitz, J.; Del Rio, C.; et al. Epidemiology of Human Immunodeficiency Virus (HIV) Drug Resistance in HIV Patients with Virologic Failure of First-Line Therapy in the Country of Georgia. *J. Med. Virol.* **2019**, *91*, 235–240. [CrossRef]
32. Armenia, D.; Bouba, Y.; Gagliardini, R.; Gori, C.; Bertoli, A.; Borghi, V.; Gennari, W.; Micheli, V.; Callegaro, A.P.; Gazzola, L.; et al. Evaluation of Virological Response and Resistance Profile in HIV-1 Infected Patients Starting a First-Line Integrase Inhibitor-Based Regimen in Clinical Settings. *J. Clin. Virol.* **2020**, *130*, 104534. [CrossRef]
33. El-Khatib, Z.; Ekstrom, A.M.; Ledwaba, J.; Mohapi, L.; Laher, F.; Karstaedt, A.; Charalambous, S.; Petzold, M.; Katzenstein, D.; Morris, L. Viremia and Drug Resistance among HIV-1 Patients on Antiretroviral Treatment: A Cross-Sectional Study in Soweto, South Africa. *AIDS* **2010**, *24*, 1679–1687. [CrossRef]
34. Hoffmann, C.J.; Ledwaba, J.; Li, J.-F.; Johnston, V.; Hunt, G.; Fielding, K.L.; Chaisson, R.E.; Churchyard, G.J.; Grant, A.D.; Johnson, J.A.; et al. Resistance to Tenofovir-Based Regimens during Treatment Failure of Subtype C HIV-1 in South Africa. *Antivir. Ther.* **2013**, *18*, 915–920. [CrossRef] [PubMed]
35. Mziray, S.R.; Kumburu, H.H.; Assey, H.B.; Sonda, T.B.; Mahande, M.J.; Msuya, S.E.; Kiwelu, I.E. Patterns of Acquired HIV-1 Drug Resistance Mutations and Predictors of Virological Failure in Moshi, Northern Tanzania. *PLoS ONE* **2020**, *15*, e0232649. [CrossRef] [PubMed]
36. Neogi, U.; Engelbrecht, S.; Claassen, M.; Jacobs, G.B.; van Zyl, G.; Preiser, W.; Sonnerborg, A. Mutational Heterogeneity in P6 Gag Late Assembly (L) Domains in HIV-1 Subtype C Viruses from South Africa. *AIDS Res. Hum. Retrovir.* **2016**, *32*, 80–84. [CrossRef] [PubMed]
37. Riddler, S.A.; Haubrich, R.; DiRienzo, A.G.; Peeples, L.; Powderly, W.G.; Klingman, K.L.; Garren, K.W.; George, T.; Rooney, J.F.; Brizz, B.; et al. Class-Sparing Regimens for Initial Treatment of HIV-1 Infection. *N. Engl. J. Med.* **2008**, *358*, 2095–2106. [CrossRef] [PubMed]
38. Rosen-Zvi, M.; Altmann, A.; Prosperi, M.; Aharoni, E.; Neuvirth, H.; Sönnerborg, A.; Schülter, E.; Struck, D.; Peres, Y.; Incardona, F.; et al. Selecting Anti-HIV Therapies Based on a Variety of Genomic and Clinical Factors. *Bioinformatics* **2008**, *24*, i399–i406. [CrossRef]
39. Svärd, J.; Mugusi, S.; Mloka, D.; Neogi, U.; Meini, G.; Mugusi, F.; Incardona, F.; Zazzi, M.; Sönnerborg, A. Drug Resistance Testing through Remote Genotyping and Predicted Treatment Options in Human Immunodeficiency Virus Type 1 Infected Tanzanian Subjects Failing First or Second Line Antiretroviral Therapy. *PLoS ONE* **2017**, *12*, e0178942. [CrossRef]
40. Vergani, B.; Cicero, M.L.; Vigano', O.; Sirianni, F.; Ferramosca, S.; Vitiello, P.; Di Vincenzo, P.; Pia De Pasquale, M.; Galli, M.; Rusconi, S. Evolution of the HIV-1 Protease Region in Heavily Pretreated HIV-1 Infected Patients Receiving Atazanavir. *J. Clin. Virol.* **2008**, *41*, 154–159. [CrossRef]
41. Abecasis, A.B.; Deforche, K.; Snoeck, J.; Bacheler, L.T.; McKenna, P.; Carvalho, A.P.; Gomes, P.; Camacho, R.J.; Vandamme, A.-M. Protease Mutation M89I/V Is Linked to Therapy Failure in Patients Infected with the HIV-1 Non-B Subtypes C, F or G. *AIDS* **2005**, *19*, 1799–1806. [CrossRef]
42. Gong, Y.F.; Robinson, B.S.; Rose, R.E.; Deminie, C.; Spicer, T.P.; Stock, D.; Colonno, R.J.; Lin, P.F. In Vitro Resistance Profile of the Human Immunodeficiency Virus Type 1 Protease Inhibitor BMS-232632. *Antimicrob. Agents Chemother.* **2000**, *44*, 2319–2326. [CrossRef]
43. Malan, D.R.N.; Krantz, E.; David, N.; Yang, R.; Mathew, M.; Iloeje, U.H.; Su, J.; McGrath, D.; 089 Stuy Group. 96-Week Efficacy and Safety of Atazanavir, with and without Ritonavir, in a HAART Regimen in Treatment-Naive Patients. *J. Int. Assoc. Physicians AIDS Care* **2010**, *9*, 34–42. [CrossRef]
44. Molina, J.-M.; Andrade-Villanueva, J.; Echevarria, J.; Chetchotisakd, P.; Corral, J.; David, N.; Moyle, G.; Mancini, M.; Percival, L.; Yang, R.; et al. Once-Daily Atazanavir/Ritonavir versus Twice-Daily Lopinavir/Ritonavir, Each in Combination with Tenofovir and Emtricitabine, for Management of Antiretroviral-Naive HIV-1-Infected Patients: 48 Week Efficacy and Safety Results of the CASTLE Study. *Lancet* **2008**, *372*, 646–655. [CrossRef]
45. Rosenbloom, D.I.S.; Hill, A.L.; Rabi, S.A.; Siliciano, R.F.; Nowak, M.A. Antiretroviral Dynamics Determines HIV Evolution and Predicts Therapy Outcome. *Nat. Med.* **2012**, *18*, 1378–1385. [CrossRef] [PubMed]
46. Stockdale, A.J.; Saunders, M.J.; Boyd, M.A.; Bonnett, L.J.; Johnston, V.; Wandeler, G.; Schoffelen, A.F.; Ciaffi, L.; Stafford, K.; Collier, A.C.; et al. Effectiveness of Protease Inhibitor/Nucleos(t)Ide Reverse Transcriptase Inhibitor-Based Second-Line Antiretroviral Therapy for the Treatment of Human Immunodeficiency Virus Type 1 Infection in Sub-Saharan Africa: A Systematic Review and Meta-Analysis. *Clin. Infect. Dis.* **2018**, *66*, 1846–1857. [CrossRef] [PubMed]
47. Colonno, R.J.; Thiry, A.; Limoli, K.; Parkin, N. Activities of Atazanavir (BMS-232632) against a Large Panel of Human Immunodeficiency Virus Type 1 Clinical Isolates Resistant to One or More Approved Protease Inhibitors. *Antimicrob. Agents Chemother.* **2003**, *47*, 1324–1333. [CrossRef]
48. Rhee, S.-Y.; Taylor, J.; Fessel, W.J.; Kaufman, D.; Towner, W.; Troia, P.; Ruane, P.; Hellinger, J.; Shirvani, V.; Zolopa, A.; et al. HIV-1 Protease Mutations and Protease Inhibitor Cross-Resistance. *Antimicrob. Agents Chemother.* **2010**, *54*, 4253–4261. [CrossRef]
49. Yanchunas, J.; Langley, D.R.; Tao, L.; Rose, R.E.; Friborg, J.; Colonno, R.J.; Doyle, M.L. Molecular Basis for Increased Susceptibility of Isolates with Atazanavir Resistance-Conferring Substitution I50L to Other Protease Inhibitors. *Antimicrob. Agents Chemother.* **2005**, *49*, 3825–3832. [CrossRef]
50. Rhee, S.-Y.; Shafer, R.W. Geographically-Stratified HIV-1 Group M Pol Subtype and Circulating Recombinant Form Sequences. *Sci. Data* **2018**, *5*, 180148. [CrossRef]

51. Stanford HIV Drug Resistance Database HIV Drug Resistance Database. Available online: https://hivdb.stanford.edu/pages/documentPage/PI_mutationClassification.html (accessed on 2 March 2022).
52. Rhee, S.-Y.; Sankaran, K.; Varghese, V.; Winters, M.A.; Hurt, C.B.; Eron, J.J.; Parkin, N.; Holmes, S.P.; Holodniy, M.; Shafer, R.W. HIV-1 Protease, Reverse Transcriptase, and Integrase Variation. *J. Virol.* **2016**, *90*, 6058–6070. [CrossRef]
53. Holm, S. A Simple Sequentially Rejective Multiple Test Procedure. *Scand. J. Stat.* **1979**, *6*, 65–70.
54. Rhee, S.-Y.; Liu, T.F.; Holmes, S.P.; Shafer, R.W. HIV-1 Subtype B Protease and Reverse Transcriptase Amino Acid Covariation. *PLoS Comput. Biol.* **2007**, *3*, e87. [CrossRef]
55. Scutari, M. Learning Bayesian Networks with the Bnlearn R Package. *J. Stat. Soft.* **2010**, *35*, 1–22. [CrossRef]
56. Almende, B.V.; Benoit, T.; Titouan, R. VisNetwork: Network Visualization Using "vis.Js" Library. Available online: https://CRAN.R-project.org/package=visNetwork (accessed on 2 March 2022).

pathogens

MDPI

Review

Probe Capture Enrichment Methods for HIV and HCV Genome Sequencing and Drug Resistance Genotyping

Chantal Munyuza [1], Hezhao Ji [1,2] and Emma R. Lee [1,*]

[1] National HIV and Retrovirology Laboratories, National Microbiology Laboratory at JC Wilt Infectious Diseases Research Centre, Public Health Agency of Canada, Winnipeg, MB R3E 3R2, Canada; chantal.munyuza@phac-aspc.gc.ca (C.M.); hezhao.ji@phac-aspc.gc.ca (H.J.)

[2] Department of Medical Microbiology and Infectious Diseases, University of Manitoba, Winnipeg, MB R3E 0J9, Canada

* Correspondence: emma.r.lee@phac-aspc.gc.ca; Tel.: +1-204-789-6512

Abstract: Human immunodeficiency virus (HIV) infections remain a significant public health concern worldwide. Over the years, sophisticated sequencing technologies such as next-generation sequencing (NGS) have emerged and been utilized to monitor the spread of HIV drug resistance (HIVDR), identify HIV drug resistance mutations, and characterize transmission dynamics. Similar applications also apply to the Hepatitis C virus (HCV), another bloodborne viral pathogen with significant intra-host genetic diversity. Several advantages to using NGS over conventional Sanger sequencing include increased data throughput, scalability, cost-effectiveness when batched sample testing is performed, and sensitivity for quantitative detection of minority resistant variants. However, NGS alone may fail to detect genomes from pathogens present in low copy numbers. As with all sequencing platforms, the primary determinant in achieving quality sequencing data is the quality and quantity of the initial template input. Samples containing degraded RNA/DNA and/or low copy number have been a consistent sequencing challenge. To overcome this limitation probe capture enrichment is a method that has recently been employed to target, enrich, and sequence the genome of a pathogen present in low copies, and for compromised specimens that contain poor quality nucleic acids. It involves the hybridization of sequence-specific DNA or RNA probes to a target sequence, which is followed by an enrichment step via PCR to increase the number of copies of the targeted sequences after which the samples are subjected to NGS procedures. This method has been performed on pathogens such as bacteria, fungus, and viruses and allows for the sequencing of complete genomes, with high coverage. Post NGS, data analysis can be performed through various bioinformatics pipelines which can provide information on genetic diversity, genotype, virulence, and drug resistance. This article reviews how probe capture enrichment helps to increase the likelihood of sequencing HIV and HCV samples that contain low viral loads and/or are compromised.

Keywords: HIV; HCV; probe capture; enrichment; next-generation sequencing

Citation: Munyuza, C.; Ji, H.; Lee, E.R. Probe Capture Enrichment Methods for HIV and HCV Genome Sequencing and Drug Resistance Genotyping. *Pathogens* **2022**, *11*, 693. https://doi.org/10.3390/pathogens11060693

Academic Editor: Wenyu Lin

Received: 27 April 2022
Accepted: 14 June 2022
Published: 16 June 2022

1. Introduction

After four decades of intense efforts from all relevant fields across the world, HIV/AIDS remains a significant global public health concern. According to the Joint United Nations Programme on HIV/AIDS (UNAIDS), approximately 38 million people were living with HIV and an estimated 1.7 million people were newly infected with HIV in 2020 worldwide [1,2]. UNAIDS has set ambitious targets for the elimination of HIV/AIDS by 2030 [3]. The UNAIDS 95-95-95 targets stipulate that 95% of people living with HIV (PLWH) should be aware of their HIV status, 95% of people who are aware of their status should be receiving treatment, and 95% of people on treatment should be virally suppressed [3]. Likewise, hepatitis C virus (HCV) is another major bloodborne pathogen of significant public health concern. An estimated 58 million people currently live with chronic HCV infection, and approximately 1.5 million new HCV infections occur each year [4]. In 2016, the World Health Organization (WHO) developed the Global Health Sector Strategy on Viral Hepatitis. This strategy aims to treat 80% of HCV infections, reduce new viral hepatitis infections by 90%, and reduce deaths caused by viral hepatitis infection by 65% by 2030 [4]. HIV and HCV share commonalities in that both are enveloped viruses with a positive-sense, single-stranded RNA genome. In addition, both viruses are featured by their significant genetic diversity, resulting largely from their rapid replication rates and the error-prone reverse transcriptases they rely on [5–7]. Effective HIV and HCV strain and drug resistance monitoring facilitated by genome sequencing and drug resistance (DR) genotyping help monitor the progress towards these elimination targets.

Conventional Sanger sequencing has been the primary technology applied in genome sequencing and genotypic DR testing for HIV and HCV [8,9]. Since 2005, next-generation sequencing (NGS) technologies have revolutionized the sequencing methodology, with significantly improved scalability, data throughput, sensitivity for minority resistant variants, and cost-effectiveness when batched sample testing is performed [10–13]. Nevertheless, the concentration and integrity of the input viral RNA or DNA templates determine the success of viral genotyping, regardless of the sequencing technology applied. Low viral load (VL) and low integrity often pose a significant challenge when sequencing samples collected from patients on antiviral therapy or those with severe RNA degradation [14,15].

Probe capture enrichment (also called target enrichment sequencing or hybridization capture) is a fairly recent methodology used to sequence samples containing low genomic copy numbers of a particular pathogen versus the host or from samples that have been compromised [16]. Hybridization capture involves the hybridization of sequence-specific DNA or RNA probes to a target fragment of DNA [17]. Probes are often custom-designed, targeting specific regions of interest within the template genome. For example, HIV probes can be designed to capture all major subtypes or to target particular subtypes such as subtype B of HIV-1 [18,19]. This method when performed prior to NGS would allow for complete genomes to be reconstructed directly from clinical samples. Whole genome sequencing data could then have various applications such as phylogenetics, epidemiology, and drug resistance testing [16]. Implementing this method in clinical diagnostic settings would have a direct effect on patient care as the information provided can guide patient treatment plans.

This promising method has been used successfully in a wide array of pathogens, including the parasite *Plasmodium falciparum* [20], fungi such as *Candida albicans* [21], bacteria such as *Mycobacterium tuberculosis* [22], and *Chlamydia trachomatis* [23] and viral pathogens such as HIV [18,19,24–29], HCV [24,28] and SARS-CoV-2 [30]; however, currently there is no consensus /standardized target enrichment protocol for HIV or HCV [16,31]. In this review, the various aspects of probe capture enrichment protocols used on HIV, and in some cases HCV, will be presented.

2. Overview of Experimental Methods

Hybridization capture protocols all include the same general steps [32]. The first step is nucleic acid extraction from a sample (DNA and/or RNA). This is followed by library preparation which will differ depending on the target organism, the quality and quantity of sample, and the library preparation kit being used. Target enrichment will occur after the library preparation. This process involves steps to hybridize the probes to the target sequence, enrich the probe-target complex, and elution to obtain the enriched fragment of interest. PCR-amplification will then be conducted to prepare the NGS library before sequencing on an NGS platform. The NGS data can then be processed using a professional bioinformatics platform for further analysis and alignment of the reads (Figure 1).

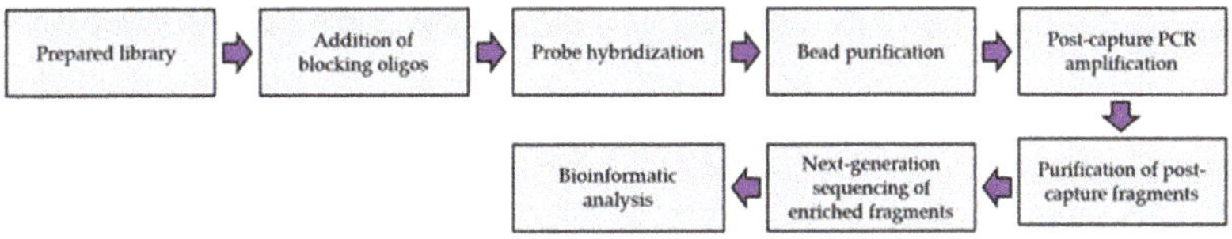

Figure 1. Overview of target-enrichment NGS procedure.

3. Extraction Method

Sequencing projects typically begin by extracting nucleic acid from a given sample. The steps involved in the extraction of DNA or RNA include cell lysis, removal of membrane lipids (or other nucleic acids), purification, and concentration of the nucleic acid [33]. The most common methodologies for nucleic acid extraction include full automation or manually conducted kits. Target enrichment protocols mainly use spin columns or an automated liquid-handling robot. These two nucleic acid extraction methods were evaluated for their advantages and disadvantages by N. Ali et al. [33]. They found that column-based nucleic acid extraction is one of the best techniques used as it is fast and its results are easily reproducible. The main drawback is that it requires a small centrifuge that can generate aerosols and lead to a slight chance of cross-contamination. Conversely, automated liquid handling robots offer precise handling of reagents and samples, reducing sample loss and artificial errors. However, the main drawback to this method would be the high cost of the equipment.

The nucleic acid extraction methods used in some target enrichment protocols are summarized in Table 1. Another consideration involved in nucleic acid extraction is the starting material. Nucleic acid extraction from whole blood, plasma, and serum is typically more successful than extraction from dried blood spots (DBS) [33–35]. With its easiness of sample collection and relieved requirements for transportation and storage, DBS is becoming a popular, cost-effective alternative to plasma, serum, or whole blood for HIV-1 genotyping and VL monitoring in resource-limited settings [15,36]. However, one primary limitation of DBS for such molecular assays is that the nucleic acid integrity can be significantly compromised, making downstream PCR amplification difficult [15,36]. Although further studies are warranted, the probe capture methodology could be a solution to salvage samples of poor viral RNA integrity for molecular assays.

Table 1. Summary of nucleic acid extraction methods used in reported target enrichment protocols.

Virus	Samples Tested	Extraction Method	Ref
HIV	HIV-1 (plasma)	m2000sp RNA protocol (Abbott Laboratories)	[19]
HIV	HIV-1 (subtype B) from HIV-1-infected latent cell lines	DNeasy Blood and Tissue Kit (Qiagen)	[25]
HIV	HIV-1-infected cell line (ACH-2)	DNeasy Blood and Tissue Kit (Qiagen)	[26]
HCV	Clinical HCV samples (plasma)	NucliSENS Magnetic Extraction System (bioMérieux)	[24]
HIV	HIV-1 infected cell lines (ACH-2, J-Lat)	Gentra Puregene cell kit (Qiagen)	[27]
HCV	Clinical HCV samples (plasma), In vitro RNA transcipts, assay controls (plasma)	Agencourt RNAdvance blood kit (Beckman Coulter), QIAamp viral RNA minikit (Qiagen), NucliSENS magnetic extration system (bioMérieux)	[28]
HIV	Clinical HIV samples (plasma)	NucliSENS easyMAG system (bioMérieux)	[18]
HIV	Clinical HIV samples from peripheral blood mononuclear cells	EZ1 Virus Mini Kit v2.0 (Qiagen)	[29]

A successful library can be prepared from nucleic acid extracted from various sample types with either a manual or an automated protocol. Therefore, the primary considerations in choosing an extraction protocol for target enrichment will depend upon cost expectations and the availability of the required equipment.

4. Library Preparation Method

For any NGS-based project, the library preparation method is of utmost importance. The ability to generate a high-quality library is necessary for obtaining successful sequencing data. NGS library preparation is when the DNA fragments are prepared for sequencing via the addition of specific adapter sequences onto the ends of the DNA fragments (Figure 2) [37]. Several different library preparation kits and protocols can be used to produce a library, some of which are compiled in Table 2. While these kits may differ regarding their particular protocol and the amount of sample input required, most kits involve enzymatical or mechanical DNA fragmentation followed by tagmentation and incorporation of adapter sequences to the ends of the fragments. The derived libraries are then amplified and quantified prior to sequencing.

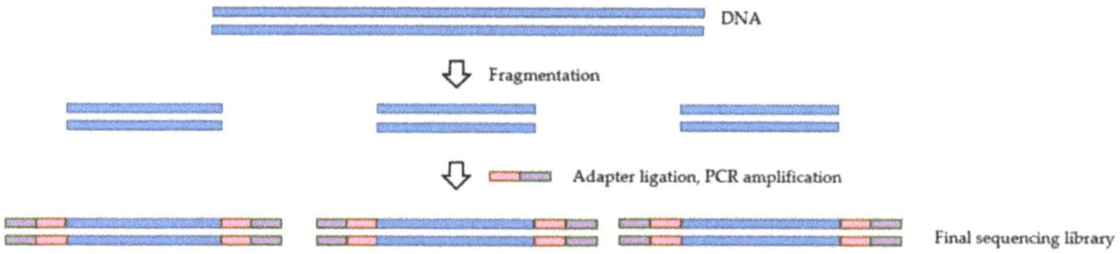

Figure 2. Overview of the library preparation process.

Table 2. Summary of library preparation methods used in target enrichment protocol.

Virus	Library Preparation Method	Ref
HIV	Nextera XT Kit (Illumina)	[19,29]
HIV	NEBNext UltraDNA II library preparation kit and NEBNExt multiplex oligos for Illumina (New England BioLabs)	[25,26]
HCV	NEBNext® UltraTM Directional RNA Library Prep Kit for Illumina® (New England Biolabs)	[24]
HIV	SPRI-TE nucleic acid extractor automated library preparation (Beckman Coulter) with NEXTflex adapters (Bioo Scientific)	[27]
HCV	KAPA Library Preparation Kit with index tagging using KAPA HiFi HotStart (KAPA Biosystems) and NEBNext multiplex oligos for Illumina Index Primer Sets 1 and 2 (New England BioLabs), SureSelect^{XT} Target Enrichment (Aligent), NEBNext Ultra Directional RNA Library Prep kit for Illumina (New England BioLabs)	[28]
HIV	SMARTer Stranded Total RNA-Seq Kit V2—Pico Input Mammalian (Clontech, Takara Bio)	[18]

The fragmentation step is vital to the target enrichment process as it influences its outcome. Shorter fragments are captured with higher specificity than longer pieces [38]. An additional consideration when selecting a library preparation kit for target enrichment is the number of PCR amplification steps. PCR amplification can introduce bias when DNA fragments are not all amplified with the same efficiency. A negative influence of PCR amplification on the uniformity of enrichment was noted in a study conducted by Mamanova et al. [38]. This negative influence was due to the bias introduced in PCRs before and after hybridization.

Fragments that are either G-C rich or A-T rich are often underrepresented in the library preparations in comparison to G-C neutral fragments, which are amplified more efficiently [37]. One possible solution to this issue could be eliminating the PCR amplification step before hybridization, thus preventing the introduction of bias. However, while this may be possible when dealing with intact DNA available in large quantities, it lacks robustness in low-integrity samples [38]. As a result, this could be a concern when dealing with samples such as DBS, which may contain viral templates of low integrity, rendering the PCR amplification step inevitable. A mitigation solution in such cases could be to reduce the number of PCR cycles rather than remove the step entirely in order to reduce some of the bias while also generating a robust library from low integrity samples [38]. Additionally, Van Dijk et al. [37] have suggested several library preparation methods for reducing bias in NGS, including the use of Kapa HiFi polymerase instead of the standard Phusion polymerase used in Illumina library preparation.

5. Target Enrichment

Several target enrichment protocols, including xGen Lockdown probe protocol (IDT, Coralville, IA, USA), NimbleGen Seq Cap EZ system (Roche, Indianapolis, IN, USA), and the SureSelect Target Enrichment System (Agilent Technologies, Santa Clara, CA, USA), all operate using the same general procedure (Figure 3). However, the IDT xGen Lockdown probe protocol appears to be the most commonly used [39]. This protocol recommends using 500 ng of each prepared library as the input. Enrichment steps include combining DNA with the blocking oligos, after which the mixture is dried using a SpeedVac system. Blocking oligos are short oligonucleotide sequences that are added to decrease the possibility of hybridization between library adapters and capture probes during the target enrichment process [39]. The hybridization reaction can then be performed by combining the biotinylated probes with the dried DNA. Following hybridization, streptavidin-coated beads are added to pull down the probe-target complexes. Non-target fragments with no probe binding will then be washed off, and post-capture PCR amplification will follow to amplify the target fragment further. The final step involves purification of the post-capture PCR amplicons, after which the enriched library may be quantified and validated for sequencing on a NGS instrument. Some of the commercially available probe capture enrichment kits are listed in Table 3.

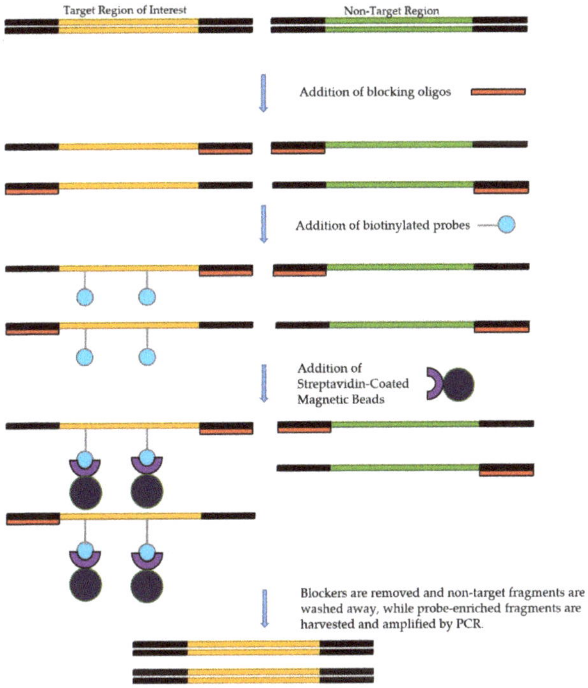

Figure 3. Overview of the target enrichment process.

Table 3. Commercially available probe capture enrichment kits.

Company	Kit	Compatible NGS Platforms	Type of Baits	Ref
Agilent Technologies	SureSelect^{XT} Target Enrichment System	HiSeq, MiSeq, NextSeq 500, NovaSeq 6000	Pre-designed or custom designed DNA probes	[40]
Agilent Technologies	SureSelect^{XT} RNA Target Enrichment System	HiSeq, MiSeq, NextSeq 500	Pre-designed or custom designed RNA probes	[41]
Arbor Biosciences	myBaits Hybridization Capture for Targeted NGS	Illumina platforms, Ion Torrent, PacBio, Oxford Nanopore Technologies	Pre-designed or custom designed RNA or DNA probes	[42]
Integrated DNA Technologies (IDT)	xGen™ NGS Hybridization Capture	Illumina platforms	Pre-designed or custom designed DNA probes	[43]
Lucigen	NxSeq HybCap Target Enrichment Kit	Illumina platforms, Ion Torrent	Custom designed RNA probes	[44]
Roche	NimbleGen Seq Cap EZ system	Illumina platforms	Pre-designed or custom designed DNA probes	[45]

The probes used in target enrichment are either DNA or RNA explicitly designed for the genomic region of interest. Probes are designed to the desired tiling density across the target region. The tiling density refers to the extent of the coverage of the target region by the probes. For example, 1× tiling density means that the probes cover the region of interest one time. In contrast, 2× tiling density means that the region of interest would be covered twice using a series of overlapping probes. Figure 4 depicts the differences between 1× and 2× tiling densities. The probes are often approximately 120 nt in length; however, this could differ, and are labeled by 5′ terminal biotinylation. Once the desired probes have been designed, they can then be synthesized by a biotechnology company for use in enrichment studies. Table 4 summarizes various probe design methods that have been used in reported target enrichment studies.

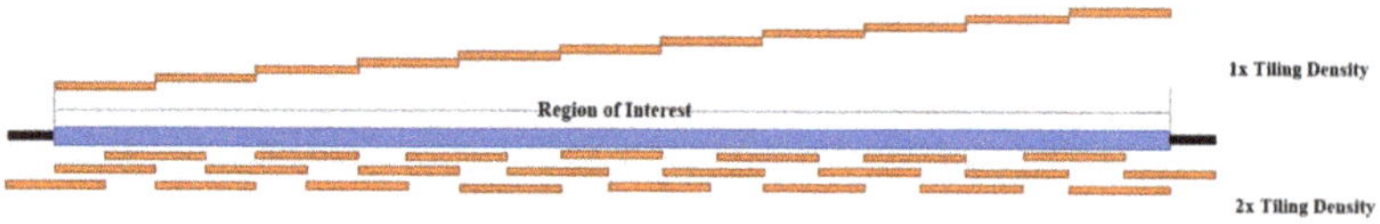

Figure 4. Comparison of 1× and 2× Tiling Density (Adapted from IDT).

Table 4. Summary of probe design methods used in target enrichment protocols.

Virus	Probe Design/Enrichment Method	Sequencing Platform	Ref
HIV	120 nt biotinylated DNA probes based on consensus sequences of HIV-1 and HIV-2 (xGen Lockdown probes and reagents, Integrated DNA Technologies)	MiSeq (Illumina)	[19]
HIV	120 nt biotinylated DNA probes based on HXB2 reference sequence (xGen Lockdown probes and reagents, Integrated DNA Technologies)	MiSeq or NextSeq (Illumina)	[25]
HIV	120 nt biotinylated DNA probes based on HXB2 reference sequence (xGen Lockdown probes, Integrated DNA Technologies) with SeqCap EZ Hybridization and Wash Kit (Roche NimbleGen)	MiSeq or NextSeq (Illumina)	[26]
HCV	120 nt DNA oligonucleotide probes (xGen Lockdown probes, Integrated DNA Technologies) and xGen® Lockdown® protocol (Integrated DNA Technologies)	MiSeq (Illumina)	[24]

Table 4. *Cont.*

Virus	Probe Design/Enrichment Method	Sequencing Platform	Ref
HIV	120 nt DNA oligonucleotide probes (xGen Lockdown probes, Integrated DNA Technologies) with Dynabeads MyOne Streptavidin T1 (Life Technologies), PCR enrichment with Kapa HiFi DNA polymerase	MiSeq (Illumina)	[27]
HCV	120 nt RNA probes spanning 953 GenBank HCV reference genomes. Enrichment using xGen Lockdown protocol (Integrated DNA Technologies), NimbleGen Seq Cap EZ system (Roche), SureSelect Target Enrichment System (Agilent), or SureSelect^{XT} Target Enrichment (Agilent)	MiSeq (Illumina)	[28]
HIV	Custom HIV-specific biotinylated 120 nt probe set (XGen Lockdown Probes, Integrated DNA Technologies) with SeqCap EZ hybridization and wash kit (Roche)	MiSeq (Illumina)	[18]
HIV	Custom HIV-specific 120 nt probes (Arbor Biosciences) used with the myBaits target capture kit (Arbor Bioesceinces)	MiSeq (Illumina)	[29]

In studies focusing on a highly diversified virus such as HIV or HCV, probe design takes careful consideration if attempting to be inclusive of all subtypes and groups. In order to design probes to variable sequences such as those present in the different subtypes of HIV, one strategy is to first design the probes based on a consensus sequence and then subsequently design probes that will cover the variable regions for each subtype to be covered [19]. Alternatively, probes can be designed to be specific to one subtype rather than inclusive of all subtypes [26].

While the IDT xGen Lockdown probe protocol appears to be the most commonly used target enrichment protocol, an alternative protocol that has recently been gaining attention is the myBaits Hybridization Capture Kit by Arbour Biosciences (Ann Arbor, MI, USA). The myBaits protocol involves using pools of in-solution biotinylated RNA/DNA probes that are provided with reagents and allow for targeted sequencing on NGS platforms such as Illumina (San Diego, CA, USA), Ion Torrent, PacBio (Menlo Park, CA, USA), and Nanopore [42]. This kit also allows the user to use custom-designed probes with the kit.

The specific design of the probes will be influenced by the particular goal of the laboratory investigation. Additionally, the choice between RNA and DNA probes may depend on factors such as cost, storage requirements, and stability of the probes. A big advantage of using DNA probes is their stability as they can be safely stored at −20 °C, whereas RNA probes are sensitive to freeze-thaw cycles and need to be held at −80 °C for long-term storage [46]. RNA probes are often used due to the increased stability and hybridization efficiency of RNA-DNA duplexes compared to DNA-DNA duplexes [46].

6. Next-Generation Sequencing

After target enrichment, samples are sequenced on an NGS platform [47]. Although several NGS platforms are available, the MiSeq and NextSeq systems by Illumina have been most commonly used in target enrichment studies [19,25]. Both the MiSeq and the NextSeq operate using sequencing by synthesis technology in which the addition of fluorescently labeled nucleotides is tracked as the DNA chain is copied [47]. This process occurs in a massively parallel fashion, with the number of cycles determining the read length. The main difference between the two platforms is the read length and data output. MiSeq generates a maximum read length of 600 bp with a maximum output of 13.2–15 Gb compared to a maximum read length of 300 bp reads and output of 32.5–39 Gb with the NextSeq [48]. Both the MiSeq and NextSeq have been used successfully in target enrichment studies, so the choice of which sequencing platform to use will depend on the specifics of the research project itself and the availability of sequencing instruments.

7. Post-Sequencing Analysis (Bioinformatics)

After completion of sequencing on an NGS instrument, the data from the sequencing run should be analyzed using sophisticated bioinformatics tools. Both MiSeq and NextSeq systems provide read information in a fastq file, which can then be imported into bioanalytic software for analysis. Regardless of the platform, many researchers apply the same procedures to refine their sequencing data. This includes an initial data cleaning up by discarding reads of low quality scores. Adapter sequences are then removed from the reads. The remaining good quality reads are then mapped to a reference sequence available from GenBank or even a custom-defined reference. Once the reads have been aligned, a consensus sequence can be derived and the final alignment determined for further downstream applications [19,25,26]. A summary of the bioinformatics tools that have been used in target enrichment studies of HIV and HCV viruses can be found in Table 5.

Table 5. Summary of bioinformatics platforms used in target enrichment protocols.

Virus	Bioinformatic Platforms Used	Ref
HIV	CLC Genomics Workbench 9.0 (CLC Bio) for analysis of reads, phylogenetic analysis using SIMPLOT	[19]
HIV	In-house Pearl script for selection of paired-reads and cleaning of the reads, BWA-MEM algorithm for alignment to reference, Samtools program and Picard command line tools to remove multiply aligned reads and duplicates, final aligned files visualized with Integrative Genomics Viewer (IGV)	[25]
HIV	BWA-MEM algorithm for mapping, Picard tool for the removal of PCR duplicates, Strand NGS (Strand Life Science) for the visualization of mapped data, Low Frequency Variant Detection Tool (CLC Genomics Workbench 7.5 software, CLC Bio) for error correction	[26]
HCV	QUASR v7.01 & CutAdapt v1.7.1 for trimming sequences, Bowtie v2.2.4 for comparision to human reference, BLASTn database for screenning reads, Vicuna v1.3 & V-FAT v1.0 for de novo assembly, Mosaik v2.2.28 for mapping reads back to assembly, V-Phaser v2.0 for calling variants, V-Profiler v1.0 for examining intra-host diversity	[24]
HIV	BWA-MEM algorithm for alignment, sambamba for marking duplicate alignments, Gene SeT AnaLysis Toolkit for gene ontology analysis	[27]
HCV	FastQC, Tanoti, in-house resistance mutation tools, de novo assembly using MetAmos Genome mapping, assembly, and finishing using CLC Genomics Workbench, DAA analysis using in-house script QUASR v7.01 & CutAdapt v1.7.1 for trimming sequences, Bowtie v2.2.4 for comparision to human reference, BLASTn database for screenning reads, Vicuna v1.3 & V-FAT v1.0 for de novo assembly, Mosaik v2.2.28 for mapping reads back to assembly, V-Phaser v2.0 for calling variants, V-Profiler v1.0 for examining intra-host diversity	[28]
HIV	Kraken for processing raw sequences, Trimmomatic for trimming sequences, SPAdes, metaSPAdes for assembly into contigs, cd-hit-est for cluster generation, shiver for mapping reads, Kallisto for mapping reads with no contigs assembled, phyloscanner for identifying and removing contaminant reads, Stanford drug resistance tool for determining consensus and minority drug resisitance levels	[18]
HIV	CLC Genomics Workbench software (CLC Bio/Qiagen) for analysis of reads and assembly by mapping to the HIV genome (HIV-1 Strain HXB2) from GenBank	[29]

8. Target Enrichment Performance

The success of target enrichment protocols has been demonstrated in studies comparing sequencing data from a run without enrichment and a run with enrichment prior to sequencing. In a study by P. Miyazato et al. [26], libraries prepared in the absence of enrichment resulted in 1.9% of the total reads mapping to the provirus. When the same libraries were enriched the total number of reads mapping to the provirus was increased from 1.9% to 99%. Similarly, in a study by S. Iwase et al. [25], DNA-capture sequencing was tested in HIV-1 infected latent cell lines. In the absence of target enrichment, from a total of 1.6×10^6 reads, only three mapped to the provirus. This number increased in a subsequent experiment involving target enrichment prior to sequencing. In this case, out of 560,000 mapped reads, there were 28,000 reads aligning with the provirus [25]. This target enrichment protocol provided information that allowed researchers to characterize the provirus using a new method and authors indicated its applications to other experiments aiming to treat HIV-1 infection.

In addition, target enrichment has also been shown in an HIV study by J. Yamaguchi et al. [19], to aid in the sequencing of low titer samples. They found that the genomes obtained from samples with VLs between log 4 and 5 copies/mL were still incomplete in the absence of the enrichment protocol procedure. In addition, when using samples at even a lower titer of log 3.5 copies/mL sequencing without the enrichment steps resulted in 20–50% coverage only. In comparison, sequencing the same low titer samples (log 3.5 copies/mL) using the enrichment protocol resulted in full genome sequences. This result is important as it indicates that low titer specimens, such as those present in patients undergoing antiretroviral therapy, may be characterized using the probe capture enrichment method.

9. Limitations

Despite the potential benefit target enrichment procedures could have in the study of highly diverse pathogens, like HIV and HCV, there are limitations to its implementation in a clinical diagnostic setting. A major drawback to using this method is the elevated cost of the target enrichment procedure which would make it difficult to implement in low-income settings. The estimated cost per sample from extraction to NGS is approximately $65 US although the cost may be lower if the probes are diluted, and a larger number of samples are pooled during hybridization [46]. In addition to the cost, target enrichment procedures often involve lengthy and complex protocols which would require skilled individuals who are knowledgeable about the various components of the protocols. These factors would make it difficult for a target enrichment procedure to be implemented in a clinical setting where results are required in a timely manner, especially in cases where novel pathogens are of interest [16].

10. Conclusions

Next-generation sequencing-based viral genome sequencing is crucial to understanding the ever-changing dynamics of HIV and HCV. The ability to generate quality sequencing data from samples with low viral titre or samples with poor nucleic acid integrity is important. Target enrichment has emerged as a potential solution to the problems of sequencing difficult samples and can potentially enable complete viral genome sequence even for low-quality clinical specimens. Increased adoption of such technology in research and development fields for HIV, HCV, and other pathogens is foreseeable.

Author Contributions: Conceptualization, E.R.L. and H.J.; Methodology, C.M. and E.R.L.; Writing—Original Draft Preparation, C.M.; Writing—Review & Editing, C.M., H.J. and E.R.L.; Supervision, H.J.; Project Administration, E.R.L. All co-authors made substantial contributions to this work. All authors have read and agreed to the published version of the manuscript.

Funding: This research received no external funding.

Institutional Review Board Statement: Not applicable.

Informed Consent Statement: Not applicable.

Data Availability Statement: Not applicable.

Acknowledgments: This work is funded by the National Microbiology Laboratory branch of the Public Health Agency of Canada, to which all co-authors are affiliated.

Conflicts of Interest: The authors declare no conflict of interest. The funder played no role in the design of the study; in the collection, analyses, or interpretation of data; in the writing of the manuscript, or in the decision to publish the results.

References

1. HIV/AIDS. UNAIDS Data 2020. 432 Geneva, Switzerland. 2020. Available online: https://www.unaids.org/en/resources/documents/2020/unaids-data (accessed on 25 March 2022).
2. World Health Organization. Available online: https://www.who.int/news-room/fact-sheets/detail/hiv-aids (accessed on 9 March 2022).
3. UNAIDS. Fast-Track- Ending the AIDs Epidemic by 2030. Available online: https://www.unaids.org/sites/default/files/media_asset/JC2686_WAD2014report_en.pdf (accessed on 10 March 2022).
4. World Health Organisation. Available online: https://www.who.int/news-room/fact-sheets/detail/hepatitis-c (accessed on 9 March 2022).
5. Tough, R.H.; Tough, R.H.; McLaren, P.J.; McLaren, P.J.; Tough, R.H.; Tough, R.H.; McLaren, P.J.; McLaren, P.J. Interaction of the Host and Viral Genome and Their Influence on HIV Disease. *Front. Genet.* **2019**, *9*, 720. [CrossRef] [PubMed]
6. Gobran, S.T.; Ancuta, P.; Shoukry, N.H. A Tale of Two Viruses: Immunological Insights Into HCV/HIV Coinfection. *Front. Immunol.* **2021**, *12*, 726419. [CrossRef] [PubMed]
7. Martinez, M.A.; Nevot, M.; Jordan-Paiz, A.; Franco, S. Similarities between Human Immunodeficiency Virus Type 1 and Hepatitis C Virus Genetic and Phenotypic Protease Quasispecies Diversity. *J. Virol.* **2015**, *89*, 9758–9764. [CrossRef]
8. Manyana, S.; Gounder, L.; Pillay, M.; Manasa, J.; Naidoo, K.; Chimukangara, B. HIV-1 Drug Resistance Genotyping in Resource Limited Settings: Current and Future Perspectives in Sequencing Technologies. *Viruses* **2021**, *13*, 1125. [CrossRef] [PubMed]
9. Raj, V.S.; Hundie, G.B.; Schürch, A.; Smits, S.L.; Pas, S.D.; Le Pogam, S.; Janssen, H.L.A.; De Knegt, R.J.; Osterhaus, A.D.M.E.; Najera, I.; et al. Identification of HCV Resistant Variants against Direct Acting Antivirals in Plasma and Liver of Treatment Naïve Patients. *Sci. Rep.* **2017**, *7*, 4688. [CrossRef]
10. Simen, B.; Simons, J.F.; Hullsiek, K.H.; Novak, R.M.; MacArthur, R.D.; Baxter, J.D.; Huang, C.; Lubeski, C.; Turenchalk, G.S.; Braverman, M.S.; et al. Low-Abundance Drug-Resistant Viral Variants in Chronically HIV-Infected, Antiretroviral Treatment–Naive Patients Significantly Impact Treatment Outcomes. *J. Infect. Dis.* **2009**, *199*, 693–701. [CrossRef] [PubMed]
11. Margulies, M.; Egholm, M.; Altman, W.E.; Attiya, S.; Bader, J.S.; Bemben, L.A.; Berka, J.; Braverman, M.S.; Chen, Y.-J.; Chen, Z.; et al. Genome sequencing in microfabricated high-density picolitre reactors. *Nature* **2005**, *437*, 376–380. [CrossRef] [PubMed]
12. Inzaule, S.C.; Ondoa, P.; Peter, T.; Mugyenyi, P.N.; Stevens, W.S.; de Wit, T.F.R.; Hamers, R.L. Affordable HIV drug-resistance testing for monitoring of antiretroviral therapy in sub-Saharan Africa. *Lancet Infect. Dis.* **2016**, *16*, e267–e275. [CrossRef]
13. Masquelier, B. Low-Frequency HIV-1 Drug Resistance Mutations and Risk of NNRTI-Based Antiretroviral Treatment Failure. *JAMA* **2011**, *305*, 1327–1335. [CrossRef]
14. Fitzpatrick, A.H.; Rupnik, A.; O'Shea, H.; Crispie, F.; Keaveney, S.; Cotter, P. High Throughput Sequencing for the Detection and Characterization of RNA Viruses. *Front. Microbiol.* **2021**, *12*, 621719. [CrossRef]
15. Aitken, S.C.; Wallis, C.L.; Stevens, W.; de Wit, T.R.; Schuurman, R. Stability of HIV-1 Nucleic Acids in Dried Blood Spot Samples for HIV-1 Drug Resistance Genotyping. *PLoS ONE* **2015**, *10*, e0131541. [CrossRef] [PubMed]
16. Gaudin, M.; Desnues, C. Hybrid Capture-Based Next Generation Sequencing and Its Application to Human Infectious Diseases. *Front. Microbiol.* **2018**, *9*, 2924. [CrossRef] [PubMed]
17. Shih, S.Y.; Bose, N.; Gonçalves, A.B.R.; Erlich, H.A.; Calloway, C.D. Applications of Probe Capture Enrichment Next Generation Sequencing for Whole Mitochondrial Genome and 426 Nuclear SNPs for Forensically Challenging Samples. *Genes* **2018**, *9*, 49. [CrossRef] [PubMed]
18. Bonsall, D.; Golubchik, T.; De Cesare, M.; Limbada, M.; Kosloff, B.; MacIntyre-Cockett, G.; Hall, M.; Wymant, C.; Ansari, M.A.; Abeler-Dörner, L.; et al. A Comprehensive Genomics Solution for HIV Surveillance and Clinical Monitoring in Low-Income Settings. *J. Clin. Microbiol.* **2020**, *58*, e00382-20. [CrossRef] [PubMed]
19. Yamaguchi, J.; Olivo, A.; Laeyendecker, O.; Forberg, K.; Ndembi, N.; Mbanya, D.; Kaptue, L.; Quinn, T.C.; Cloherty, G.A.; Rodgers, M.A.; et al. Universal Target Capture of HIV Sequences from NGS Libraries. *Front. Microbiol.* **2018**, *9*, 2150. [CrossRef] [PubMed]
20. Melnikov, A.; Galinsky, K.; Rogov, P.; Fennell, T.; Van Tyne, D.; Russ, C.; Daniels, R.; Barnes, K.G.; Bochicchio, J.; Ndiaye, D.; et al. Hybrid selection for sequencing pathogen genomes from clinical samples. *Genome Biol.* **2011**, *12*, R73. [CrossRef]
21. Amorim-Vaz, S.; Tran, V.D.T.; Pradervand, S.; Pagni, M.; Coste, A.T.; Sanglard, D. RNA Enrichment Method for Quantitative Transcriptional Analysis of Pathogens In Vivo Applied to the Fungus Candida albicans. *mBio* **2015**, *6*, e00942-15. [CrossRef]
22. Brown, A.C.; Bryant, J.M.; Einer-Jensen, K.; Holdstock, J.; Houniet, D.T.; Chan, J.Z.M.; Depledge, D.P.; Nikolayevskyy, V.; Broda, A.; Stone, M.J.; et al. Rapid Whole-Genome Sequencing of Mycobacterium tuberculosis Isolates Directly from Clinical Samples. *J. Clin. Microbiol.* **2015**, *53*, 2230–2237. [CrossRef]
23. Christiansen, M.T.; Brown, A.C.; Kundu, S.; Tutill, H.J.; Williams, R.; Brown, J.R.; Holdstock, J.; Holland, M.J.; Stevenson, S.; Dave, J.; et al. Whole-genome enrichment and sequencing of Chlamydia trachomatisdirectly from clinical samples. *BMC Infect. Dis.* **2014**, *14*, 591. [CrossRef]
24. Bonsall, D.; Ansari, M.A.; Ip, C.L.; Trebes, A.; Brown, A.; Klenerman, P.; Buck, D.S.; Piazza, P.; Barnes, E.; Bowden, R.; et al. ve-SEQ: Robust, unbiased enrichment for streamlined detection and whole-genome sequencing of HCV and other highly diverse pathogens. *F1000Research* **2015**, *4*, 1062. [CrossRef]
25. Iwase, S.C.; Miyazato, P.; Katsuya, H.; Islam, S.; Yang, B.T.J.; Ito, J.; Matsuo, M.; Takeuchi, H.; Ishida, T.; Matsuda, K.; et al. HIV-1 DNA-capture-seq is a useful tool for the comprehensive characterization of HIV-1 provirus. *Sci. Rep.* **2019**, *9*, 12326. [CrossRef] [PubMed]

26. Miyazato, P.; Katsuya, H.; Fukuda, A.; Uchiyama, Y.; Matsuo, M.; Tokunaga, M.; Hino, S.; Nakao, M.; Satou, Y. Application of targeted enrichment to next-generation sequencing of retroviruses integrated into the host human genome. *Sci. Rep.* **2016**, *6*, 28324. [CrossRef] [PubMed]
27. Sunshine, S.; Kirchner, R.; Amr, S.S.; Mansur, L.; Shakhbatyan, R.; Kim, M.; Bosque, A.; Siliciano, R.F.; Planelles, V.; Hofmann, O.; et al. HIV Integration Site Analysis of Cellular Models of HIV Latency with a Probe-Enriched Next-Generation Sequencing Assay. *J. Virol.* **2016**, *90*, 4511–4519. [CrossRef] [PubMed]
28. Thomson, E.; Vattipally, B.S.; Badhan, A.; Christiansen, M.T.; Adamson, W.; Ansari, M.A.; Bibby, D.; Breuer, J.; Brown, A.; Bowden, R.; et al. Comparison of Next-Generation Sequencing Technologies for Comprehensive Assessment of Full-Length Hepatitis C Viral Genomes. *J. Clin. Microbiol.* **2016**, *54*, 2470–2484. [CrossRef]
29. Colson, P.; Dhiver, C.; Tamalet, C.; Delerce, J.; Glazunova, O.O.; Gaudin, M.; Levasseur, A.; Raoult, D. Dramatic HIV DNA degradation associated with spontaneous HIV suppression and disease-free outcome in a young seropositive woman following her infection. *Sci. Rep.* **2020**, *10*, 2548. [CrossRef]
30. Charre, C.; Ginevra, C.; Sabatier, M.; Regue, H.; Destras, G.; Brun, S.; Burfin, G.; Scholtes, C.; Morfin, F.; Valette, M.; et al. Evaluation of NGS-based approaches for SARS-CoV-2 whole genome characterisation. *Virus Evol.* **2020**, *6*, veaa075. [CrossRef]
31. Martínez-Puchol, S.; Itarte, M.; Rusiñol, M.; Forés, E.; Mejías-Molina, C.; Andrés, C.; Antón, A.; Quer, J.; Abril, J.F.; Girones, R.; et al. Exploring the diversity of coronavirus in sewage during COVID-19 pandemic: Don't miss the forest for the trees. *Sci. Total Environ.* **2021**, *800*, 149562. [CrossRef]
32. Berg, M.G.; Yamaguchi, J.; Alessandri-Gradt, E.; Tell, R.W.; Plantier, J.-C.; Brennan, C.A. A Pan-HIV Strategy for Complete Genome Sequencing. *J. Clin. Microbiol.* **2016**, *54*, 868–882. [CrossRef]
33. Ali, N.; Rampazzo, R.; Costa, A.D.T.; Krieger, M.A. Current Nucleic Acid Extraction Methods and Their Implications to Point-of-Care Diagnostics. *BioMed Res. Int.* **2017**, *2017*, 9306564. [CrossRef]
34. Cornelissen, M.; Gall, A.; Vink, M.; Zorgdrager, F.; Binter, Š.; Edwards, S.; Jurriaans, S.; Bakker, M.; Ong, S.H.; Gras, L.; et al. From clinical sample to complete genome: Comparing methods for the extraction of HIV-1 RNA for high-throughput deep sequencing. *Virus Res.* **2017**, *239*, 10–16. [CrossRef]
35. Guichet, E.; Serrano, L.; Laurent, C.; Eymard-Duvernay, S.; Kuaban, C.; Vidal, L.; Delaporte, E.; Ngole, E.M.; Ayouba, A.; Peeters, M. Comparison of different nucleic acid preparation methods to improve specific HIV-1 RNA isolation for viral load testing on dried blood spots. *J. Virol. Methods* **2017**, *251*, 75–79. [CrossRef] [PubMed]
36. Singh, D.; Dhummakupt, A.; Siems, L.; Persaud, D. Alternative Sample Types for HIV-1 Antiretroviral Drug Resistance Testing. *J. Infect. Dis.* **2017**, *216*, S834–S837. [CrossRef] [PubMed]
37. van Dijk, E.L.; Jaszczyszyn, Y.; Thermes, C. Library preparation methods for next-generation sequencing: Tone down the bias. *Exp. Cell Res.* **2014**, *322*, 12–20. [CrossRef] [PubMed]
38. Mamanova, L.; Coffey, A.J.; Scott, C.E.; Kozarewa, I.; Turner, E.; Kumar, A.; Howard, E.; Shendure, J.; Turner, D.J. Target-enrichment strategies for next-generation sequencing. *Nat. Methods* **2010**, *7*, 111–118. [CrossRef] [PubMed]
39. Integrated DNA Technologies IDT. Available online: https://www.idtdna.com (accessed on 18 January 2022).
40. Agilent Technologies. Available online: https://www.agilent.com/cs/library/usermanuals/public/G7530-90000.pdf (accessed on 25 March 2022).
41. Agilent Technologies. Available online: https://www.agilent.com/cs/library/usermanuals/Public/G9691-90000.pdf (accessed on 25 March 2022).
42. Arbor Biosciences. Available online: https://arborbiosci.com/genomics/targeted-sequencing/mybaits/ (accessed on 11 March 2022).
43. Integrated DNA Technologies IDT. Available online: https://www.idtdna.com/pages/products/next-generation-sequencing/workflow/xgen-ngs-hybridization-capture?utm_source=google&utm_medium=cpc&utm_campaign=ga_ngs&utm_content=ad_group_hyb_capture&gclid=EAIaIQobChMI3feYsL7i9gIVshbUAR1G9AFyEAAYASAAEgJrsvD_BwE (accessed on 18 January 2022).
44. Lucigen. Available online: https://www.lucigen.com/nxseq-hybcap-target-enrichment-kit/ (accessed on 11 March 2022).
45. Roche. Available online: https://www.roche.com/ (accessed on 11 March 2022).
46. Hale, H.; Gardner, E.M.; Viruel, J.; Pokorny, L.; Johnson, M.G. Strategies for reducing per-sample costs in target capture sequencing for phylogenomics and population genomics in plants. *Appl. Plant Sci.* **2020**, *8*, e11337. [CrossRef]
47. Slatko, B.E.; Gardner, A.F.; Ausubel, F.M. Overview of Next-Generation Sequencing Technologies. *Curr. Protoc. Mol. Biol.* **2018**, *122*, e59. [CrossRef]
48. Goodwin, S.; McPherson, J.D.; McCombie, W.R. Coming of age: Ten years of next-generation sequencing technologies. *Nat. Rev. Genet.* **2016**, *17*, 333–351. [CrossRef]

pathogens

MDPI

Commentary

Point-of-Care Tests for HIV Drug Resistance Monitoring: Advances and Potentials

Rayeil J. Chua [1], Rupert Capiña [1] and Hezhao Ji [1,2,*]

[1] National Microbiology Laboratory at JC Wilt Infectious Diseases Research Centre, Public Health Agency of Canada, Winnipeg, MB R3E 3R2, Canada; rayeil.chua@phac-aspc.gc.ca (R.J.C.); rupert.capina@phac-aspc.gc.ca (R.C.)

[2] Max Rady College of Medicine, University of Manitoba, Winnipeg, MB R3E 0J9, Canada

* Correspondence: hezhao.ji@phac-aspc.gc.ca; Tel.: +1-204-789-6521

Abstract: HIV/AIDS is a global public health crisis that is yet to be contained. Effective management of HIV drug resistance (HIVDR) supported by close resistance monitoring is essential in achieving the WHO 95-95-95 targets, aiming to end the AIDS epidemic by 2030. Point-of-care tests (POCT) enable decentralized HIVDR testing with a short turnaround time and minimal instrumental requirement, allowing timely initiation of effective antiretroviral therapy (ART) and regimen adjustment as needed. HIVDR POCT is of particular significance in an era when ART access is scaling up at a global level and enhanced HIVDR monitoring is urgently needed, especially for low-to-middle-income countries. This article provides an overview of the currently available technologies that have been applied or potentially used in HIVDR POCT. It may also benefit the continued research and development efforts toward more innovative HIVDR diagnostics.

Keywords: HIV; drug resistance; point-of-care test; resource-limited setting

Citation: Chua, R.J.; Capiña, R.; Ji, H. Point-of-Care Tests for HIV Drug Resistance Monitoring: Advances and Potentials. *Pathogens* **2022**, *11*, 724. https://doi.org/10.3390/pathogens11070724

Academic Editor: Thibault Mesplède

Received: 17 May 2022
Accepted: 22 June 2022
Published: 25 June 2022

1. Introduction

The HIV/AIDS epidemic has spread to all populated continents in the past four decades, with no sign of ending in the foreseeable future. HIV has infected 79.3 million people since it was identified in the early 1980s, and approximately 36.3 million people have died from AIDS-related illnesses thus far [1]. In 2014, UNAIDS declared ambitious new targets (95-95-95) to end the HIV epidemic by 2030 [2,3]. However, a challenge that hinders the elimination of HIV is its ability to constantly mutate genetically and antigenically [4]. The high variability of HIV causes the emergence of drug-resistant variants, reducing the effectiveness of available antiretroviral (ARV) drugs [4,5]. As access to antiretroviral therapy continues to scale up globally, HIV drug resistance (HIVDR) has become an imminent danger that threatens the substantial strides taken by UNAIDS and impairs the maximization of antiretroviral therapy (ART) benefits [5].

HIV infections are treated with drugs that target viral proteins essential for their replication, such as protease (PR), reverse transcriptase (RT), and integrase (IN). Nucleoside and non-nucleoside reverse transcriptase inhibitors (NRTI and NNRTIs) prevent the reverse transcription of HIV RNA to proviral DNA. In contrast, protease inhibitors (PIs) prevent the cleavage of HIV polyproteins, and integrase inhibitors (INIs) interrupt viral integration into the host genome. The rise of HIV drug resistance mutations (HIVDRMs) may render these drugs inefficient in virological suppression for all available ART agents. As such, genotypic HIVDR typing aims to examine the presence of known HIVDRMs, qualitatively or semi-quantitatively [6]. HIV RNA and proviral DNA represents replication-competent viruses and archived/historical viral populations respectively. Therefore, the detection of HIVDRM(s) in HIV RNA and DNA may have different clinical application values. For instance, HIVDRMs in HIV DNA may only inform the treatment initiation with proper ARV drugs, while HIVDRM detection in HIV RNA benefits both ART initiation and subsequent regimen adjustment.

To minimize the impacts of HIVDR variants, the WHO recommends routine surveillance of HIVDR to monitor ART and pre-exposure prophylaxis (PrEP) distribution [4]. The information obtained can also be facilitated by countries when forming their national treatment guidelines to optimize patient outcomes [4]. Since most infections occur in the developing world, an ideal HIVDR assay should be accountable and readily accessible/operable in resource-limited settings (RLS) [7]. Point-of-care tests (POCT) are vital for de-centralized HIVDR monitoring, which offers lower testing costs, broader test access, shorter turnaround time, and timely initiation of effective ARV treatment and regimen adjustment as needed [8]. In addition, an ideal POCT should meet the ASSURED (**A**ffordable, **S**ensitive, **S**pecific, **U**ser-friendly, **R**apid, **E**quipment-free, and **D**eliverable) criteria endorsed by WHO (Geneva, Switzerland) [7].

POCT has been of great interest to HIVDR professionals for decades. It is acknowledged that the topic of HIVDR POCT had previously been reviewed by others [8–10]. While minimizing the overlap with the previous literature, we focus in this article on the recent advances in the previously examined POCTs, newly emerged technologies that have recently been attempted for HIVDR and also those assays with great POCT potentials but yet to be validated for HIVDR.

2. Technologies Attempted for HIVDR POCT

Conventional genotypic HIVDR typing relies on Sanger sequencing of target HIV genes and examines the presence of all known HIVDRMs within collectively. In contrast, while the mechanisms vary, all attempted HIVDR POCTs thus far target single or multiple selected known HIVDRMs only. Described below are several near-POCTs attempted for HIVDR testing thus far.

2.1. Oligonucleotide Ligation Assays (OLA)

OLA is a point mutation test initially developed by Landegren et al. to detect mutations associated with sickle cell anemia [11,12]. The assay was devised based on the premise that two adjacent oligonucleotide probes hybridized to a specific DNA sequence could be covalently bonded with a ligase that will discriminate against mismatched bases [11,13]. Frenkel et al. modified the OLA to detect HIVDR mutations in the HIV-1 *pol* gene with colorimetry or spectrophotometry [14–16]. OLA is the most-studied POCT for HIVDR. It has been implemented to detect HIVDR mutations associated with NNRTIs and NRTIs in Thailand, Zimbabwe, and Kenya [17–20]. Panpradist et al. recognized the need to improve the detection step, which proved too extensive and complex [12]. As a result, they created the OLA-Simple, allowing ligated products to be viewed as colored lines on a lateral flow strip either with a scanner or by plain sight [12,21,22].

The latest version of the OLA-Simple is capable of detecting HIVDRMs across multiple HIV-1 subtypes (A, B, C, D, and CRF01_AE) using different specimen types (dried blood spots, peripheral blood mononuclear cells, and plasma) [21]. There are four main steps involved in OLA-Simple, as illustrated in Figure 1A: (1) acquirement of a cDNA/DNA template, (2) PCR amplification, (3) ligation of oligonucleotide probes that identify single mutations, and (4) lateral flow detection [12,22]. In the ligation step, a genotype (mutation or wild-type) specific probe coupled with a reporter molecule and a common probe with biotin will bind adjacent to one another to a complementary sequence on the template [14,15]. The ligated products are then captured with immobilized antibodies on the lateral flow strip and detected with anti-biotin antibodies conjugated with gold nanoparticles to generate lines on the strip [21].

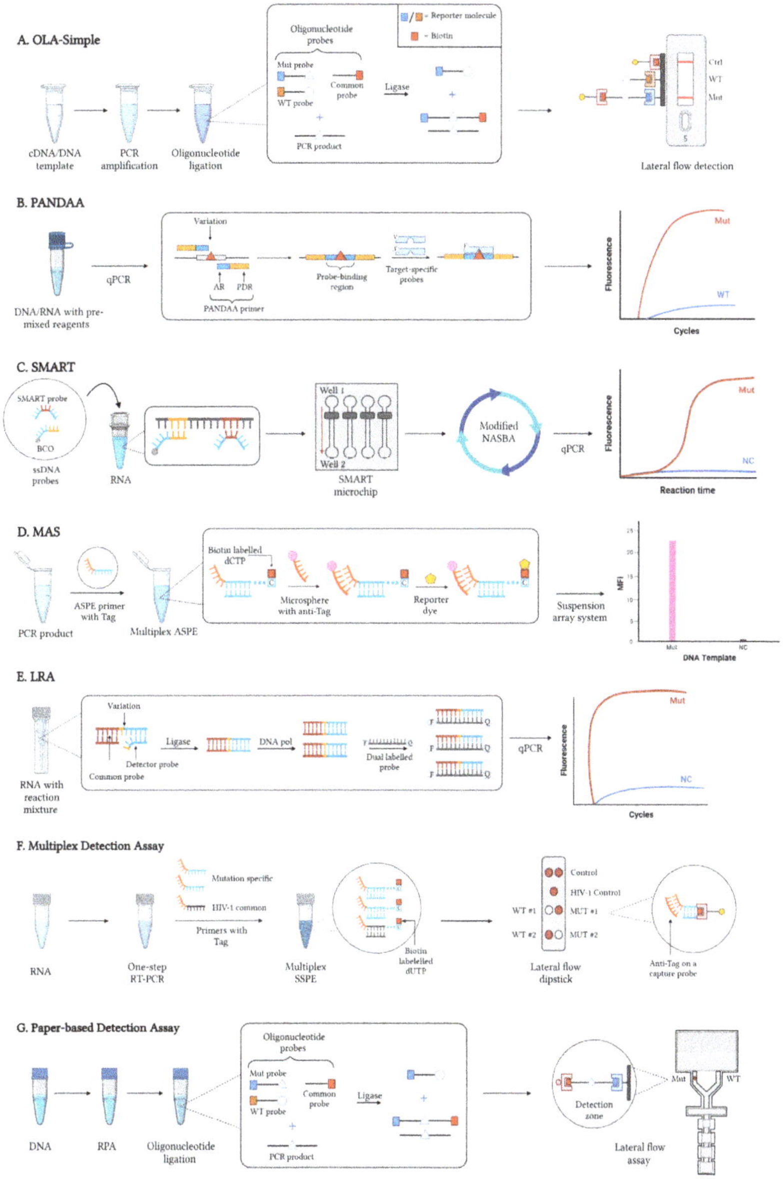

Figure 1. Simplified workflow of the exemplar POCTs. (**A**) In the OLA-Simple workflow, using pre-made dry reagents, RNA is used to make PCR products that will undergo oligonucleotide ligation. In this step, mutant (Mut)/wild-type (WT) probes with a reporter molecule will bind adjacent to a common probe with biotin to a complementary sequence on the template. The ligation products are eventually visualized using a lateral flow device; (**B**) PANDAA workflow, displaying how primers and probes bind to their specific target to determine the mutation of interest. Starting with the binding of PANDAA primers, qPCR will generate a homogenous population with a probe-binding region, followed by the annealing of a target-specific probe with FAM fluorophore (F) to detect the single nucleotide polymorphism. Wild-type specific probes are labelled with VIC fluorophore (V) for comparison.

(**C**) The SMART assay combines molecular biology with microfluidics. The ssDNA probes are first added to RNA, where the SMART probe will bind to the mutation sequence and the BCO binds to a conserved sequence. Next, a SMART microchip will facilitate the separation of bound and unbound probes from well 1 to 2. This step is followed by a modified NASBA that will amplify probes and generate a sequence for a molecular beacon to identify the presence or absence of a mutation. (NC = negative control). (**D**) The MAS assay utilizes ASPE primers labelled with Tag to discriminate against a mutation. Primers are first added to a PCR product, and multiplex ASPE ensues. While amplification proceeds, biotin is incorporated into the final product and the Tag/anti-Tag sequences will bind to one another. After, a reporter dye will find biotin and detect hybridized products using a suspension array system. Data is then recorded by measuring the mean fluorescence intensity (MFI). (**E**) The LRA assay starts with adding RNA template to a reaction mixture containing ligases, DNA polymerases and oligonucleotide primers. Ligation occurs between a common probe that is complementary to the RNA template and a detector probe that is complementary to the variant. DNA polymerase will then become activated, and qPCR will amplify ligated products using dual-labelled probes with fluorophore (F) and quencher (Q) for detection. (**F**) Multiplex detection assay that uses specific primers with a Tag sequence and a lateral flow dipstick to detect mutations. PCR samples undergo a multiplex SSPE, and biotin is incorporated into the extended products. As amplicons flow through the dipstick, they bind to a complementary anti-Tag and anti-biotin antibodies with gold nanoparticles will produce red dots for identification. (**G**) A paper-based assay that combines different techniques to detect HIVDRM. It starts with RPA, followed by oligonucleotide ligation at the site of interest. Products are then applied to an ELISA lateral flow assay, where fixed antibodies will hybridize with reporter molecules. Then streptavidin conjugated with horseradish peroxidase binds to biotin to produce brown precipitates for signal detection.

OLA-Simple has been successfully applied in detecting HIVDRMs across multiple major HIV-1 subtypes using specimens from Kenya, South Africa, Peru, Thailand, and Mexico. High concordances were obtained between the results from OLA-Simple and those from Sanger sequencing and even high-sensitivity HIVDR assays such as Next Generation Sequencing (NGS) with a mutation frequency cut-off at 1% [21,22]. The significant advantages of this assay include the use of lyophilized reagents for fast and accurate setup and the elimination of purification between steps [21,22]. The major equipment required to complete this assay includes a thermocycler and an office scanner linked to instructional software [21].

OLA-Simple is the best-developed near-POCT HIVDR thus far that has been validated for multiple key HIVDRMs from different HIV-1 subtypes. The instructional software by the assay developers also ensures the user-friendliness of performing OLA-Simple assay by inexperienced lab personnel, especially in RLS. Despite the promising approach of the OLA-Simple, it needs extra machinery to generate a DNA template, electricity to operate, and storage for lyophilized reagents. Proper training may also be necessary to avoid cross-contamination between different steps.

2.2. *Pan-Degenerate Amplification and Adaptation (PANDAA)*

Allele-specific PCR is one of the most widely used tests for HIVDR identification using quantitative PCR (qPCR) and is one of the many foundations of current POCTs. PANDAA is a point mutation assay developed by MacLeod et al. to tolerate the diversity of nucleotide sequences flanking the target mutation site, which showed a 96.9% sensitivity and 97.5% specificity for quantifying HIVDRMs present at $\geq$5% [23]. In a traditional qPCR reaction, the binding of probes that are not in perfect complementation to the template are unstable and can produce false-negative results. In contrast, the PANDAA assay addresses high sequence variability through normalization of probe-binding regions, as seen in Figure 1B. PANDAA primers have two main features: (1) a pan-degenerate region (PDR) containing degenerate bases to account for nucleotide variability and (2) an adaptor region (AR) that matches the probe-binding regions flanking the mutation of interest [24].

PANDAA requires no separate cDNA synthesis or PCR procedures, and the starting materials could be RNA or DNA. During the initial qPCR cycles, site-directed mutagenesis will occur to generate a population of homogenous amplicons with similar probe-binding regions complementary to the probes. This step removes any secondary polymorphisms that interfere with probe hybridization in a traditional qPCR. A target-specific probe will bind in the next stage, and qPCR results will differentiate between a mutant and a wild-type. While these primers were created by combining multiple HIV-1 subtypes to build a consensus sequence, the PANDAA assay can be curated to accommodate local HIV-1 sequence diversity [23]. One intrinsic limitation of PANDAA, and other allele-specific assays in general, is that a negative readout from it implies the absence of the target DRM allele. It could result from wild-type template, shown by a positive outcome from the wild-type control, or from a new allele at the target locus, which may render negative results for both wild-type and mutation-specific reactions.

Kouamou et al. assessed the diagnostic accuracy of PANDAA against plasma samples from patients in Zimbabwe that have acquired HIVDR [25]. Five HIVDRMs associated with resistance against NNRTIs and NRTIs were examined with PANDAA, and the results were compared against data from Sanger sequencing. The results demonstrated that PANDAA rendered excellent sensitivity (95~98%) and specificity (83~100%), although the readouts fluctuated among assays targeting different HIVDRMs. Maraupala et al. conducted another study to test the diagnostic accuracy of PANDAA against Sanger in a cohort of patients from Botswana to use the assay as an alternative approach for rapid HIVDR test, and high concordance was observed between the data obtained from the two compared assays [24]. This positions PANDAA as a promising assay for HIVDR, although further refinement is required to meet the ASSURED criteria [7].

PANDAA requires a qPCR machine, but there is no need for bioinformatics support in data interpretation [26]. One significant advantage of PANDAA is that it mitigates the impacts of sequence diversity in the flanking region, which would inevitably affect the probe binding and reduce assay sensitivity and accuracy. Still, it requires either RNA/DNA as a starting material, which indicates an extra step on top of the assay.

2.3. SMART (Simple Method for Amplifying RNA Targets)

The prevalence of influenza prompted McCalla et al. to develop a method to amplify RNA with engineered ssDNA probes [27]. They reasoned that the availability of rapid POCT diagnostics would aid the healthcare community in containing known infections and preventing antiviral misuse. Their research found nucleic acid sequence-based amplification (NASBA) assays advanced with the incorporation of microfluidic devices showed a positive response. McCalla's methodology realized the benefit of this combination and made crucial modifications to NASBA to remove RNA secondary structures that hindered the assay and presented the SMART assay. Morabito et al. then repurposed the assay to detect HIVDR mutation from HIV-1 samples [28].

The SMART technique uses two ssDNA probes that will bind to a specific RNA target sequence: (1) biotinylated capture oligonucleotide (BCO) attached to a streptavidin-coated magnetic bead (SMB) binds to a conserved region and (2) a SMART probe binds to the mutated region (Figure 1C). The two probes are added to the solution to bind to the RNA target. The solution is then added to the SMART microchip, where it will pass through a microfluidic channel from one well to the other while a magnet separates bound and unbound structures. Afterwards, the modified NASBA will isothermally amplify the probes and molecular beacons will quantify data in real-time [27–29].

In this assay, amplification and detection rely on the specific hybridization of the SMART probe rather than the target RNA. The SMART probe can be engineered to have favourable or unfavourable binding energies to ensure it does not bind to other oligonucleotides. Additional benefits are the use of microfluidics, which provide a close, efficient, automated system that reduces hands-on time, human error, and probable contamination. To complete this assay, a microfluidic device and a qPCR are the main components needed [27–29]. Limitations in this assay consist of the absence of an extraction step to obtain an RNA template and qPCR, which utilizes molecular beacons. Concerns may also arise as to proper laboratory operation and the requirement of technicians to be trained. Again, a laboratory space will be essential in implementing this method. Moreover, this preliminary study has only tested a single NNRTI mutation, and the lack of real-world studies hinders the determination of feasibility of the assay, although it holds great promise for POCT application.

2.4. Multiplex Allele-Specific (MAS) Assay

This assay was developed by Zhang et al. to address issues with existing POCTs only detecting one or few mutations per test. Based on a suspension array technology, they produced the MAS assay that would allow simultaneous detection of multiple major HIV-DRs [30–33]. In their study, allele-specific primer extension (ASPE) primers were designed to target HIVDRMs associated with NNRTIs, NRTIs, and PIs in HIV-1 subtype C [31,33]. The ASPE primers are further designed so that the 3′ end contains an allele-specific nucleotide, while its 5′ end has a Tag sequence [31].

The assay begins with adding ASPE primers to a reaction tube with a reagent mixture and the templates (Figure 1D). Primer extension occurs and biotin-labelled dCTP is incorporated into the derived amplicon. Afterwards, hybridization occurs where microspheres containing an anti-Tag anneal to the extended DNA fragment through complementary Tag sequence. A reporter molecule will then bind to the biotin and record the mean fluorescence intensity of each microsphere based on its unique internal dye.

In a follow-up study, Zhang et al. adapted the assay for subtype B by altering ASPE primers and applied it to dried blood spot specimens collected from patients on antiretroviral therapy [33]. For both HIV-1 subtypes B and C, MAS assays showed high concordance and comparability when compared to conventional Sanger sequencing [31,33]. The flexibility of the suspension array technology allows MAS assay to be easily adapted to create any ASPE primer and corresponding microspheres. Unlike sequencing, the results can be easily interpreted and reported right away [31]. The sensitivity of MAS assay ranged from 1.56% to 12.5% depending on the HIVDRM being examined [33].

The extreme variation among HIV-1 sequences warrants the need for specific primers to be made. In addition, as a PCR product is the starting material, raw material will have to be processed to obtain a template. There is also the requirement for a suspension array system to perform the assay and, as previously mentioned, such equipment comes with an extra burden. Considering the logistic and operational constraints as the assay is now, more development efforts are warranted to apply MAS in practice for HIVDR POCT.

2.5. Ligation on RNA Amplification (LRA)

A preliminary study by Barany exhibited a ligase-mediated detection technique to distinguish between mismatched and complementary bases [34]. This process joins two oligonucleotides together when they bind to a complementary sequence on a template. The products then undergo cyclic amplification with another set of oligos complementary to the original ones. In the presence of a mismatch, ligation and amplification are inhibited, suggesting the presence of a variation. This method has been adapted to anneal two DNA probes using miRNA as a template [35–37]. Zhang et al. noted the valuable role this assay played and the part it could have in HIVDR testing. After some modifications, one being the exclusion of cDNA production, which eliminated the risk of nucleotide misincorporation, the LRA assay was formed [38].

The LRA assay is a one-step, single-buffer scheme to detect point mutations from RNA. In a single tube with optimized buffer, ligase, hot-start DNA polymerase, and oligonucleotide primers are added (Figure 1E). The reaction has three phases: (1) ligation, (2) polymerase activation, and (3) quantitative PCR. The temperature is set low during the first stage, allowing ligase to be the only active enzyme. In this step, a common probe that fully complements the RNA target and a detector probe that is complementary only to the variant are hybridized adjacent to one another by a ligase. In the next stage, the ligase enzyme is inactivated and DNA polymerase is activated instead, signalling the start of the amplification phase. Ligated probes are then amplified with dual-labelled probes during qPCR for detection [38].

This method separates the ligation and qPCR reaction by exploiting hot-start polymerases. By doing so, only one reaction is active at a time, thereby achieving maximum sensitivity, which for K103N was determined as 1%. The results showed that this assay outperformed allele-specific PCR and pyrosequencing in detecting mutant specificity [38]. To perform this assay, a qPCR is needed, suggesting that it needs the minimum requirements of a laboratory.

Zhang et al. had only presented a proof of principle for this assay. The RNA template used had mutations introduced into the pol gene of the HIV-1 genome through site-directed mutagenesis. Further follow-up study and validation of this assay to examine different HIV-1 subtypes and HIVDRMs other than the K103N mutation they studied remain to be completed and are necessary before its potential for HIVDR POCT can be better assessed.

2.6. Multiplex Detection Assay

Gomez et al. first developed a novel method for rapid genotyping of blood groups using a lateral flow biosensor to prevent alloimmunization, a major complication during blood transfusions [39]. Using whole blood sample, multiplex PCR was performed, and amplicons were transferred onto a lateral flow strip. Products were then captured with probes and red dots appeared for blood group deduction. Combining strategies that were previously used for genetic diseases and cancer, they adapted the assay to detect HIVDRM [40–42].

The study executed a proof-of-concept test on HIV-1 subtype B plasma specimens to rapidly detect mutations that cause resistance in NNRTIs. The assay has two major components: (1) a rapid multiplex detection system utilizing sequence-specific primer extension (SSPE) primers containing a Tag sequence and (2) a dry reagent lateral flow dipstick that generates red dots (Figure 1F). As the sample migrates on the dipstick, the products are captured by probes with an anti-Tag sequence. Then, an anti-biotin antibody conjugated with gold nanoparticles will cause the generation of red dots for easy visual recognition. On the membrane, wild-types can be detected on the left, while mutants can be found on the right [43]. This assay was shown to have a limit of detection of 100 copies of plasmid DNA, while its sensitivity for mutation detection was determined as 10~20% depending on the HIVDRMs being examined. Notably, these findings remain to be validated using clinical specimens.

Besides the OLA-Simple, Multiplex Detection Assay is another methodology claimed to be near-point-of-care assay [43]. It proves to be versatile as primers and probes of this assay can be tailored to detect known or new HIVDR mutations prevalent in an area. It is specific, and no cross-reaction has occurred between sequences from different subtypes or between wild-type and variant sequences. Compared to Sanger, which has a lower detection limit of 200 copies per assay, the study achieved a lower detection limit of 20 copies per assay, demonstrating higher sensitivity. To perform this assay, some of the instruments required include a thermal cycler and a drying oven. Regardless of the positive indications of this assay, an extraction step is needed. Also, much like the LRA, it fails to provide much real-life evidence to showcase its practicality.

2.7. Paper-Based Detection Assay

This proof-of-concept assay builds on multiple techniques and previous work done by researchers. Bui et al. found success when they joined PCR with OLA to detect drug resistance in *Streptococcus pneumonia*. As discussed earlier, Panpradist et al. made significant strides in modifying the OLA-Simple [21,44]. Based on these findings, Natoli et al. established a technique that would isothermally amplify HIV products and detect drug resistance through a lateral flow [45].

The assay starts with using recombinase polymerase amplification (RPA) to amplify a portion of the HIV-1 pol region (Figure 1G). Afterwards, an oligonucleotide assay, akin to the OLA-Simple, is used to discriminate against wild-type, and visualization occurs through the paper-based ELISA. In the lateral flow membrane, antibodies corresponding to reporter molecules are immobilized on each side of the fork and will each capture ligated products as they flow through the membrane. Brown precipitates will then appear if ligated products are present. The detection limit of this assay was determined as 10^3 copies of pre-amplification template while mutant templates were present at 20% [45].

RPA not only isothermally amplifies DNA in a short time, but it also tolerates impure samples, which is favorable in places where contamination is unavoidable. Reagents of this amplification technique can also be in lyophilized form, shortening preparation time. Additionally, the assay design proves to be specific as the fork in the membrane limits the aggregation of OLA products. To complete this assay, a heat block and a tabletop centrifuge is necessary for the RPA step prior to proceeding to OLA [45].

Although this assay can merely detect one mutation per test, it can be adapted to detect other high-impact mutations. At its current state, the assay is yet to have sample preparation as an integrated step, and more hands-on time is required when adding ELISA reagents to the membrane. Furthermore, gBlocks stocks were used as DNA template and the membrane design lacks a control region, lowering the validity of this assay. More research is needed to advance this technology towards POCT.

HIV patients often elude clinics after a one-time visit because of stigma, inconvenience, travel costs, or other socio-economic factors. It is then essential for physicians to diagnose and treat the patients on the same day. POCTs for HIVDR will aid physicians when determining the best drug regimen to start with or switch to in order to achieve suppressed viral loads. Table 1 provides an overview of some general features and requirements of these assays. The estimates of the assay costs and assay time was excluded as these numbers can vary depending on manufacturers and number of samples, respectively.

Table 1. An overview of current technologies promising for HIVDR POCT.

POCTs	Starting Material	Subtype Specificity	Major Equipment Required	Validated against Sanger	Refs.
OLA-Simple	DNA or RNA	HIV-1 (A, B, C, D, AE)	Thermocycler, Office scanner	✓	[16]
PANDAA	DNA or RNA	Subtype independent	qPCR machine	✓	[23]
SMART	RNA	HIV-1 (any subtype with a K103N region)	Microfluidic device, qPCR machine	×	[27]
MAS	DNA	HIV-1 (B, C)	Compact suspension array system	✓	[31,33]
LRA	RNA	HIV-1 (any subtype with a K103N region)	qPCR machine	×	[38]
Multiplex Detection Assay	RNA	HIV-1 (B)	Thermocycler, Dry oven	✓	[43]
Paper-based Detection Assay	DNA	HIV-1 (B)	Heat block, Thermocycler, Tabletop centrifuge	×	[45]

3. Other Potential POCT Technologies

As new methods arise, so do more opportunities for creating an ideal test for RLS. In this section, we explore two new technologies with the potential for simplified HIVDR typing.

3.1. Multiplex Solid-Phase Melt Curve Analysis

This melt curve analysis platform is a genotypic resistance assay that measures the hybridization, capture, and dissociation of multiple nucleic acid targets to and from surface-bound oligonucleotide probes. The probes have two parts: (1) a complementary sequence to HIV-1 strains and (2) a nucleotide triplet complementary to a codon at a drug resistance mutation. First, fluorescently labelled DNA is added to the oligonucleotide microarray at one temperature (i.e., 55 °C). Then, the concentration of labelled DNA captured is monitored in real-time by the probes as the solution temperature progressively increases. A time-series data is generated that defines duplex stability, which is used to identify the correct codon at the position of a drug resistance mutation. In vitro experiments were performed with HIV-1 plasma samples and culture supernatants, containing HIV-1 subtype A, B, C, D, CRF01_AE, and CRF02_AG [46]. Although this is a promising approach, operation in a closed-tube format and removing the wash step are essential. Multiplex PCR will need to be executed to detect the entire set of known HIVDRMs. Lastly, a production version of a prototype chip was used to detect fluorescence, so it is unsure how this would translate in real-world settings [46].

3.2. μBAR Platform

Myers et al. have developed the Microfluidic Biomolecular Amplification Reader (μBAR) in an attempt to combine electronics, optics, microfluidics, and molecular biology. The μBAR is a battery-powered, portable instrument capable of isothermal amplification of multiple markers with the use disposable microfluidic assay cartridges. First, the sample (i.e., blood, sputum, or saliva) is loaded onto a disposable microfluidic cartridge, where the system uses a loop-mediated isothermal amplification (LAMP) technique. The cartridge is then inserted into the μBAR, where it will control assay temperature, illuminate the chip, and monitor real-time fluorescence signals from individual reaction chambers [47,48].

Previously, the LAMP assay was verified to detect HIV and malaria from blood samples and TB drug resistance from sputum samples. Myers et al. have also exhibited use of the LAMP assay on the μBAR platform in detecting the HIV integrase gene. The platform also has GPS and cellphone connectivity for healthcare delivery in remote locations and epidemiological surveillance. The chip contains six inlets, meaning multiple samples can be loaded simultaneously. In its current form, the μBAR requires more work to modify for HIVDR detection [48].

3.3. Oxford Nanopore MinION (ONT) Sequencing

The increase in using NGS technologies to detect HIVDR have been on the rise. It is noteworthy that most of available NGS platforms are not even close to the bedside POCT considering their prohibitive instrument and reagent costs, demanding technical operation and complexity in data interpretation. One exception could be the MinION platform, developed by the Oxford Nanopore Technologies (https://nanoporetech.com/, accessed on 16 June 2022). MinION is thus far the only portable device that execute NGS on DNA or RNA templates with minimal requirement for additional instrumental and technical support.

Gonzalez et al. pioneered applying MinION sequencing to HIVDR analysis. HIV RNA was first extracted from plasma samples followed by PCR amplification. PCR products were then prepared for MinION library preparation and a sequencing library was generated to load into a flow cell. Good concordance was observed between the MinION consensus sequences and the Sanger sequencing outputs from the same patients, regarding both the sequence identity and HIVDR profiling [49]. While their findings support the usage of ONT in decentralized laboratories, the scarcity of supporting data from other labs warrants further investigation on the full potentials of MinION technologies in HIVDR POCT.

The technologies listed in this section are but a snippet of potential and relevant assays. For example, techniques that use GeneXpert, Clustered Regularly Interspaced Short Palindromic Repeats (CRISPR), and High-Resolution Melting (HRM) have also been implemented in drug resistance detection for varying pathogens. Perhaps these methods, coupled with the rise in technological advancement, may inspire new HIVDR POCTs.

4. Conclusions

The expansion of ART access comes with a growing concern for the rise in HIVDR. HIVDR monitoring is essential for effective HIV/AIDS management at individual and population levels. Conventional Sanger sequencing-based HIVDR genotyping may not be readily assessable, especially in RLS, for logistical and operational reasons. POCT offers a quick and affordable solution administered at or near patient care. The assays explored here show the progression of each test, where they stand, and adjustments that need to be made. Although the work that has been done is impressive, no such assay entirely embodies the ASSURED criteria. A fully validated POCT that satisfies the set standards and meets all the needs for HIVDR diagnostics, especially in RLS, has yet to be developed. More research still needs to be done as POCTs are indispensable in controlling the spread of drug-resistant HIV.

Author Contributions: Conceptualization, H.J.; Methodology, R.J.C., R.C. and H.J.; Writing—Original Draft Preparation, R.J.C.; Writing—Review & Editing, R.J.C., R.C. and H.J.; Supervision, H.J.; Project Administration, H.J. All co-authors made substantial contributions to this work. All authors have read and agreed to the published version of the manuscript.

Funding: This work is funded, APC included, by the National Microbiology Laboratory Branch of the Public Health Agency of Canada, to which all co-authors are affiliated.

Conflicts of Interest: The authors declare no conflict of interest. The funder had no role in the design of the study; in the collection, analyses, or interpretation of data; in the writing of the manuscript, or in the decision to publish the results.

References

1. UNAIDS. *Global HIV & AIDS Statistics—Fact Sheet*; UNAIDS: Geneva, Switzerland, 2022.
2. UNAIDS. *Understanding Fast-Track Acceleratiing Action to End the AIDS Epidemic by 2030*; UNAIDS: Geneva, Switzerland, 2015.
3. UNAIDS. *Prevailing against Pandemics by Putting People at the Center _World AIDS Day Report*; UNAIDS: Geneva, Switzerland, 2020.
4. World Health Organization. *HIV Drug Resistance Report 2021*; WHO: Geneva, Switzerland, 2021.
5. World Health Organization. *Global Action Plan on HIV Drug Resistance 2017–2021*; WHO: Geneva, Switzerland, 2017.
6. Inzaule, S.C.; Hamers, R.L.; Paredes, R.; Yang, C.; Schuurman, R.; Rinke de Wit, T.F. The Evolving Landscape of HIV Drug Resistance Diagnostics for Expanding Testing in Resource-Limited Settings. *AIDS Rev.* **2017**, *19*, 219–230. [PubMed]
7. Land, K.J.; Boeras, D.I.; Chen, X.S.; Ramsay, A.R.; Peeling, R.W. REASSURED diagnostics to inform disease control strategies, strengthen health systems and improve patient outcomes. *Nat. Microbiol.* **2019**, *4*, 46–54. [CrossRef]
8. Duarte, H.A.; Panpradist, N.; Beck, I.A.; Lutz, B.; Lai, J.; Kanthula, R.M.; Kantor, R.; Tripathi, A.; Saravanan, S.; MacLeod, I.J.; et al. Current Status of Point-of-Care Testing for Human Immunodeficiency Virus Drug Resistance. *J. Infect. Dis.* **2017**, *216*, S824–S828. [CrossRef] [PubMed]
9. Inzaule, S.C.; Ondoa, P.; Peter, T.; Mugyenyi, P.N.; Stevens, W.S.; de Wit, T.F.R.; Hamers, R.L. Affordable HIV drug-resistance testing for monitoring of antiretroviral therapy in sub-Saharan Africa. *Lancet Infect. Dis.* **2016**, *16*, e267–e275. [CrossRef]
10. Noguera-Julian, M. HIV drug resistance testing—The quest for Point-of-Care. *EBioMedicine* **2019**, *50*, 11–12. [CrossRef] [PubMed]
11. Landegren, U.; Kaiser, R.; Sanders, J.; Hood, L. A ligase-mediated gene detection technique. *Science* **1988**, *241*, 1077–1080. [CrossRef]
12. Panpradist, N.; Beck, I.A.; Chung, M.H.; Kiarie, J.N.; Frenkel, L.M.; Lutz, B.R. Simplified Paper Format for Detecting HIV Drug Resistance in Clinical Specimens by Oligonucleotide Ligation. *PLoS ONE* **2016**, *11*, e0145962. [CrossRef]
13. Beck, I.A.; Crowell, C.; Kittoe, R.; Bredell, H.; Machaba, M.; Willamson, C.; Janssens, W.; Jallow, S.; van der Groen, G.; Shao, Y.; et al. Optimization of the oligonucleotide ligation assay, a rapid and inexpensive test for detection of HIV-1 drug resistance mutations, for non-North American variants. *J. Acquir. Immune Defic. Syndr.* **2008**, *48*, 418–427. [CrossRef]
14. Beck, I.A.; Mahalanabis, M.; Pepper, G.; Wright, A.; Hamilton, S.; Langston, E.; Frenkel, L.M. Rapid and sensitive oligonucleotide ligation assay for detection of mutations in human immunodeficiency virus type 1 associated with high-level resistance to protease inhibitors. *J. Clin. Microbiol.* **2002**, *40*, 1413–1419. [CrossRef]
15. Edelstein, R.E.; Nickerson, D.A.; Tobe, V.O.; Manns-Arcuino, L.A.; Frenkel, L.M. Oligonucleotide ligation assay for detecting mutations in the human immunodeficiency virus type 1 pol gene that are associated with resistance to zidovudine, didanosine, and lamivudine. *J. Clin. Microbiol.* **1998**, *36*, 569–572. [CrossRef]

16. Frenkel, L.M.; Wagner, L.E.; Atwood, S.M.; Cummins, T.J.; Dewhurst, S. Specific, sensitive, and rapid assay for human immunodeficiency virus type 1 pol mutations associated with resistance to zidovudine and didanosine. *J. Clin. Microbiol.* **1995**, *33*, 342–347. [CrossRef] [PubMed]
17. Chung, M.H.; Beck, I.A.; Dross, S.; Tapia, K.; Kiarie, J.N.; Richardson, B.A.; Overbaugh, J.; Sakr, S.R.; John-Stewart, G.C.; Frenkel, L.M. Oligonucleotide ligation assay detects HIV drug resistance associated with virologic failure among antiretroviral-naive adults in Kenya. *J. Acquir. Immune Defic. Syndr.* **2014**, *67*, 246–253. [CrossRef] [PubMed]
18. Jourdain, G.; Wagner, T.A.; Ngo-Giang-Huong, N.; Sirirungsi, W.; Klinbuayaem, V.; Fregonese, F.; Nantasen, I.; Techapornroong, M.; Halue, G.; Nilmanat, A.; et al. Association between detection of HIV-1 DNA resistance mutations by a sensitive assay at initiation of antiretroviral therapy and virologic failure. *Clin. Infect. Dis.* **2010**, *50*, 1397–1404. [CrossRef] [PubMed]
19. Mutsvangwa, J.; Beck, I.A.; Gwanzura, L.; Manhanzva, M.T.; Stranix-Chibanda, L.; Chipato, T.; Frenkel, L.M. Optimization of the oligonucleotide ligation assay for the detection of nevirapine resistance mutations in Zimbabwean Human Immunodeficiency Virus type-1 subtype C. *J. Virol. Methods* **2014**, *210*, 36–39. [CrossRef]
20. Van Dyke, R.B.; Ngo-Giang-Huong, N.; Shapiro, D.E.; Frenkel, L.; Britto, P.; Roongpisuthipong, A.; Beck, I.A.; Yuthavisuthi, P.; Prommas, S.; Puthanakit, T.; et al. A comparison of 3 regimens to prevent nevirapine resistance mutations in HIV-infected pregnant women receiving a single intrapartum dose of nevirapine. *Clin. Infect. Dis.* **2012**, *54*, 285–293. [CrossRef]
21. Panpradist, N.; Beck, I.A.; Vrana, J.; Higa, N.; McIntyre, D.; Ruth, P.S.; So, I.; Kline, E.C.; Kanthula, R.; Wong-On-Wing Lim, J.; et al. OLA-Simple: A software-guided HIV-1 drug resistance test for low-resource laboratories. *EBioMedicine* **2019**, *50*, 34–44. [CrossRef]
22. Panpradist, N.; Beck, I.A.; Ruth, P.S.; Avila-Rios, S.; Garcia-Morales, C.; Soto-Nava, M.; Tapia-Trejo, D.; Matias-Florentino, M.; Paz-Juarez, H.E.; Del Arenal-Sanchez, S.; et al. Near point-of-care, point-mutation test to detect drug resistance in HIV-1: A validation study in a Mexican cohort. *AIDS* **2020**, *34*, 1331–1338. [CrossRef]
23. MacLeod, I.J.; Rowley, C.F.; Essex, M. PANDAA intentionally violates conventional qPCR design to enable durable, mismatch-agnostic detection of highly polymorphic pathogens. *Commun. Biol.* **2021**, *4*, 227. [CrossRef]
24. Maruapula, D.; MacLeod, I.J.; Moyo, S.; Musonda, R.; Seatla, K.; Molebatsi, K.; Leteane, M.; Essex, M.; Gaseitsiwe, S.; Rowley, C.F. Use of a mutation-specific genotyping method to assess for HIV-1 drug resistance in antiretroviral-naive HIV-1 Subtype C-infected patients in Botswana. *AAS Open Res.* **2020**, *3*, 50. [CrossRef]
25. Kouamou, V.; Manasa, J.; Katzenstein, D.; McGregor, A.M.; Ndhlovu, C.E.; Makadzange, T. Diagnostic Accuracy of Pan-Degenerate Amplification and Adaptation Assay for HIV-1 Drug Resistance Mutation Analysis in Low- and Middle-Income Countries. *J. Clin. Microbiol.* **2020**, *58*, e01045-20. [CrossRef]
26. Chung, M.H.; McGrath, C.J.; Beck, I.A.; Levine, M.; Milne, R.S.; So, I.; Andersen, N.; Dross, S.; Coombs, R.W.; Chohan, B.; et al. Evaluation of the management of pretreatment HIV drug resistance by oligonucleotide ligation assay: A randomised controlled trial. *Lancet HIV* **2020**, *7*, e104–e112. [CrossRef]
27. McCalla, S.E.; Ong, C.; Sarma, A.; Opal, S.M.; Artenstein, A.W.; Tripathi, A. A simple method for amplifying RNA targets (SMART). *J. Mol. Diagn.* **2012**, *14*, 328–335. [CrossRef] [PubMed]
28. Morabito, K.; Kantor, R.; Tai, W.; Schreier, L.; Tripathi, A. Detection of HIV-1 minority variants containing the K103N drug-resistance mutation using a simple method to amplify RNA targets (SMART). *J. Mol. Diagn.* **2013**, *15*, 401–412. [CrossRef] [PubMed]
29. Wang, J.; Tai, W.; Angione, S.L.; John, A.R.; Opal, S.M.; Artenstein, A.W.; Tripathi, A. Subtyping clinical specimens of influenza A virus by use of a simple method to amplify RNA targets. *J. Clin. Microbiol.* **2013**, *51*, 3324–3330. [CrossRef] [PubMed]
30. Dunbar, S.A. Applications of Luminex xMAP technology for rapid, high-throughput multiplexed nucleic acid detection. *Clin. Chim. Acta* **2006**, *363*, 71–82. [CrossRef]
31. Zhang, G.; Cai, F.; Zhou, Z.; DeVos, J.; Wagar, N.; Diallo, K.; Zulu, I.; Wadonda-Kabondo, N.; Stringer, J.S.; Weidle, P.J.; et al. Simultaneous detection of major drug resistance mutations in the protease and reverse transcriptase genes for HIV-1 subtype C by use of a multiplex allele-specific assay. *J. Clin. Microbiol.* **2013**, *51*, 3666–3674. [CrossRef]
32. Houser, B. Bio-Rad's Bio-Plex(R) suspension array system, xMAP technology overview. *Arch. Physiol. Biochem.* **2012**, *118*, 192–196. [CrossRef]
33. Zhang, G.; Cai, F.; de Rivera, I.L.; Zhou, Z.; Zhang, J.; Nkengasong, J.; Gao, F.; Yang, C. Simultaneous Detection of Major Drug Resistance Mutations of HIV-1 Subtype B Viruses from Dried Blood Spot Specimens by Multiplex Allele-Specific Assay. *J. Clin. Microbiol.* **2016**, *54*, 220–222. [CrossRef]
34. Barany, F. Genetic disease detection and DNA amplification using cloned thermostable ligase. *Proc. Natl. Acad. Sci. USA* **1991**, *88*, 189–193. [CrossRef]
35. Nilsson, M.; Antson, D.O.; Barbany, G.; Landegren, U. RNA-templated DNA ligation for transcript analysis. *Nucleic Acids Res.* **2001**, *29*, 578–581. [CrossRef]
36. Yan, J.; Li, Z.; Liu, C.; Cheng, Y. Simple and sensitive detection of microRNAs with ligase chain reaction. *Chem. Commun.* **2010**, *46*, 2432–2434. [CrossRef] [PubMed]
37. Cheng, Y.; Zhang, X.; Li, Z.; Jiao, X.; Wang, Y.; Zhang, Y. Highly sensitive determination of microRNA using target-primed and branched rolling-circle amplification. *Angew. Chem. Int. Ed. Engl.* **2009**, *48*, 3268–3272. [CrossRef] [PubMed]
38. Zhang, L.; Wang, J.; Coetzer, M.; Angione, S.; Kantor, R.; Tripathi, A. One-Step Ligation on RNA Amplification for the Detection of Point Mutations. *J. Mol. Diagn.* **2015**, *17*, 679–688. [CrossRef] [PubMed]

39. Gomez-Martinez, J.; Silvy, M.; Chiaroni, J.; Fournier-Wirth, C.; Roubinet, F.; Bailly, P.; Bres, J.C. Multiplex Lateral Flow Assay for Rapid Visual Blood Group Genotyping. *Anal. Chem.* **2018**, *90*, 7502–7509. [CrossRef]
40. Fountoglou, N.; Petropoulou, M.; Iliadi, A.; Christopoulos, T.K.; Ioannou, P.C. Tauwo-panel molecular testing for genetic predisposition for thrombosis using multi-allele visual biosensors. *Anal. Bioanal. Chem.* **2016**, *408*, 1943–1952. [CrossRef]
41. Petropoulou, M.; Poula, A.; Traeger-Synodinos, J.; Kanavakis, E.; Christopoulos, T.K.; Ioannou, P.C. Multi-allele DNA biosensor for the rapid genotyping of 'nondeletion' alpha thalassaemia mutations in HBA1 and HBA2 genes by means of multiplex primer extension reaction. *Clin. Chim. Acta* **2015**, *446*, 241–247. [CrossRef]
42. Papanikos, F.; Iliadi, A.; Petropoulou, M.; Ioannou, P.C.; Christopoulos, T.K.; Kanavakis, E.; Traeger-Synodinos, J. Lateral flow dipstick test for genotyping of 15 beta-globin gene (HBB) mutations with naked-eye detection. *Anal. Chim. Acta* **2012**, *727*, 61–66. [CrossRef]
43. Gomez-Martinez, J.; Foulongne, V.; Laureillard, D.; Nagot, N.; Montes, B.; Cantaloube, J.F.; Van de Perre, P.; Fournier-Wirth, C.; Moles, J.P.; Bres, J.C. Near-point-of-care assay with a visual readout for detection of HIV-1 drug resistance mutations: A proof-of-concept study. *Talanta* **2021**, *231*, 122378. [CrossRef]
44. Bui, M.H.; Stone, G.G.; Nilius, A.M.; Almer, L.; Flamm, R.K. PCR-oligonucleotide ligation assay for detection of point mutations associated with quinolone resistance in Streptococcus pneumoniae. *Antimicrob. Agents Chemother.* **2003**, *47*, 1456–1459. [CrossRef]
45. Natoli, M.E.; Rohrman, B.A.; De, S.C.; van Zyl, G.U.; Richards-Kortum, R.R. Paper-based detection of HIV-1 drug resistance using isothermal amplification and an oligonucleotide ligation assay. *Anal. Biochem.* **2018**, *544*, 64–71. [CrossRef]
46. Clutter, D.S.; Mazarei, G.; Sinha, R.; Manasa, J.; Nouhin, J.; LaPrade, E.; Bolouki, S.; Tzou, P.L.; Hannita-Hui, J.; Sahoo, M.K.; et al. Multiplex Solid-Phase Melt Curve Analysis for the Point-of-Care Detection of HIV-1 Drug Resistance. *J. Mol. Diagn.* **2019**, *21*, 580–592. [CrossRef] [PubMed]
47. Myers, F.B.; Henrikson, R.H.; Xu, L.; Lee, L.P. A point-of-care instrument for rapid multiplexed pathogen genotyping. *Annu. Int. Conf. IEEE Eng. Med. Biol. Soc.* **2011**, *2011*, 3668–3671. [PubMed]
48. Myers, F.B.; Henrikson, R.H.; Bone, J.M.; Lee, L.P. A handheld point-of-care genomic diagnostic system. *PLoS ONE* **2013**, *8*, e70266. [CrossRef]
49. Gonzalez, C.; Gondola, J.; Ortiz, A.Y.; Castillo, J.; Pascale, J.M.; Martinez, A.A. Barcoding analysis of HIV drug resistance mutations using Oxford Nanopore MinION (ONT) sequencing. *bioRxiv* **2018**. [CrossRef]

pathogens

MDPI

Review

Overview of the Analytes Applied in Genotypic HIV Drug Resistance Testing

Hezhao Ji [1,2,*] and Paul Sandstrom [1,2]

1 National Microbiology Laboratory at JC Wilt Infectious Diseases Research Centre, Public Health Agency of Canada, Winnipeg, MB R3E 3R2, Canada; paul.sandstrom@phac-aspc.gc.ca
2 Max Rady College of Medicine, University of Manitoba, Winnipeg, MB R3E 0J9, Canada
* Correspondence: hezhao.ji@phac-aspc.gc.ca; Tel.: +1-204-789-6521

Abstract: The close monitoring of HIV drug resistance using genotypic HIV drug resistance testing (HIVDRT) has become essential for effective HIV/AIDS management at both individual and population levels. Over the years, a broad spectrum of analytes or specimens have been applied or attempted in HIVDRT; however, the suitability and performance of these analytes in HIVDRT and the clinical relevance of the results from them may vary significantly. This article provides a focused overview of the performance, strengths, and weaknesses of various analytes while used in HIVDRT, which may inform the optimal analytes selection in different application contexts.

Keywords: HIV; drug resistance; testing; analytes; specimens; performance

Citation: Ji, H.; Sandstrom, P. Overview of the Analytes Applied in Genotypic HIV Drug Resistance Testing. *Pathogens* **2022**, *11*, 739. https://doi.org/10.3390/pathogens11070739

Academic Editor: Ayalew Mergia

Received: 27 April 2022
Accepted: 28 June 2022
Published: 29 June 2022

1. Introduction

Human immunodeficiency virus (HIV) and the acquired immunodeficiency syndrome (AIDS) it causes, pose significant public health concern at a global level. With the enhanced access and improved efficacy of antiretroviral therapy (ART), HIV/AIDS has become a manageable chronic reaction in resource-permitted settings [1]. ART improves the lives of people living with HIV, and it also plays a vital role in reducing HIV transmission and HIV incidence [2]. However, HIV drug resistance (HIVDR) significantly decreases the ART efficacy and undermines its benefits. Over 27.5 million people were receiving ART globally by the end of 2020, but up to 24% of pre-treatment patients and 50~90% of patients failing ART may harbor ART-resistant variants [3,4]. Among many recommendations from the 2017 World Health Organization (WHO) Global Action Plan on HIVDR are the expanded coverage and improved effectiveness of genotypic HIVDR testing (HIVDRT) for surveillance and clinical purposes [4]. Any strategy that promotes the access, affordability, sensitivity, and accuracy of HIVDRT would benefit HIVDR management globally. The appropriate selection of clinical specimen or analyte plays a vital role in the assay performance and subsequent HIVDR data interpretation and application.

Current HIVDRTs examine the presence of drug resistance-associated mutation (DRM) either via allele-specific assays targeting specific viral mutation(s) or by HIVDR genotyping, which sequences the ART-targeted HIV-1 genes and analyzes all potential DRMs collectively. Any HIV-positive specimen or analyte that contains HIV ribonucleic acid (RNA) or deoxyribonucleic acid (DNA) for the target HIV gene(s) could be used for HIVDRT. Unsurprisingly, a broad spectrum of analytes has been applied or attempted in HIVDRT. Most of such analytes are also applicable for other HIV molecular assays, such as viral load (VL) determination. This HIVDR thematic article provides a focused overview of various analytes' performance, strengths, and weaknesses while applied in HIVDRT.

2. Varied Analytes for HIVDRT

The commonly-used analytes are summarized as below: (Table 1).

2.1. Plasma

Plasma is the supernatant after the cellular components of the anti-coagulated blood are removed after centrifugation. Plasma specimens are usually collected for molecular assays such as HIVDR testing, which examines the HIV viral RNA it contains. Plasma has the highest viral RNA concentration among all analytes applied in HIVDRT. The viral population in plasma best represents the cell-free, replication-competent, circulating HIV viruses in the patients. HIV viral RNA in plasma remains stable in ambient temperature and long-term storage under freezing conditions [5–7].

Plasma is the gold standard analyte most commonly used for HIVDRT [8]. It serves all clinical, surveillance, and research HIVDRT needs. All breakthroughs in HIVDRT assay development and validation were first established using plasma and then applied to other analytes. The prevention of blood clotting maximizes the number of viral templates available in plasma for HIV genotyping. This is particularly important for specimens collected from ART-treated individuals whose VLs could be extremely low. It is noteworthy that ethylenediaminetetraacetic acid (EDTA), but not heparin, should be used as the anti-coagulant if a molecular assay such as HIVDRT is to be performed on the derived plasma. This is due to the inhibitory effect of heparin in the downstream polymerase chain reaction (PCR) amplifications [9,10].

2.2. Serum

Serum is the fluid left after whole blood is naturally clotted. The compositions of plasma and serum are nearly identical except for fibrinogen, which is present in plasma but naturally removed from serum during clotting. Serum is the most commonly used substitute for plasma in molecular HIV assays. While plasma is always the preferred analyte, serum is often used for serological HIV diagnosis. The suitability of serum versus plasma for HIVDRT testing varies largely depending on the availability of centrifugation devices and the usage of anti-coagulant during the sample collection. However, remnant frozen sera from diagnostic testing are often utilized in retrospective HIVDR surveillance and research projects [8].

While applied in HIV molecular assays, another notable difference between plasma and serum analytes is the concentration of HIV contents. A small portion of HIV particles or viral RNA can be trapped in the blood coagulum during clotting, rendering lower VLs in serum than in plasma [11,12]. There is no evidence showing different HIVDR profiles as determined using plasma or serum, implying that the HIV viral RNA loss resulting from clotting is non-selective. However, precautions should still be taken if serum specimens are used for HIVDRT and viral diversity analysis, especially when next generation sequencing (NGS) technologies are used. NGS resolves the intra-host viral diversity and DRMs of lower abundance with a significantly higher resolution than conventional population-based Sanger sequencing [13,14]. Moreover, serum might not be an ideal analyte for patients with lower expected VLs, such as those currently on ART.

The advantages of plasma and serum analytes in HIVDRT are apparent. However, their limitations are also evident. Both analytes require well-trained phlebotomists, skilled lab personnel, stringent cold-chain transportation, and low-temperature storage conditions to maintain the specimen quality and HIV template integrity. These requirements limit the suitability and feasibility of plasma and serum for applications in remote or resource-limited settings (RLS) [15,16]. Searching for ideal alternative analytes or specimen collection metrics has been an everlasting interest for HIVDR professionals.

Table 1. Varied analytes applied in HIV drug resistance test.

Specimens	Specimen Collection/Preparation	Applications	Pros	Cons
Plasma	• The supernatant harvested after centrifugation of anti-coagulated whole blood.	• Conventional analyte for HIVDRT. • Suitable for HIVDRT serving all relevant clinical, surveillance, and research needs.	• Representing actively circulating HIV population. • Maximal recovery of cell-free viral RNA in blood. • Low RNA degradation/high template integrity. • Suitable for varied assays.	• Needs for phlebotomy, centrifugation, and low-temperature transportation and storage. • Poor HIV amplification when VL is low.
Serum	• The fluid left after natural clotting of whole blood.	• Suitable for HIVDR test serving all relevant clinical, surveillance and research needs. • Remnant sera from diagnosis often used in HIVDR surveillance or research projects.	• Closest substitute to plasma. • Representing actively circulating HIV population. • No need for centrifuging device. • Suitable for varied assays.	• Needs for phlebotomy, low-temperature transportation and storage. • Lower template concentration than plasma. • Poor HIV amplification when VL is low.
Whole blood	• Anti-coagulated whole blood collected via venipuncture.	• Depending on the nucleic acid extracts used, it supports HIVDR analysis of circulating HIV viruses (RNA), archival proviruses (DNA), or general (TNA).	• Covering circulating and integrated viruses. • No need for centrifugation device. • Short-term storage at ambient is acceptable. • Good HIV amplification even when VL is low.	• Needs for phlebotomy. • Discordant HIVDR profiling to plasma. • Not ideal for clinical HIVDR monitoring. • Poor reproducibility.
PBMCs	• Mononuclear cells isolated from anti-coagulated whole blood by density gradient centrifugation.	• DNA from PBMCs is occasionally used for HIVDRT, primarily in research projects. • Substitute when RNA test is not feasible. • Retrospective HIVDR analysis in which the order of DRM occurrence is less a concern.	• Proviral DNA in PBMCs is stable. • High HIV amplification rates from patients with even undetectable plasma VL.	• Needs for phlebotomy. • Discordant HIVDR readout to plasma and limited reflection on circulating HIV population, limiting its value for clinical monitoring.

Table 1. *Cont.*

Specimens	Specimen Collection/Preparation	Applications	Pros	Cons
Dried filter paper analytes				
DBS	• Spotting and drying blood drops onto filter paper cards.	• Applied primarily in HIVDR surveillance testing and research studies, rarely for clinical monitoring.	• Easy to collect, transport, and store. • Good HIV amplification if TNA is applied. • No strict requirement for venipuncture. • Suitable for pediatric patients.	• Low sensitivity due to small volume and viral RNA degradation. • Discordant HIVDR profiling to plasma, not suitable for clinical monitoring.
DPS	• Spotting and drying plasma drops onto a filter paper card.	• Applicable for clinical monitoring when the VL is high, i.e., prior to ART initiation. • HIVDR surveillance testing or research use.	• Closely mimics plasma in representing circulating virus. • Concordant to plasma for HIVDR profiling, if successfully genotyped.	• As compared to DBS: • Lower viral RNA integrity, lower HIV amplification; • Shorter storage, lower ambient temperature, and shorter transportation is required; • Needs for phlebotomy.
DSS	• Spotting and drying serum drops onto a filter paper card.	• Occasionally applied in surveillance testing. • Attempted for centralized HIVDRT in RLS.		
Dried analytes collected with the newer generation of devices				
HemaSpot	• Loading and drying blood drops onto a HemaSpot device.	• Research use only thus far. • May facilitate HIVDRT in RLS.	• Easy to collect, transport, and store. • No strict requirement for venipuncture.	• Low sensitivity likely due to suboptimal viral RNA integrity. • Preservation of viral RNA/DNA remains to be better determined. • More validation studies needed before broader adoption in HIVDRT.
ViveST™	• Loading and drying liquid specimen onto ViveST matrix.	• Research use only thus far. • May facilitate HIVDRT in RLS.	• Easy to collect, transport, and store. • Applicable for different liquid specimens. • Holds larger volume of liquid.	

2.3. Whole Blood

Besides plasma and serum, anticoagulated whole blood (WB) is another commonly-used laboratory analyte. WB is widely used when the isolation of plasma/serum is not feasible, but nucleic acid extraction from WB on time is doable. HIV RNA may retain its integrity for 72 h in WB at an ambient temperature of 25 °C [17]. Therefore, WB could be a suitable substitute for HIV molecular assays targeting HIV viral RNA. Despite this, most WB-based HIVDR studies employed only the DNA extracts.

While plasma and serum both contain HIV viral RNA primarily, the HIV-infected cellular components in WB carry HIV proviral DNA. Depending on the nucleic acid extraction strategies applied, the HIV genetic materials recovered from WB could include viral RNA, proviral HIV DNA, or a combination of both if total nucleic acid (TNA) is extracted. Likewise, the application values of the WB specimens vary depending on the HIV templates used in further HIVDRT. Using RNA extract from WB may approximate the results from plasma/serum reflecting the circulating HIV population. In contrast, data from the DNA extracts may convey the information from HIV proviruses, a distinct archival viral population that is not as informative for patient management.

Steegen et al. assessed the feasibility of HIVDRT using DNA extracted from WB and compared it with results from plasma viral RNA [18]. High genotyping success rates were achieved for all specimens with detectable viral loads from plasma viral RNA and DNA from WB. Moreover, HIV protease (PR) and reverse transcriptase (RT) genes were successfully amplified from 67.7% and 61.3% of WB DNA preparations from patients with undetectable plasma VL [18]. While the viral DNA from WB boosts the HIV amplification rates, HIVDR data from such DNA extracts were often discordant with RNA extracts, confirming that they reflect different viral populations [19]. In addition, HIVDR data from DNA extracts showed poor reproducibility, implying a possible founder effect [18]. Furthermore, defective proviruses that harbor stop codons in the HIVDRT target genes are not rare, and excluding such defective proviruses from the whole blood DNA-based HIVDR data would significantly improve its clinical application value [20].

To overcome the limitations of DNA from WB, using RNA or TNA from WB for HIVDRT may be beneficial. Saracino et al. demonstrated that combining viral RNA and DNA in HIVDR typing might help identify more DRMs in the patients and assist in a more informed, effective ART regimen selection [21]. Targeted extraction of the RNA or DNA components from WB by enzymatically removing the other is always an option if fewer confounding data are expected. However, this will inevitably reduce the net HIV application rates.

While WB sampling still requires phlebotomy, this analyte eliminates the need for centrifugation devices unavailable in many decentralized health facilities. Skipping the centrifugation step also reduces professional HIV exposure, artificial errors, or contaminations associated with plasma/serum sample processing. The relative stability of HIV RNA in WB at an ambient temperature also enables centralized lab testing if such specimens could be quickly transferred from the collection site to the testing lab, even in the absence of a cold chain [17].

2.4. Peripheral Blood Mononuclear Cells (PBMCs)

PBMCs consist of lymphocytes and monocytes isolated from the anti-coagulated whole blood by density gradient centrifugation. DNA extraction is usually performed on PBMCs to recover the cellular DNA containing proviral HIV DNA that is integrated into the HIV-infected cells' genome. The derived DNA can then be used for HIVDRT. The genetic discordance between plasma HIV RNA and proviral HIV DNA from PBMCs has been well-documented [22–25]. Bi et al. showed that plasma viral RNA-based genotyping could detect HIV DRMs up to 425 days earlier than PBMC DNA when the plasma VL was less than 104 copies/mL [26]. It further highlights the slow turnover of the proviral population and the drastic distinction between the HIV proviruses and the circulating viral population in plasma [26]. A higher comparability of data from plasma and PBMCs was achievable only when the HIV duration is ≤2 years, the sample VLs are ≥5000 copies/mL, or when the patient is treatment naïve or off ART [27,28].

Depending on the ultimate HIVDRT objectives, proviral DNA from PBMC may have added value for comprehensive HIVDR profiling when HIV DRMs from HIV proviruses are considered [29]. PBMCs could be an alternative analyte for HIVDRT when using plasma viral RNA is not feasible or unsuccessful [30]. While conventional plasma RNA-based HIVDRT performs poorly on samples of low VLs, proviral DNA can be readily recovered from PBMCs in these patients for an extended period [31–33]. Therefore, PBMC may also satisfy the needs for retrospective HIVDR analysis or population-level surveillance, in which the order of DRM occurrence is less of a consideration.

Interestingly, Armenia et al. showed that, combined with low nadir CD4 counts and a short-term viral suppression history, PBMC-based HIVDR profiling could help predict the potential viral rebound after the ART regimen switch [34]. A bit counterintuitively, one recent study by Peng et al. reported that HIVDR mutants emerges in PBMS DNA months before they could be detected in plasma, suggesting that PBMC DNA could be an effective tool for early HIVDR detection [35]. Notably, this was from studying a single patient infected by HIV-1 CRF01_AE and experienced multiple ART failure episodes [35]. The validation of these findings in larger studies remains to be conducted. Moreover, Moraka et al. recently showed that HIV DRMs identified in PBMCs are often associated with defective proviral genomes among early-treatment children [36]. It could lead to an overestimated HIVDR profiling if such PBMC DNA-based HIVDR data were applied in patient care.

2.5. Dried Fluid Analytes

As a more affordable and practical sampling option, dried fluid analytes are increasingly applied in HIVDRT, especially in low- to middle-income countries where the HIV/AIDS pandemic hits the most but optimal sample collection and storage are not always feasible [37]. In such cases, dried fluid specimens collected/dried with different matrices or devices may be collected from peripheral clinics, community sites, or even self-collected from patients' homes and then transferred under natural ambient conditions to laboratories for centralized testing.

HIV genetic materials in such dried analytes remain relatively stable over an extended period under a wide range of ambient temperatures and suboptimal shipping and storage conditions. However, the reduced assay sensitivity, consistency, and reproducibility due to the small sample volume and the inevitable RNA degradation are primary concerns when such dried analytes are applied in HIVDRT. Refining the preparation of such specimens, improving the integrity of the HIV templates they contain, and boosting the analytical sensitivity of such analytes for HIVDRT are all everlasting topics in this field of work.

Several dried fluid analytes that have been applied in HIVDR studies thus far are overviewed below. This list is by no means exhaustive, and more developments in this field should come up in the foreseeable future (Table 1).

2.5.1. Dried Filter Paper Analytes (DFPAs)

DFPAs have been applied in diagnostic tests for decades, mainly due to the low cost and the ease of sample collection, transportation, and storage. The use of filter paper for blood collection dates back to the early 1960s, when dried blood spots (DBS) were first used for phenylketonuria diagnosis in pediatric patients [38]. Since then, filter paper has been used as a collection matrix for different body fluids, and DFPAs have been used for a broad spectrum of laboratory assays.

Depending on the fluids used, DFPAs for HIVDRT consist of conventional DBS, dried plasma spots (DPS), and dried serum spots (DSS). While the integrity of HIV templates in DFPAs inevitably decreases, HIVDRT with such analytes has often been reported, although their performance varies significantly [37,39].

DBS

DBS is the foremost DFPA option for HIVDRT. DBS is prepared by spotting and drying whole blood onto absorbent filter paper cards [40,41]. The blood could be from phlebotomy or a simple lancet-prick that even patients themselves can do. The small sample volume it requires (50~75 μL per spot) and no stringent need for phlebotomy make DBS an attractive option peculiarly for pediatric patients. The technical, practical, and operational advantages of DBS are evident. DBS can be naturally dried, packed, shipped in a regular envelope and stored at ambient temperature using zip-lock plastic bags with desiccant for days to weeks before processing. It helps avoid the requirement for cold-chain transportation while posing minimal biohazard peril to the ambience.

The performance of DBS in HIVDRT has been well-documented in varied contexts, and DBS is proven to be an accountable analyte for HIVDRT in most cases. Well-established DBS-based HIVDRT guidelines have been implemented [16]. With the proven success of DBS usage in HIVDRT from many studies, DBS is currently the WHO-recommended blood sampling method in low- to middle-income countries [16,42,43].

Although DBS is considered a suitable alternate analyte for HIVDRT, DBS has its intrinsic limitations. Like WB, the presence of proviral DNA in DBS renders a higher success rate for HIV amplification than DPS or DSS. However, such proviral DNA contribution also limits its capacity to manifest the HIVDR status of circulating replication-active HIV viruses. Studies have shown that proviral DNA in the DBS may contribute to up to 80% of the application success rates of these samples [44,45]. Steegen et al. successfully genotyped HIV PR and RT genes from 54.8% and 58.1% DBS DNA preparations from patients with undetectable plasma VL [18]. The comparability of DNased-treated extracts from DBS and DPS in HIV PCR success rates further confirms the proviral DNA contribution to the DBS-based HIV genotyping [45]. HIVDR profiling data from DBS and matching plasma are concordant only when the VL is ≥5000 copies/mL, and/or the patients have no ART experience, and/or the duration of HIV infection is short [27]. This restricts the DBS application in clinical HIVDR monitoring, for which low VL specimens from ART-treated patients are unavoidable.

DBS has been applied primarily in HIVDR surveillance and research studies. Occasionally, DBS was assessed for centralized HIVDR monitoring in which DBS specimens were collected from RLS where clinical monitoring is required, but DBS is the only feasible sampling option. Regardless of the success rate of HIVDRT in such studies, DBS is not an ideal option for HIVDR monitoring purposes. However, one exception is for HIV-infected pediatric patients, from whom collecting large blood volume via venipuncture is often impractical and unrealistic. With nearly half of the HIV-infected infants/children carrying HIVDR variants even before ART initiation in Sub-Saharan Africa, where HIV/AIDS hits the hardest, the advantage of DBS could be of particular significance in this patient category [3].

DPS

By spotting and drying plasma drops onto a filter paper card, DPS can be prepared similar to DBS. Rottinghaus et al. compared the performance of DBS and DPS against plasma in HIV VL determination and HIVDRT. Their data showed that DBS, not DPS specimens, rendered VL readouts comparable to plasma, and that DPS had a significantly lower HIVDRT success rate as compared to DBS (38.9% vs. 100%) for specimens with VL ≥1000 copies/mL [46]. The high concordance of VL determination and PCR amplification results between DPS and DNase-treated DBS specimens confirms the proviral DNA contribution to the DBS-based HIVDR data [45]. It also necessitates a shorter storage time, a lower ambient temperature, and a shorter transportation for DPS than DBS due to reduced RNA stability [47].

While DPS consistently produces lower VL values, DPS-derived HIVDR data are highly comparable with those derived from plasma of the same patients [39], implying that the RNA degradation-induced HIV template loss in DPS is non-selective and HIVDR variants are not affected disproportionally. It makes DPS a better option than DBS for clinical HIVDR monitoring. The trade-off of the additional spotting and drying procedures is the relief of the stringent shipping and storage requirements for the fresh plasma specimens, which could be advantageous in certain circumstances.

DSS

DSS can be prepared by spotting and drying serum drops onto a filter paper card. While other dried spot analytes are often applied in HIVDRT, DSS usage is rarely reported, even though the suitability of DSS for HIVDRT has been confirmed [48–51]. HIV PR and RT gene amplification was achieved from >86% of DSS specimens with VL >10,000 copies/mL [49]. DSS showed a good consistency under conditions representative of field conditions [48]. These support DSS as an alternative specimen for scaled HIVDR surveillance or even centralized HIVDR monitoring tests in RLS. Similar to DPS, the lack of a more stable HIV proviral DNA component in DSS compared to DBS results in a lower success rate of HIVDR typing. However, the DSS-based HIVDR profiling is expected to be comparable with plasma or serum. Strategies that may improve the long-term HIV viral RNA stability in DPS and DSS specimens would significantly improve the suitability of such analytes for more broad HIV molecular assays, including HIVDRT. In addition, a modified experimental design with shorter amplicons also enhances the robustness of DSS or DPS-based HIVDRT [52].

2.5.2. Dried Analytes Collected with the Newer Generation of Devices

Besides the filter paper card, a newer generation of dried specimen collection devices has been developed since the early 2010s. Two exemplary product series of this category, HemaSpot^{TM} and ViveST^{TM}, are described below:

HemaSpot^{TM}

Hemaspot^{TM} is a product series designed explicitly for dried blood specimen collection offered by Spot on Sciences (San Francisco, CA, USA), founded in 2010 (https://www.spotonsciences.com/, accessed on 20 March 2022). The HemaSpot HF device has been tested in HIVDR assays. The HemaSpot HF device is a moisture-tight cartridge containing a circular chamber. A spoked absorbent filter paper pad, a descant ring, and an application disk are layered from the bottom up. Once the fluid drops are loaded, the cartridge can be closed immediately. The built-in desiccant dries the sample in minutes, and the sample is then ready for shipment. Samples collected with HemaSpot devices closely mimic the DFPAs while easing the requirement for additional drying procedures and holding up to 200 µL of original liquid specimens. The moisture-tight design and the tamper-resistant latch on the cartridge also help minimize the ambience's impact and retain the stability of the dried analyte it holds. Upon analysis, each spoke on the dried fluid pad can be plucked individually for multiple assays without punching, minimizing the risk of cross-contamination.

Dried blood analytes collected with HemaSpot have been applied as an alternative to DBS for serologic tests for several human viral pathogens [53–56]. While HemaSpot appears to be a promising technology, data on the usage of HemaSpot specimens for HIV molecular assays are scarce. Hirshfield et al. first confirmed the feasibility of using self-collected HemaSpot blood specimens for HIV VL monitoring [57]. Brooks et al. pioneered applying dried whole blood prepared with HemaSpot devices in HIVDRT in 2016 [58]. They evaluated the performance of HemaSpot specimens prepared from either fresh blood at various VL dilutions and a storage time up to 4 weeks at room temperature, or thawed frozen whole blood, both at 100 µL. For all specimens at VL >1000 copies /mL, HIV typing was successful in 79% and 58% of HemaSpot specimens prepared from fresh and frozen-thaw blood, respectively. The genotyping success rates improved significantly with a shorter storage period and higher VLs. The HIV PR and RT gene sequences derived from HemaSpot specimens show >96% identity compared to those from matching plasmas. In addition, the HIVDR profiling concordance between the paired HemaSpot specimens and plasma was determined as 86% [58]. Considering the intrinsic differences between plasma and DBS analytes described above, such discrepancies are expectable. Nonetheless, this study showed that the HemaSpot is a promising dried blood sample collection technology that may promote expanded HIVDRT in RLS.

With the scarcity of follow-up studies on this technology, the findings from this pilot study remain to be confirmed by more comprehensive evaluations regarding its sensitivity, accuracy, and consistency. These may include verifying the findings from Brooks' study on dried whole blood and assessing the performance of dried plasma or serum specimens collected with the HemaSpot device in HIV molecular assays. Notably, the HemaSpot SE product is designed to separate and dry the cellular components and serum onto the same absorbent membrane, which may serve different analysis needs targeting serum/plasma or cellular components of blood with one analyte. Comprehensive studies on the suitability of specimens from HemaSpot SE device for HIV molecular assays remain to be conducted.

ViveST™

ViveST™, formerly called SampleTanker™ (ST), is another dried sample storage and transportation device marketed by ViveBio Scientific (Alpharetta, GA, USA) since 2013 (https://vivebio.com/, accessed on 15 June 2022). The ST tubes have a proprietary, non-paper-based absorbent matrix attached to the tube cap and a descant block at the bottom. The biological substance, such as proteins and nucleic acids, in the original liquid specimens can be retained on the matrix while the water part is evaporated during the drying process. The matrix can be rehydrated for downstream lab assays using molecular-grade water, and the reconstituted sample can then be recovered. Compared to 50~75 μL per DFPA spot and ~200 μL for the HemaSpot device, up to 1.5 mL of biological fluid can be loaded and dried onto the ST matrix and then stored or transported at ambient temperature. It is a revolutionary solution for collecting, storing, and transporting liquid specimens from the field. It aims to expand the decentralized collection of any liquid biological samples, including blood, plasma, serum, and other body fluid analytes.

Dried plasma specimens collected with the ST device have been validated for VL assays for HIV, hepatitis B virus (HBV), and hepatitis C virus (HCV) [59–62], implying the application value of this new device in viral molecular assays. Lloyd et al. first reported ST application in HIVDRT during the XIII International HIV Drug Resistance Workshop in 2004 [60]. While lower VL readouts were obtained consistently from the ST plasma compared with frozen plasma, which was expected, the HIVDR mutations identified from the two compared analytes were concordant for all examined HIV-1 gene fragments. These observations were confirmed in an expanded study by this research group, which further demonstrated that the HIV viral RNA in ST plasma retained good integrity throughout the eight weeks of storage at 23 °C, 37 °C, and −80 °C [59].

In contrast, less optimistic findings were reported by Diallo et al., who assessed the application of the ST device for HIVDRT in RLS. They collected the whole blood or plasma specimens using the ST device and stored them at ambient temperature for 2 or 4 weeks. The performance of these two new analytes were compared against frozen plasma. Compared to 96% from frozen plasma specimens, both of the two new analytes performed poorly with significantly lower genotyping rates (48.98% and 42.85% for ST whole blood specimens stored for 2 and 4 weeks; 36% and 36% for ST plasma specimens stored for 2 and 4 weeks, respectively). Although the nucleotide sequence identities and the HIVDR profiles are highly concordant with the matching frozen plasmas for the successfully genotyped specimens, the low amplification rates from both ST specimens suggest that the ST device may not be ideal for HIVDRT sample collection in RLS [63]. Similar conclusions were also drawn from a study by Kantor et al. in which the performance of two ST processed specimen types (ST™-plasma (STP) and ST™-blood (STB)) in HIV genotyping were assessed [64]. The HIVDRT success rates using STP and STB in the Kantor study were 32% and 12%, compared to 82% from matching frozen plasmas [64]. While the specimens in these studies varied, the unfavorable outcomes from the two newer studies raise concerns over the preservation of HIV RNA/DNA integrity in the samples collected with ST tubes [63,64]. The further assessment of ViveST analytes for HIVDRT is warranted.

3. Application Considerations on HIVDRT Analytes

As described above, the quantity and quality of the HIV viral contents vary significantly among different analytes. The suitability of these analytes for the HIVDRT differ. The sensitivity, consistency, and accuracy vary considerably among the analytes due to the distinct nature of clinical analytes and the integrity of the HIV RNA or DNA templates they contain. Data collected from different analytes may hold differing values as applied to subsequent HIVDR interpretation. While plasma is the preferred analyte, it is not always available, especially in RLS, and alternative analytes are often required.

The suitability of an analyte for HIVDRT primarily depends on the resource availability for sample collection and transfer and downstream data application. One factor often neglected in HIVDRT analyte selection is the requirements from the downstream experimental procedures and data interpretation, which may differ significantly. Genotypic HIVDRT examines the presence of HIV DRMs either individually by allele-specific assays or collectively by sequencing using Sanger sequencing or NGS. Allele-specific assays target narrow viral genetic regions on which the impact from HIV RNA/DNA degradation is minimal. This is especially advantageous when a poorer HIV template quality is expected, such as the DFPAs and other dried analytes. In contrast, sequencing-based HIVDRT usually requires longer templates, making them more susceptible to HIV RNA/DNA degradation. One strategy to mitigate the limitation of degraded analytes, such as DFTAs, for HIVDRT is to implement modified protocols that generate shorter PCR amplicons or sequencing libraries. Compared to HIV RNA, a higher PCR amplification and sequencing success rate are expectable if DNA extracts from PBMC are used, especially when the VL is low. If targeting longer HIV genomic region(s) by long-range PCR or long-template NGS sequencing, fresh plasma/serum specimens with minimal HIV RNA/DNA degradation or HIV DNA extracts from PBMCs are always preferred.

4. Conclusions

In conclusion, although many analytes can be applied for HIVDR genotyping, their performance varies. Each analyte has its pros and cons from practicability and applicability perspectives. No single analyte could satisfy all requirements and applications. The suitability of an analyte for HIVDRT depends on: (1) the resource availability and accessibility; (2) the target viral population (circulating cell-free HIV viral particle vs. cell-associated HIV provirus); (3) the ease and convenience of the specimen acquisition, transportation, and storage; (4) the expected assay sensitivity, precision, and reproducibility; and (5) the downstream application (i.e., clinical monitoring vs surveillance) of the data obtained from the HIVDR assay. The optimal analyte selection always relies on the trade-off between test accountability and logistical capacity. A combined application of all such analytes is inevitable when varied application needs and requirements are present. Although their performance varies, all analytes contribute to the enhanced HIVDR management in unique ways, especially in RLS.

Author Contributions: Conceptualization, H.J.; Writing—Original Draft Preparation, H.J.; Writing—Review and Editing, H.J. and P.S. Both co-authors have read and approved this submitted version of the manuscript for publication. All authors have read and agreed to the published version of the manuscript.

Funding: This research received no external funding.

Institutional Review Board Statement: Not applicable.

Informed Consent Statement: Not applicable.

Acknowledgments: This work is fully funded by the National Microbiology Laboratory Branch of the Public Health Agency of Canada, to which both co-authors are affiliated.

Conflicts of Interest: The authors declare no conflict of interest. The funder had no role in the design of the study; in the collection, analyses, or interpretation of data; in the writing of the manuscript, or in the decision to publish the results.

References

1. Menendez-Arias, L.; Delgado, R. Update and latest advances in antiretroviral therapy. *Trends Pharmacol. Sci.* **2022**, *43*, 16–29. [CrossRef] [PubMed]
2. Yombi, J.C.; Mertes, H. Treatment as Prevention for HIV Infection: Current Data, Challenges, and Global Perspectives. *AIDS Rev.* **2018**, *20*, 131–140. [CrossRef] [PubMed]
3. World Health Organization. *HIV Drug Resistance Report 2021*; WHO: Geneva, Switzerland, 2021.
4. World Health Organization. *Global Action Plan on HIV Drug Resistance 2017–2021*; WHO: Geneva, Switzerland, 2017.
5. Sebire, K.; McGavin, K.; Land, S.; Middleton, T.; Birch, C. Stability of human immunodeficiency virus RNA in blood specimens as measured by a commercial PCR-based assay. *J. Clin. Microbiol.* **1998**, *36*, 493–498. [CrossRef] [PubMed]
6. Hardie, D.; Korsman, S.; Ameer, S.; Vojnov, L.; Hsiao, N.Y. Reliability of plasma HIV viral load testing beyond 24 hours: Insights gained from a study in a routine diagnostic laboratory. *PLoS ONE* **2019**, *14*, e0219381. [CrossRef]
7. Amellal, B.; Murphy, R.; Maiga, A.; Brucker, G.; Katlama, C.; Calvez, V.; Marcelin, A.G. Stability of HIV RNA in plasma specimens stored at different temperatures. *HIV Med.* **2008**, *9*, 790–793. [CrossRef]
8. World Health Organization. *WHO/HIVResNet HIV Drug Resistance Laboratory Strategy*; WHO: Geneva, Switzerland, 2010.
9. Yokota, M.; Tatsumi, N.; Nathalang, O.; Yamada, T.; Tsuda, I. Effects of heparin on polymerase chain reaction for blood white cells. *J. Clin. Lab. Anal.* **1999**, *13*, 133–140. [CrossRef]
10. Imai, H.; Yamada, O.; Morita, S.; Suehiro, S.; Kurimura, T. Detection of HIV-1 RNA in heparinized plasma of HIV-1 seropositive individuals. *J. Virol. Methods* **1992**, *36*, 181–184. [CrossRef]
11. Rodriguez, R.J.; Dayhoff, D.E.; Chang, G.; Cassol, S.A.; Birx, D.L.; Artenstein, A.W.; Michael, N.L. Comparison of serum and plasma viral RNA measurements in primary and chronic human immunodeficiency virus type 1 infection. *J. Acquir. Immune Defic. Syndr. Hum. Retrovirol.* **1997**, *15*, 49–53. [CrossRef]
12. Lew, J.; Reichelderfer, P.; Fowler, M.; Bremer, J.; Carrol, R.; Cassol, S.; Chernoff, D.; Coombs, R.; Cronin, M.; Dickover, R.; et al. Determinations of levels of human immunodeficiency virus type 1 RNA in plasma: Reassessment of parameters affecting assay outcome. TUBE Meeting Workshop Attendees. Technology Utilization for HIV-1 Blood Evaluation and Standardization in Pediatrics. *J. Clin. Microbiol.* **1998**, *36*, 1471–1479. [CrossRef]
13. Avila-Rios, S.; Parkin, N.; Swanstrom, R.; Paredes, R.; Shafer, R.; Ji, H.; Kantor, R. Next-Generation Sequencing for HIV Drug Resistance Testing: Laboratory, Clinical, and Implementation Considerations. *Viruses* **2020**, *12*, 617. [CrossRef]
14. Van, L.K.; Theys, K.; Vandamme, A.M. HIV-1 genotypic drug resistance testing: Digging deep, reaching wide? *Curr. Opin. Virol.* **2015**, *14*, 16–23.
15. Crowe, S.; Turnbull, S.; Oelrichs, R.; Dunne, A. Monitoring of human immunodeficiency virus infection in resource-constrained countries. *Clin. Infect. Dis.* **2003**, *37*, S25–S35. [CrossRef]
16. World Health Organization. *WHO Manual for HIV Drug Resistance Testing Using Dried Blood Spot Specimens*, 3rd ed.; WHO: Geneva, Switzerland, 2020.
17. Bonner, K.; Siemieniuk, R.A.; Boozary, A.; Roberts, T.; Fajardo, E.; Cohn, J. Expanding access to HIV viral load testing: A systematic review of RNA stability in EDTA tubes and PPT beyond current time and temperature thresholds. *PLoS ONE* **2014**, *9*, e113813.
18. Steegen, K.; Luchters, S.; Demecheleer, E.; Dauwe, K.; Mandaliya, K.; Jaoko, W.; Plum, J.; Temmerman, M.; Verhofstede, C. Feasibility of detecting human immunodeficiency virus type 1 drug resistance in DNA extracted from whole blood or dried blood spots. *J. Clin. Microbiol.* **2007**, *45*, 3342–3351. [CrossRef]
19. Sotillo, A.; Sierra, O.; Martinez-Prats, L.; Gutierrez, F.; Zurita, S.; Pulido, F.; Rubio, R.; Delgado, R. Analysis of drug resistance mutations in whole blood DNA from HIV-1 infected patients by single genome and ultradeep sequencing analysis. *J. Virol. Methods* **2018**, *260*, 1–5. [CrossRef] [PubMed]
20. Allavena, C.; Rodallec, A.; Leplat, A.; Hall, N.; Luco, C.; Le, G.L.; Bernaud, C.; Bouchez, S.; Andre-Garnier, E.; Boutoille, D.; et al. Interest of proviral HIV-1 DNA genotypic resistance testing in virologically suppressed patients candidate for maintenance therapy. *J. Virol. Methods* **2018**, *251*, 106–110. [CrossRef] [PubMed]
21. Saracino, A.; Gianotti, N.; Marangi, M.; Cibelli, D.C.; Galli, A.; Punzi, G.; Monno, L.; Lazzarin, A.; Angarano, G. Antiretroviral genotypic resistance in plasma RNA and whole blood DNA in HIV-1 infected patients failing HAART. *J. Med. Virol.* **2008**, *80*, 1695–1706. [CrossRef]
22. Smith, M.S.; Koerber, K.L.; Pagano, J.S. Zidovudine-resistant human immunodeficiency virus type 1 genomes detected in plasma distinct from viral genomes in peripheral blood mononuclear cells. *J. Infect. Dis.* **1993**, *167*, 445–448. [CrossRef]
23. Kaye, S.; Comber, E.; Tenant-Flowers, M.; Loveday, C. The appearance of drug resistance-associated point mutations in HIV type 1 plasma RNA precedes their appearance in proviral DNA. *AIDS Res. Hum. Retrovir.* **1995**, *11*, 1221–1225. [CrossRef]

24. Pessoa, R.; Watanabe, J.T.; Calabria, P.; Felix, A.C.; Loureiro, P.; Sabino, E.C.; Busch, M.P.; Sanabani, S.S. Deep sequencing of HIV-1 near full-length proviral genomes identifies high rates of BF1 recombinants including two novel circulating recombinant forms (CRF) 70_BF1 and a disseminating 71_BF1 among blood donors in Pernambuco, Brazil. *PLoS ONE* **2014**, *9*, e112674. [CrossRef]
25. Turriziani, O.; Bucci, M.; Stano, A.; Scagnolari, C.; Bellomi, F.; Fimiani, C.; Mezzaroma, I.; D'Ettorre, G.; Brogi, A.; Vullo, V.; et al. Genotypic resistance of archived and circulating viral strains in the blood of treated HIV-infected individuals. *J. Acquir. Immune Defic. Syndr.* **2007**, *44*, 518–524. [CrossRef] [PubMed]
26. Bi, X.; Gatanaga, H.; Ida, S.; Tsuchiya, K.; Matsuoka-Aizawa, S.; Kimura, S.; Oka, S. Emergence of protease inhibitor resistance-associated mutations in plasma HIV-1 precedes that in proviruses of peripheral blood mononuclear cells by more than a year. *J. Acquir. Immune Defic. Syndr.* **2003**, *34*, 1–6. [CrossRef] [PubMed]
27. Ji, H.; Li, Y.; Liang, B.; Pilon, R.; MacPherson, P.; Bergeron, M.; Kim, J.; Graham, M.; Van, D.G.; Sandstrom, P.; et al. Pyrosequencing dried blood spots reveals differences in HIV drug resistance between treatment naive and experienced patients. *PLoS ONE* **2013**, *8*, e56170. [CrossRef] [PubMed]
28. Huruy, K.; Mulu, A.; Liebert, U.G.; Maier, M. HIV-1C proviral DNA for detection of drug resistance mutations. *PLoS ONE* **2018**, *13*, e0205119.
29. Montejano, R.; Dominguez-Dominguez, L.; de Miguel, R.; Rial-Crestelo, D.; Esteban-Cantos, A.; Aranguren-Rivas, P.; Garcia-Alvarez, M.; Alejos, B.; Bisbal, O.; Santacreu-Guerrero, M.; et al. Detection of archived lamivudine-associated resistance mutations in virologically suppressed, lamivudine-experienced HIV-infected adults by different genotyping techniques (GEN-PRO study). *J. Antimicrob. Chemother.* **2021**, *76*, 3263–3271. [CrossRef]
30. Khairunisa, S.Q.; Megasari, N.L.A.; Indriati, D.W.; Kotaki, T.; Natalia, D.; Nasronudin Kameoka, M. Identification of HIV-1 subtypes and drug resistance mutations among HIV-1-infected individuals residing in Pontianak, Indonesia. *Germs* **2020**, *10*, 174–183. [CrossRef]
31. Hirsch, M.S.; Brun-Vezinet, F.; D'Aquila, R.T.; Hammer, S.M.; Johnson, V.A.; Kuritzkes, D.R.; Loveday, C.; Mellors, J.W.; Clotet, B.; Conway, B.; et al. Antiretroviral drug resistance testing in adult HIV-1 infection: Recommendations of an International AIDS Society-USA Panel. *JAMA* **2000**, *283*, 2417–2426. [CrossRef]
32. Chun, T.W.; Stuyver, L.; Mizell, S.B.; Ehler, L.A.; Mican, J.A.; Baseler, M.; Lloyd, A.L.; Nowak, M.A.; Fauci, A.S. Presence of an inducible HIV-1 latent reservoir during highly active antiretroviral therapy. *Proc. Natl. Acad. Sci. USA* **1997**, *94*, 13193–13197. [CrossRef]
33. Finzi, D.; Hermankova, M.; Pierson, T.; Carruth, L.M.; Buck, C.; Chaisson, R.E.; Quinn, T.C.; Chadwick, K.; Margolick, J.; Brookmeyer, R.; et al. Identification of a reservoir for HIV-1 in patients on highly active antiretroviral therapy. *Science* **1997**, *278*, 1295–1300. [CrossRef]
34. Armenia, D.; Zaccarelli, M.; Borghi, V.; Gennari, W.; Di, C.D.; Giannetti, A.; Forbici, F.; Bertoli, A.; Gori, C.; Fabeni, L.; et al. Resistance detected in PBMCs predicts virological rebound in HIV-1 suppressed patients switching treatment. *J. Clin. Virol.* **2018**, *104*, 61–64. [CrossRef]
35. Peng, X.; Xu, Y.; Huang, Y.; Zhu, B. Intrapatient Development of Multi-Class Drug Resistance in an Individual Infected with HIV-1 CRF01_AE. *Infect. Drug Resist.* **2021**, *14*, 3441–3448. [CrossRef] [PubMed]
36. Moraka, N.O.; Garcia-Broncano, P.; Hu, Z.; Ajibola, G.; Bareng, O.T.; Pretorius-Holme, M.; Maswabi, K.; Maphorisa, C.; Mohammed, T.; Gaseitsiwe, S.; et al. Patterns of pretreatment drug resistance mutations of very early diagnosed and treated infants in Botswana. *AIDS* **2021**, *35*, 2413–2421. [CrossRef] [PubMed]
37. Hamers, R.L.; Smit, P.W.; Stevens, W.; Schuurman, R.; Rinke de Wit, T.F. Dried fluid spots for HIV type-1 viral load and resistance genotyping: A systematic review. *Antivir. Ther.* **2009**, *14*, 619–629. [CrossRef] [PubMed]
38. Guthrie, R.; Susi, A. A simple phenyylalanine method for detecting phenylketonuria in large populations of newborn infants. *Pediatrics* **1963**, *32*, 338–343. [CrossRef]
39. Rodriguez-Auad, J.P.; Rojas-Montes, O.; Maldonado-Rodriguez, A.; Alvarez-Munoz, M.T.; Munoz, O.; Torres-Ibarra, R.; Vazquez-Rosales, G.; Lira, R. Use of Dried Plasma Spots for HIV-1 Viral Load Determination and Drug Resistance Genotyping in Mexican Patients. *Biomed. Res. Int.* **2015**, *2015*, 240407. [CrossRef]
40. Rottinghaus, E.; Bile, E.; Modukanele, M.; Maruping, M.; Mine, M.; Nkengasong, J.; Yang, C. Comparison of Ahlstrom grade 226, Munktell TFN, and Whatman 903 filter papers for dried blood spot specimen collection and subsequent HIV-1 load and drug resistance genotyping analysis. *J. Clin. Microbiol.* **2013**, *51*, 55–60. [CrossRef]
41. Rottinghaus, E.K.; Beard, R.S.; Bile, E.; Modukanele, M.; Maruping, M.; Mine, M.; Nkengasong, J.; Yang, C. Evaluation of dried blood spots collected on filter papers from three manufacturers stored at ambient temperature for application in HIV-1 drug resistance monitoring. *PLoS ONE* **2014**, *9*, e109060. [CrossRef]
42. Bertagnolio, S.; Parkin, N.T.; Jordan, M.; Brooks, J.; Garcia-Lerma, J.G. Dried blood spots for HIV-1 drug resistance and viral load testing: A review of current knowledge and WHO efforts for global HIV drug resistance surveillance. *AIDS Rev.* **2010**, *12*, 195–208.
43. Monleau, M.; Aghokeng, A.F.; Eymard-Duvernay, S.; Dagnra, A.; Kania, D.; Ngo-Giang-Huong, N.; Toure-Kane, C.; Truong, L.X.; Chaix, M.L.; Delaporte, E.; et al. Field evaluation of dried blood spots for routine HIV-1 viral load and drug resistance monitoring in patients receiving antiretroviral therapy in Africa and Asia. *J. Clin. Microbiol.* **2014**, *52*, 578–586. [CrossRef]

44. McNulty, A.; Jennings, C.; Bennett, D.; Fitzgibbon, J.; Bremer, J.W.; Ussery, M.; Kalish, M.L.; Heneine, W.; Garcia-Lerma, J.G. Evaluation of dried blood spots for human immunodeficiency virus type 1 drug resistance testing. *J. Clin. Microbiol.* **2007**, *45*, 517–521. [CrossRef]
45. Monleau, M.; Butel, C.; Delaporte, E.; Boillot, F.; Peeters, M. Effect of storage conditions of dried plasma and blood spots on HIV-1 RNA quantification and PCR amplification for drug resistance genotyping. *J. Antimicrob. Chemother.* **2010**, *65*, 1562–1566. [CrossRef] [PubMed]
46. Rottinghaus, E.K.; Ugbena, R.; Diallo, K.; Bassey, O.; Azeez, A.; DeVos, J.; Zhang, G.; Aberle-Grasse, J.; Nkengasong, J.; Yang, C. Dried blood spot specimens are a suitable alternative sample type for HIV-1 viral load measurement and drug resistance genotyping in patients receiving first-line antiretroviral therapy. *Clin. Infect. Dis.* **2012**, *54*, 1187–1195. [CrossRef] [PubMed]
47. Garcia-Lerma, J.G.; McNulty, A.; Jennings, C.; Huang, D.; Heneine, W.; Bremer, J.W. Rapid decline in the efficiency of HIV drug resistance genotyping from dried blood spots (DBS) and dried plasma spots (DPS) stored at 37 degrees C and high humidity. *J. Antimicrob. Chemother.* **2009**, *64*, 33–36. [CrossRef] [PubMed]
48. Dachraoui, R.; Brand, D.; Brunet, S.; Barin, F.; Plantier, J.C. RNA amplification of the HIV-1 Pol and env regions on dried serum and plasma spots. *HIV Med.* **2008**, *9*, 557–561. [CrossRef]
49. Plantier, J.C.; Dachraoui, R.; Lemee, V.; Gueudin, M.; Borsa-Lebas, F.; Caron, F.; Simon, F. HIV-1 resistance genotyping on dried serum spots. *AIDS* **2005**, *19*, 391–397. [CrossRef]
50. Hauser, A.; Hofmann, A.; Hanke, K.; Bremer, V.; Bartmeyer, B.; Kuecherer, C.; Bannert, N. National molecular surveillance of recently acquired HIV infections in Germany, 2013 to 2014. *Eurosurveillance* **2017**, *22*, 30436. [CrossRef]
51. Andrea, H.; Alexandra, H.; Claudia, S.H.; Ruth, Z.; Osamah, H.; Norbert, B.; Claudia, K. Analysis of transmitted drug resistance and HIV-1 subtypes using dried serum spots of recently HIV-infected individuals in 2013 in Germany. *J. Int. AIDS Soc.* **2014**, *17*, 19670. [CrossRef]
52. Hauser, A.; Meixenberger, K.; Machnowska, P.; Fiedler, S.; Hanke, K.; Hofmann, A.; Bartmeyer, B.; Bremer, V.; Bannert, N.; Kuecherer, C. Robust and sensitive subtype-generic HIV-1 pol genotyping for use with dried serum spots in epidemiological studies. *J. Virol. Methods* **2018**, *259*, 32–38. [CrossRef]
53. Kaduskar, O.; Bhatt, V.; Prosperi, C.; Hayford, K.; Hasan, A.Z.; Deshpande, G.R.; Tilekar, B.; Vivian Thangaraj, J.W.; Kumar, M.S.; Gupta, N.; et al. Optimization and Stability Testing of Four Commercially Available Dried Blood Spot Devices for Estimating Measles and Rubella IgG Antibodies. *mSphere* **2021**, *6*, e0049021. [CrossRef]
54. Manak, M.M.; Hack, H.R.; Shutt, A.L.; Danboise, B.A.; Jagodzinski, L.L.; Peel, S.A. Stability of Human Immunodeficiency Virus Serological Markers in Samples Collected as HemaSpot and Whatman 903 Dried Blood Spots. *J. Clin. Microbiol.* **2018**, *56*, e00933-18. [CrossRef]
55. Prosperi, C.; Kaduskar, O.; Bhatt, V.; Hasan, A.Z.; Vivian Thangaraj, J.W.; Kumar, M.S.; Sabarinathan, R.; Kumar, S.; Duraiswamy, A.; Deshpande, G.R.; et al. Diagnostic Accuracy of Dried Blood Spots Collected on HemaSpot HF Devices Compared to Venous Blood Specimens To Estimate Measles and Rubella Seroprevalence. *mSphere* **2021**, *6*, e0133020. [CrossRef] [PubMed]
56. Yamamoto, C.; Nagashima, S.; Isomura, M.; Ko, K.; Chuon, C.; Akita, T.; Katayama, K.; Woodring, J.; Hossain, M.S.; Takahashi, K.; et al. Evaluation of the efficiency of dried blood spot-based measurement of hepatitis B and hepatitis C virus seromarkers. *Sci. Rep.* **2020**, *10*, 3857. [CrossRef] [PubMed]
57. Hirshfield, S.; Teran, R.A.; Downing, M.J., Jr.; Chiasson, M.A.; Tieu, H.V.; Dize, L.; Gaydos, C.A. Quantification of HIV-1 RNA Among Men Who Have Sex With Men Using an At-Home Self-Collected Dried Blood Spot Specimen: Feasibility Study. *JMIR Public Health Surveill.* **2018**, *4*, e10847. [CrossRef] [PubMed]
58. Brooks, K.; DeLong, A.; Balamane, M.; Schreier, L.; Orido, M.; Chepkenja, M.; Kemboi, E.; D'Antuono, M.; Chan, P.A.; Emonyi, W.; et al. HemaSpot, a Novel Blood Storage Device for HIV-1 Drug Resistance Testing. *J. Clin. Microbiol.* **2016**, *54*, 223–225. [CrossRef]
59. Lloyd, R.M., Jr.; Burns, D.A.; Huong, J.T.; Mathis, R.L.; Winters, M.A.; Tanner, M.; De La Rosa, A.; Yen-Lieberman, B.; Armstrong, W.; Taege, A.; et al. Dried-plasma transport using a novel matrix and collection system for human immunodeficiency virus and hepatitis C virus virologic testing. *J. Clin. Microbiol.* **2009**, *47*, 1491–1496. [CrossRef]
60. Lloyd, R.M.J.; Burns, D.A.; Thompson, A.M.; Mathis, R.L.; Holodniy, M.; Huong, J.T.; De La Rosa, A.; Yen-Lieberman, B.; Armstrong, W.; Taege, A.; et al. Comparison of HIV-1 viral load and resistance genotyping between frozen plasma and a novel dried plasma transportation matrix. *Antivir. Ther.* **2004**, *9*, S135.
61. Zanoni, M.; Cortes, R.; Diaz, R.S.; Sucupira, M.C.; Ferreira, D.; Inocencio, L.A.; Vilhena, C.; Loveday, C.; Lloyd, R.M., Jr.; Holodniy, M. Comparative effectiveness of dried plasma HIV-1 viral load testing in Brazil using ViveST for sample collection. *J. Clin. Virol.* **2010**, *49*, 245–248. [CrossRef]
62. Zanoni, M.; Giron, L.B.; Vilhena, C.; Sucupira, M.C.; Lloyd, R.M., Jr.; Diaz, R.S. Comparative effectiveness of dried-plasma hepatitis B virus viral load (VL) testing in three different VL commercial platforms using ViveST for sample collection. *J. Clin. Microbiol.* **2012**, *50*, 145–147. [CrossRef]

63. Diallo, K.; Lehotzky, E.; Zhang, J.; Zhou, Z.; de Rivera, I.L.; Murillo, W.E.; Nkengasong, J.; Sabatier, J.; Zhang, G.; Yang, C. Evaluation of a dried blood and plasma collection device, SampleTanker((R)), for HIV type 1 drug resistance genotyping in patients receiving antiretroviral therapy. *AIDS Res. Hum. Retrovir.* **2014**, *30*, 67–73. [CrossRef]
64. Kantor, R.; DeLong, A.; Balamane, M.; Schreier, L.; Lloyd, R.M., Jr.; Injera, W.; Kamle, L.; Mambo, F.; Muyonga, S.; Katzenstein, D.; et al. HIV diversity and drug resistance from plasma and non-plasma analytes in a large treatment programme in western Kenya. *J. Int. AIDS Soc.* **2014**, *17*, 19262. [CrossRef]

MDPI
St. Alban-Anlage 66
4052 Basel
Switzerland
Tel. +41 61 683 77 34
Fax +41 61 302 89 18
www.mdpi.com

Pathogens Editorial Office
E-mail: pathogens@mdpi.com
www.mdpi.com/journal/pathogens

www.ingramcontent.com/pod-product-compliance
Lightning Source LLC
LaVergne TN
LVHW070612100526
838202LV00012B/626
* 9 7 8 3 0 3 6 5 5 5 1 1 9 *